Mayo Clinic
The Essential
Diabetes Book

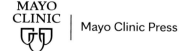 Mayo Clinic Press

MAYO CLINIC PRESS

Medical Editor | M. Regina Castro, M.D.

Publisher | Daniel J. Harke

Editor in Chief | Nina E. Wiener

Senior Editor | Karen R. Wallevand

Managing Editor | Rachel A. Haring Bartony

Art Director | Stewart J. Koski

Illustration, Photography and Production | Paul W. Honermann, Daniel J. Hubert, Joanna R. King, Michael A. King, Amanda J. Knapp, M. Alice McKinney, Steven D. Orwoll, Gunnar T. Soroos

Editorial Research Librarians | Abbie Y. Brown, Anthony J. Cook, Edward (Eddy) S. Morrow Jr., Erika A. Riggin, Katherine (Katie) J. Warner

Copy Editors | Miranda M. Attlesey, Donna L. Hanson, Nancy J. Jacoby, Julie M. Maas

Indexer | Steve Rath

Contributors | Ana L. Creo, M.D.; Donald D. Hensrud, M.D., M.S.; Anna L. Kasper, R.N., CDCES; Heather L. LaBruna; Pankaj Shah, M.D.; Vinaya Simha, M.B.B.S, M.D.; Carmen M. Terzic, M.D., Ph.D.; Laura M. Waxman; Mark D. Williams, M.D.; Gina R. Wimmer, RDN, LD

Image Credits | The individuals pictured are models, and the photos are used for illustrative purposes only. All photographs and illustrations are copyright of MFMER except for the following:
NAME: Shutterstock_125297753.psd/PAGE: 21/CREDIT: © Shutterstock NAME: Shutterstock1409211338.psd/PAGE: 41/CREDIT: © Shutterstock NAME: Shutter-stock_570006436.psd/PAGE: 49/CREDIT: © Shutterstock NAME: Shutterstock_503626594.psd/PAGE: 54/CREDIT: © Shutterstock NAME: Shutterstock_1825812650.psd/PAGE: 63/CREDIT: © Shutterstock NAME: Shutter-stock_1072994900.psd/PAGE: 85/CREDIT: © Shutterstock NAME: Shutterstock_1072994900.psd/PAGE: 87/CREDIT: © Shutterstock NAME: Shutterstock_1072994900.psd/PAGE: 97/CREDIT:© Shutterstock NAME: Shutter-stock_670209337.psd/PAGE: 101/CREDIT: © Shutterstock NAME: Shutterstock_429214114.psd/PAGE: 120/CREDIT:© Shutterstock NAME: iStock-125142926.psd/PAGE: 191/CRDIT: © Getty NAME: shutterstock_1289843290.psd/PAGE: 216/CREDIT: © Shutterstock NAME: shutter-stock_680568412.jpg/PAGE: 288/CREDIT: © Shutterstock

Published by Mayo Clinic Press

© 2022 Mayo Foundation for Medical Education and Research (MFMER)

For bulk sales to employers, member groups and health-related companies, contact Mayo Clinic, 200 First St. SW, Rochester, MN 55905 or email SpecialSalesMayoBooks@mayo.edu.

ISBN 978-1-893005-79-2

Library of Congress Control Number: 2021947773

Printed in the United States of America

Some images within this content were created prior to the COVID-19 pandemic and may not demonstrate proper pandemic protocols. Please follow all recommended CDC guidelines for masking and social distancing.

Table of Contents

10   **CHAPTER 1**
        UNDERSTANDING DIABETES

11   A visit with M. Regina Castro, M.D.
12   What is diabetes?
15   The different types
18   Signs and symptoms
20   Are you at risk?
22   Tests to detect diabetes
25   Medical emergencies
27   Long-term complications

34   **CHAPTER 2**
        DEVELOPING A HEALTHY-EATING PLAN

35   A visit with Gina R. Wimmer, RDN, LD
36   What's healthy eating?
40   Plan your meals
45   Watch your serving sizes
45   Size up your plate

46   Read food labels
47   Consider carb counting
49   The real scoop on sugar
51   Using exchange lists
53   Staying motivated

56   CHAPTER 3
ACHIEVING A HEALTHY WEIGHT

57   A visit with Donald D. Hensrud, M.D., M.S.
58   Do you need to lose weight?
62   Assess your readiness
62   Set realistic goals
65   Simple first steps
65   The Mayo Clinic healthy weight approach
70   What are your eating triggers?
73   Be a smart shopper
76   Bumps in the road: Overcoming setbacks

80   CHAPTER 4
GETTING MORE ACTIVE

81   A visit with Carmen M. Terzic, M.D., Ph.D.
82   Diabetes and exercise
82   Reduce the time you sit
83   Get more fit
100   Avoiding injury
103   Exercising safely with diabetes

106   CHAPTER 5
MONITORING YOUR BLOOD SUGAR

107   A visit with Anna L. Kasper, R.N., CDCES
108   How often and when to test
111   Performing the test
114   Recording your results
117   Staying within your range
118   Troubleshooting problems
119   Factors affecting blood glucose

123   When tests results signal an issue
123   Avoiding the highs and lows
128   Overcoming barriers

130   CHAPTER 6
MEDICAL TREATMENT

131   A visit with Pankaj Shah, M.D.
132   Diabetes medications other than insulin
140   Insulin therapy
157   Long-term benefits

158   CHAPTER 7
USING TECHNOLOGY TO MANAGE DIABETES

159   A visit with Anna L. Kasper, R.N., CDCES
160   Is diabetes technology for me?
162   What about technology for kids?
163   Technology types
173   Using technology wisely
173   Future of diabetes technology

174   CHAPTER 8
IF YOUR CHILD HAS DIABETES

175   A visit with Ana L. Creo, M.D.
176   Type 1 diabetes
179   Type 2 diabetes
182   Creating a diabetes care plan
187   Emotional and social issues
187   Good habits for staying healthy
194   Surviving sick days

196   CHAPTER 9
LIVING WELL WITH DIABETES

197   A visit with Mark D. Williams, M.D.
198   Adapting to your diagnosis

199 Navigating your relationships
205 Tending to your mental health
211 Keeping a healthy relationship with food
213 Cultivating coping skills
215 Thriving with diabetes technology
217 Empowering yourself with knowledge

220 **CHAPTER 10**
STAYING HEALTHY

221 A visit with Vinaya Simha, M.B.B.S, M.D.
222 Yearly checkups
224 Important tests
228 Caring for your eyes
233 Caring for your feet
236 Caring for your teeth
237 Getting vaccinated
239 Managing stress
245 Diabetes and pregnancy
252 Diabetes and menstruation
252 Diabetes and menopause
254 Diabetes and erectile dysfunction

256 **CHAPTER 11**
TRAVELING WITH DIABETES

257 Preparation
261 Types of travel and activities
263 Planes, trains, cars and more
265 What to pack
268 Safe travels!

270 Appendix
308 Additional resources
309 Index

Your diabetes care team

A key element of managing diabetes successfully is having the support of a knowledgeable and experienced diabetes care team. Look for professionals who will support you, educate you and help you make informed decisions in your care throughout all phases of your life. Members of your diabetes care team may include the following people:

- *Primary diabetes care provider.* This is a doctor, nurse practitioner or physician assistant who provides your basic diabetes care. This person may also be your primary care provider, who oversees all of your health care in addition to diabetes care.
- *Diabetes specialist.* If your treatment involves intensive insulin therapy, you will likely see an endocrinologist, a doctor who specializes in diabetes and other diseases related to the hormone (endocrine) system. The endocrinologist on your team oversees your insulin treatment plan and often works with your primary diabetes care provider.
- *Certified diabetes care and education specialist (CDCES).* This professional has passed a national exam focused on diabetes education and is certified to teach and empower people with diabetes to successfully manage their disease. Although a CDCES is often a registered nurse or a registered dietitian, other professionals — such as doctors, physician assistants and pharmacists — also may be certified.
- *Registered dietitian nutritionist.* A registered dietitian nutritionist works with you to develop a sustainable and customized healthy-eating plan to help manage your blood glucose levels.
- *Mental health provider.* A psychiatrist, psychologist or social worker who understands diabetes and your management needs can help you navigate the emotional challenges of living with diabetes. This person can also help with separate but related conditions such as depression or anxiety that may impact your ability to fully self-manage your diabetes.
- *Eye doctor.* An eye doctor (ophthalmologist or optometrist) who has expertise in diabetes-related eye problems can help detect early signs of eye diseases and educate you on their prevention or possible treatment options.
- *Foot doctor.* A foot doctor (podiatrist) with expertise in diabetes-related foot problems can detect and treat foot problems, such as calluses or sores, and help you prevent future problems.
- *Other professionals.* Depending on your needs, you may benefit from seeing a kidney specialist (nephrologist), nerve specialist (neurologist) or heart specialist (cardiologist). Look for professionals who have experience in caring for people with diabetes.

Preface

Most people want to live a long and healthy life. Often, the desire for longevity is motivated by a desire to achieve something — be it a personal or professional accomplishment. Maybe you want to raise a family, be a teacher or a professional athlete, travel the world, or simply spend time with those you love.

Although you may have great genes on your side, no one is guaranteed health and longevity. Today, more than ever, you have to assume responsibility for your future and play an active role in protecting your health. This is especially true if you are living with or at risk of diabetes.

The good news is that despite the challenges you may be facing, there are multiple opportunities to improve and protect your health. Our goal — mine and those of the other contributors to this book — is to help you identify and act upon those opportunities. And in encouraging this action, we hope to keep you on the path to good health.

Diabetes is serious — and increasingly common. But you can learn how to successfully manage the disease and lead a long, healthy and productive life.

In this third edition of *Mayo Clinic The Essential Diabetes Book,* we provide you with key steps to managing diabetes. This includes essential advice on how to monitor your blood sugar, how to eat better, how to become more physically active, how to lose weight and maintain a healthy weight, and how to get the most from your medications. If you have a child with diabetes, you'll also learn practical tips, including on how to recognize key signs and symptoms, involving your child in diabetes care, and coping with the emotional aspects of diabetes.

We've also added some new chapters to this latest edition. Technology is transforming diabetes management and making it easier for people to monitor their blood sugar and manage insulin therapy. But the rapid pace of technology development can be overwhelming. We aim to give you practical guidance on the pros and cons of diabetes technology and help you decide what fits best into your lifestyle.

Living with diabetes day in and day out can be emotionally draining, causing distress and burnout. Our new chapter on living well with diabetes provides tips and strategies for navigating relationships, managing stress, cultivating coping skills and finding extra help when you need it.

Finally, we've added a new chapter on traveling with diabetes because having diabetes shouldn't stop you from seeking adventure and living an active and full life.

We hope that you'll find this book helpful. Living with diabetes isn't always easy. But we believe you can do it — and do it in a way that allows you to thrive and enjoy your life. You've got this.

M. Regina Castro, M.D.
Medical Editor

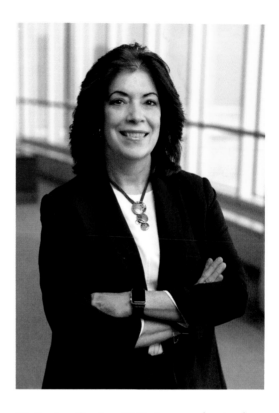

M. Regina Castro, M.D., is an endocrinologist at Mayo Clinic in Rochester, Minn., and a Professor of Medicine at Mayo Clinic College of Medicine and Science. Dr. Castro's work combines seeing patients, educating residents and fellows, and doing clinical research. She is the Director of the Endocrinology Fellowship Program at Mayo Clinic. Within the practice, her primary interests are in evaluating and treating patients living with diabetes and thyroid disorders. Her research interests include the use of technology and data to improve diabetes care, with an emphasis on machine learning algorithms.

CHAPTER 1

Understanding diabetes

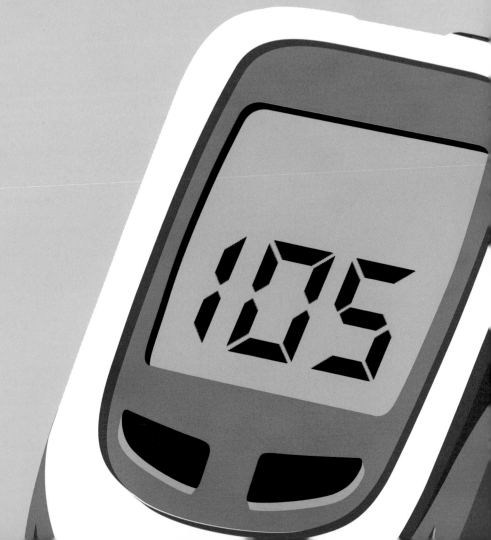

A VISIT WITH M. REGINA CASTRO, M.D.

"The threat of diabetes to our general health is significant enough that for the first time in history, younger generations may not enjoy the long lives that we have come to expect."

We seem to be involved in an uphill battle. The number of individuals diagnosed with diabetes, particularly type 2 diabetes mellitus, continues to rise.

In addition, we're seeing more young people with type 2 diabetes — many children and adolescents — as well as people of varied ethnic backgrounds and all levels of economic status.

What's driving this epidemic? Have our genes changed dramatically? No. What has changed is the way we lead our lives. Meals are often eaten on the run, high in fat and calories and low in fruits and vegetables. We've become less physically active. As a result, many of us weigh too much. This increases the risk of diabetes and predisposes us to many other serious health problems.

It's clear that we can't solve this problem in doctors' offices, clinics or hospitals — we've tried and failed. We need instead to focus on the daily decisions we make that affect our health. This requires change, and change is often hard.

When you face a big challenge, you want the best people on your side. In this book, we've recruited the help of experts who play important roles in caring for people who live with diabetes. Their advice will help you understand how small, everyday decisions can help you manage your disease and protect your health, as well as promote the health of those close to you.

As much as I believe in the importance of these changes, I know how challenging making them can be. By reading this book, you're taking a first step in empowering yourself to live a healthier life. The information here will arm you with knowledge that's easy to understand and put into action.

Identifying the obstacles that keep you from taking better care of yourself is the first step. Then recruit individuals who can help you overcome those obstacles, such as your family, friends, co-workers, and yes, your doctor. And don't forget about the people on your diabetes care team, who are there to help you succeed.

In our ever changing environment, your role in protecting your health is more important than ever. We hope you find the information available here to be a helpful tool in fulfilling that role.

TYPICAL METABOLISM

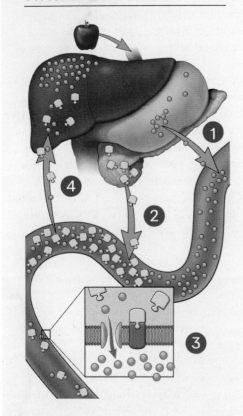

1. Glucose is broken down from the sugar in food and enters the bloodstream.
2. Insulin leaves the pancreas and enters the bloodstream.
3. Insulin "unlocks" the cell, letting glucose in to provide the cell with energy. Without insulin, glucose remains locked outside of the cells.
4. Extra glucose is stored in the liver.

Perhaps your primary care provider recently broke the news that you have diabetes or that you're very close to getting the disease. You're worried. Will you never be able to eat desserts and sweets again? Will you have to give yourself daily shots of insulin? Will you eventually face an amputation? Will diabetes kill you?

For most people with diabetes, the answer to these questions is no. Researchers have learned a great deal about how to diagnose diabetes early and how to manage it. Because of these advances, you can live well and avoid serious complications if you follow the advice of your diabetes care team regarding eating, exercise, blood sugar (glucose) monitoring and, when necessary, use of medications. You can enjoy an active and healthy life despite having diabetes, but you have to be willing to do your part.

WHAT IS DIABETES?

The term *diabetes* refers to a group of diseases that affect the way your body uses blood glucose, commonly called blood sugar. Glucose is vital to your health because it's the main source of energy for the cells that make up your muscles and tissues. It's your body's main source of fuel.

If you have diabetes — no matter which type — it means you have too much glucose in your blood, although the reasons why may differ. And too much glucose can lead to serious problems.

To understand diabetes, it helps to understand how the body typically processes blood glucose.

Processing of blood glucose

Blood glucose comes from two major sources: the food you eat and your liver. During digestion, glucose is absorbed by your bloodstream so that it can be circulated to your cells.

Your pancreas, which is sensitive to blood glucose levels, secretes a hormone called insulin into your bloodstream. This is essential because insulin gives your cells access to the glucose in your bloodstream. As insulin circulates with glucose, it acts like a key, unlocking microscopic access points that allow glucose to enter your cells. In this way, insulin helps fuel your cells and lowers the amount of glucose in your bloodstream, preventing it from reaching high levels. As your blood glucose level drops, so does the secretion of insulin from your pancreas.

Your liver acts as a glucose storage and manufacturing center. When the level of glucose in your blood is high, such as after a meal, your liver stores extra glucose as glycogen in case your cells need it later. When your glucose levels are low — for example, when you haven't eaten in a while — your liver releases stored glucose into your bloodstream to keep your blood glucose level within a standard range.

When you have diabetes

If you have diabetes, the interplay between glucose and insulin doesn't work

A NATIONAL EPIDEMIC

Due largely to the growing number of Americans who are overweight and the aging of the population, diabetes has become a major health problem in the United States. As your age and weight increase, so does your risk of the most common form of diabetes — type 2.

The latest figures from the Centers for Disease Control and Prevention show that 34 million American adults and children — or just over 10% of the population — have diabetes. Estimates also show that 88 million Americans — about 1 in 3 U.S. adults — have prediabetes, which increases the risk of diabetes. Type 2 diabetes accounts for 90% to 95% of all diabetes cases. Diabetes is the seventh-leading cause of death and contributes to more than 270,000 deaths in the United States each year. That's why it's important to treat the disease as soon as you discover you have it.

like it should. Instead of being transported into your cells, glucose builds up in your bloodstream and eventually some of it is excreted in your urine.

Too much glucose in your bloodstream usually occurs when your pancreas produces little or no insulin or your cells don't respond properly to insulin, or for both reasons.

The medical term for this condition is diabetes mellitus (MEL-lih-tuhs). *Mellitus* is a Latin word meaning "honey sweet," referring to the excess sugar in the blood and urine.

Another form of diabetes, called diabetes insipidus (in-SIP-uh-dus), is a rare condition in which the kidneys are unable to conserve water, leading to increased urination and excessive thirst. Rather than being an insulin problem, diabetes insipidus results from a different hormone disorder. In this book, the term *diabetes* refers only to diabetes mellitus.

IF I HAVE A CLOSE RELATIVE WITH TYPE 1 DIABETES, WHAT ARE MY CHANCES OF GETTING THE DISEASE?

For reasons that aren't well understood, your risk of developing diabetes varies. Note in the chart below that family history — which includes both learned behavior and genetics — along with lifestyle seems to play a larger role in the development of type 2 diabetes than type 1. Many people with type 1 diabetes have no known family history of this disease.

How does family history affect your risk of diabetes?

Type 1		Type 2	
Relatives with diabetes	Your estimated risk	Relatives with diabetes	Your estimated risk
Mother	1% to 5%	Mother	5% to 20%
Father	5% to 15%	Father	5% to 20%
Both parents	1% to 25%	Both parents	25% to 50%
Brother/sister	5% to 10%	Brother/sister	25% to 50%
Identical twin	25% to 50%	Identical twin	60% to 75%

Based on a review of medical journal articles and textbooks.

THE DIFFERENT TYPES

People often think of diabetes as a single disease. But glucose can accumulate in your blood for a number of reasons, resulting in different types of diabetes. The two most common forms are type 1 and type 2.

Type 1 diabetes

Type 1 diabetes develops when your pancreas makes little if any insulin. Without insulin circulating in your bloodstream, glucose can't get into your cells, so it remains in your blood.

Type 1 diabetes used to be called juvenile diabetes or insulin-dependent diabetes. That's because type 1 diabetes most often develops in children and teens, and daily insulin shots are needed to make up for the insulin the body doesn't produce.

However, the names juvenile diabetes and insulin-dependent diabetes aren't entirely accurate. Adults also can develop type 1 diabetes, although it's less common. And the use of insulin isn't limited to people with type 1 disease. People with other forms of diabetes also may need insulin.

Type 1 diabetes is an autoimmune disease, meaning that your own immune system is the culprit. Similar to how it attacks invading viruses or bacteria, your body's infection-fighting system attacks your pancreas, zeroing in on your beta cells, which produce insulin. Researchers aren't certain what causes your immune system to fight your own body, but they believe genetic factors, exposure to certain viruses and diet may be involved.

These attacks on your beta cells can dramatically reduce — even entirely wipe out — the insulin-making capacity of your pancreas. Between 5% and 10% of people with diabetes have type 1, with the disease occurring almost equally among males and females.

The process leading to type 1 diabetes can occur slowly, so the disease may go undetected for several months or possibly longer. More often, though, signs and symptoms come on quickly, commonly following an illness.

Type 2 diabetes

Type 2 diabetes is by far the most common form of the disease. In people older than age 20 who have diabetes, 90% to 95% have type 2 diabetes. Like type 1 diabetes, type 2 used to be called by other names: noninsulin-dependent diabetes and adult-onset diabetes. These names reflect that many people with type 2 diabetes don't need insulin shots and that the disease usually develops in adults.

As with type 1, these names aren't entirely accurate. That's because children and teenagers, as well as adults, can develop type 2 diabetes. In fact, the incidence of type 2 diabetes in children and adolescents is increasing. In addition, many people with type 2 diabetes need insulin to control their blood glucose.

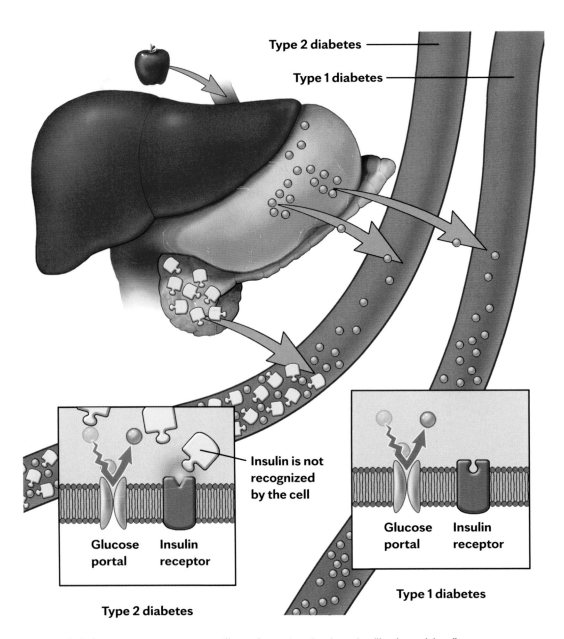

Type 2 diabetes

Type 1 diabetes

Insulin is not recognized by the cell

Glucose portal

Insulin receptor

Type 2 diabetes

Glucose portal

Insulin receptor

Type 1 diabetes

In type 2 diabetes, your pancreas still produces insulin, but the "lock-and-key" interaction between insulin and the cell's insulin receptor no longer works properly. This causes glucose to build up in your bloodstream (high blood sugar).

In type 1 diabetes, your pancreas produces little if any insulin. Without insulin to help move glucose into your cells, glucose builds up in your bloodstream.

Unlike type 1, type 2 diabetes isn't an autoimmune disease. With type 2 diabetes, your pancreas makes insulin, but your cells become resistant to insulin. So insulin can't help move glucose into your cells. As a result, most of the glucose stays in your bloodstream and accumulates. Exactly why the cells become resistant to insulin is uncertain, although excess weight and fatty tissue seem to be important factors. Most people who develop type 2 diabetes are overweight.

Some people with type 2 diabetes eventually require insulin shots. That's because the pancreas may not produce enough insulin to keep blood sugar in the standard range, or the pancreas may lose its ability to make insulin. Like people with type 1 diabetes, people with type 2 disease may become dependent on insulin.

Other types

Type 1 and type 2 are the most common forms of diabetes, and therefore they receive the most attention. The disease, however, can present in other forms.

Gestational

Gestational diabetes is the name for diabetes that develops during pregnancy. Diabetes can develop temporarily when hormones secreted during pregnancy increase the body's resistance to insulin. This happens in about 5% of pregnant women in the United States, although estimates vary. Gestational diabetes

ARE YOU AT RISK OF TYPE 2 DIABETES?

Researchers don't fully understand why some people develop prediabetes and type 2 diabetes and others don't. Certain factors do appear to increase a person's risk, however.

Place a check mark in any of the boxes below that apply to you. The more boxes that you check, the higher your risk of type 2 diabetes.

☐ Parent, brother or sister with type 2 diabetes

☐ Overweight

☐ Carry excess weight around waist or upper body (apple shape) rather than hips and thighs (pear shape)

☐ Not physically active — get little or no exercise

☐ Older than age 45

☐ Belong to certain ethnic and racial groups including African Americans, Latinos, Native Americans, Asian Americans and Pacific Islanders

☐ Gave birth to a baby who weighed more than 9 pounds

☐ Developed diabetes when pregnant (gestational diabetes)

typically develops during the second half of pregnancy — especially in the third trimester — and goes away after the baby is born. But about half of women who experience gestational diabetes develop type 2 diabetes later in life.

Most pregnant women are screened for gestational diabetes to catch the condition early. If you develop gestational diabetes, being aware of your condition and controlling your blood glucose level throughout your pregnancy can reduce complications for you and your baby.

LADA and MODY

Latent autoimmune diabetes of adults (LADA) is a form of type 1 diabetes that develops slowly over many years, usually in older adults. LADA is uncommon, but it can be mistaken for type 2 diabetes.

Maturity-onset diabetes of youth (MODY) is an uncommon form of type 2 diabetes caused by a defect in a single gene. MODY generally affects young people with a family history of the condition.

Other causes

A small number of diagnosed cases of diabetes result from conditions or medications that interfere with the production of insulin or its action. These conditions include inflammation of the pancreas (pancreatitis), surgical removal of the pancreas, adrenal or pituitary gland disorders, rare genetic defects, infection, and malnutrition.

SIGNS AND SYMPTOMS

Like many people, you may have been shocked to learn that you have diabetes because you weren't experiencing any symptoms. You felt fine.

Often there are no early symptoms. This is especially true with type 2 diabetes. Lack of symptoms and the slow emergence of the disease are the main reasons type 2 diabetes often goes undetected for years. When symptoms do develop from persistently high blood glucose, they vary.

Two classic symptoms that occur in most people with the disease are increased thirst and a frequent need to urinate.

Excessive thirst and increased urination

When you have high levels of glucose in your blood, it overwhelms your kidneys' filtering system. Your kidneys can't process all of the excess sugar. The sugar is excreted into your urine with fluids drawn from your tissues. This process leads to more-frequent urination. As a result, you feel dehydrated. To replace the fluids being drawn out, you're almost constantly drinking water or other beverages.

Flu-like feeling

Symptoms of diabetes, such as fatigue, weakness and loss of appetite, can mimic a viral illness. That's because when you have diabetes and it's not well managed, the process of using glucose for energy is impaired, affecting your body's function.

DIABETES WARNING SIGNS

Whether you have type 1 or type 2 diabetes, the classic signs and symptoms are:
- Excessive thirst
- Increased urination

Other signs and symptoms may include:
- Constant hunger
- Weakness and fatigue
- Unexplained weight loss
- Blurred vision
- Slow-healing cuts or bruises
- Tingling or loss of feeling in hands and feet
- Recurring bladder or vaginal infections
- Recurring infections of the gums or skin

Weight loss or gain

Some people, especially those with type 1 diabetes, lose weight before diagnosis. That's because some of the excess glucose in the bloodstream is being lost through urination, which leads to calorie loss. More of the body's stored fat is used for energy, and muscle tissues may not get enough glucose to generate growth. Weight loss might be less noticeable in people with type 2 diabetes because they are often overweight.

Weight gain also may precede a diagnosis of diabetes. In most people with type 2 and some people with type 1, diabetes develops after gaining additional pounds. Excess weight has a tendency to worsen insulin resistance, which makes it harder for glucose to leave the bloodstream and leads to an increase in blood sugar levels.

Blurred vision

Excessive glucose in your blood draws the fluid out of the lenses in your eyes, causing them to thin and affecting their ability to focus. Lowering your blood sugar helps restore fluid to your lenses. Your vision may remain blurry for a while as your lenses adjust to the restoration of fluid. But in time, vision typically improves.

High blood glucose can also cause the formation of tiny blood vessels in your eyes that can bleed. The blood vessels themselves don't produce symptoms, but bleeding from the vessels can cause dark spots and flashing lights in your vision, rings around lights, and even blindness.

Because diabetes-related eye changes often don't produce symptoms, it's important to see an eye specialist (ophthalmologist or optometrist) regularly. By dilating your pupils, an eye specialist can examine the blood vessels in each eye.

Slow-healing sores or frequent infections

High levels of blood glucose block your body's natural healing process and its ability to fight off infections. For women, bladder and vaginal infections are especially common.

Tingling feet and hands

High blood sugar can damage your nerves, which are nourished by your blood. Nerve damage can produce a number of symptoms. The most common are a tingling feeling and a loss of sensation that occurs mainly in your feet and hands. This results from damage to your sensory nerves. You may also experience pain in your extremities — legs, feet, arms and hands — including burning pain.

Red, swollen and tender gums

Diabetes can also weaken your mouth's ability to fight germs. This increases the risk of infection in your gums and the bones that help hold your teeth in place. Signs and symptoms of gum disease include:
- Gums that have pulled away from your teeth, exposing more of your teeth or even part of the roots
- Sores or pockets of pus in your gums
- Permanent teeth becoming loose
- Changes in the fit of your dentures

ARE YOU AT RISK?

Perhaps you've heard one of the common myths about diabetes — that it comes from eating too much sugar. That's not true. Researchers don't fully understand why some people develop the disease and others don't. It's clear, though, that your lifestyle and certain health conditions can increase your risk.

Family history

Your chance of developing either type 1 or type 2 diabetes increases if someone in your immediate family has the disease, whether that person is a parent, brother or sister (see the table on page 14). Genetics plays a role in the disease, but exactly how certain genes may cause diabetes is unknown. Scientists are studying genes that may be linked to diabetes, but tests are still under development and not available for routine clinical use.

Although people who develop diabetes may have inherited a genetic vulnerability toward the disease, some type of environmental factor usually triggers the development of the disease.

Weight

Being overweight or obese is one of the most common risk factors for type 2 diabetes. More than 80% of people living with type 2 diabetes are overweight or obese. The more fatty tissue you have, the more resistant your muscle and tissue cells become to your own insulin. This is

METABOLIC SYNDROME AND DIABETES

Metabolic syndrome (also called insulin resistance syndrome) is a cluster of metabolic disorders that makes you more likely to develop type 2 diabetes, heart disease and stroke. You may have metabolic syndrome if you have three or more of the following risk factors:

- **Large waist.** More than a 35-inch waist for women and more than a 40-inch waist for men*
- **High triglycerides.** A level of 150 milligrams per deciliter (mg/dL) of blood or above, or drug treatment for high triglycerides
- **Reduced "good" (HDL) cholesterol.** Lower than 50 mg/dL for women and lower than 40 mg/dL for men
- **Increased blood pressure.** Top number (systolic) of 130 mm Hg or above or bottom number (diastolic) of 85 mm Hg or above, or drug treatment for high blood pressure
- **Elevated fasting blood glucose.** A level of 100 mg/dL or higher, or drug treatment for high blood glucose

If you think that you have metabolic syndrome, talk with your primary care provider about tests that can help determine this. A balanced diet, a healthy weight and an increased level of physical activity can help combat metabolic syndrome and play a role in preventing diabetes and other serious diseases.

*For Asian Americans: More than a 31-inch waist for women and more than a 35-inch waist for men

Based on American Heart Association and National Heart, Lung, and Blood Institute.

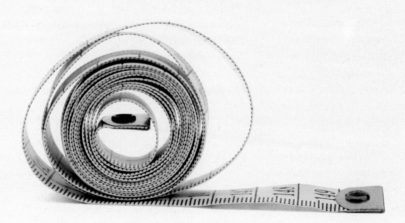

especially true if your excess weight is concentrated around your abdomen and your body is an apple shape rather than a pear shape, in which the weight is mostly on the hips and thighs.

Many people with diabetes who are overweight can improve their blood sugar levels simply by losing weight. Even a small weight loss can have beneficial effects, reducing blood sugar or allowing diabetes medications to work better.

Inactivity

The less active you are, the greater your risk of type 2 diabetes. Physical activity uses up sugar as energy, makes your cells more sensitive to insulin, increases blood flow and improves circulation. Exercise also helps build muscle mass. That's important because most of the glucose in your blood is absorbed by your muscles and burned as energy.

Age

Your risk of type 2 diabetes increases as you age, especially after age 45. At least 1 in 5 Americans age 65 and older lives with diabetes. Part of the reason is that as people grow older they tend to become less physically active, and they gradually lose muscle mass and gain weight.

Recent years have shown a dramatic rise in type 2 diabetes among people in their 30s and 40s, however. In addition, more children and teenagers are being diagnosed with type 2 diabetes.

Race and ethnicity

About 10% of the U.S. population has diabetes. Although it's unclear why, people of certain races and ethnicities are more likely to develop diabetes than are others. Type 1 diabetes is more common in white Americans, while type 2 diabetes is more prevalent among African Americans, Latinos, Native Americans, Asian Americans and Pacific Islanders.

While genetics may be a factor, it's likely that a variety of social, economic and lifestyle factors — including ease of access to health care, nutritious foods and space for physical activity — play a role.

TESTS TO DETECT DIABETES

Many people learn they have diabetes through blood tests done for another condition or as part of a physical exam. Sometimes, though, a health care provider may request tests specifically for diabetes if he or she suspects the disease, based on symptoms or risk factors.

An international committee of experts from the American Diabetes Association, the European Association for the Study of Diabetes and the International Diabetes Federation recommends that type 1 and type 2 diabetes testing include four tests.

A1C test

This blood test indicates your average blood sugar level for the past 2 to 3 months. It works by measuring what percentage of hemoglobin, the protein that carries oxygen in red blood cells, is coated with sugar. The higher your blood sugar levels, the more hemoglobin you'll have with sugar attached. An A1C level of 6.5% or higher on two separate tests indicates you have diabetes.

If the A1C test isn't available, or if you have certain conditions that can make the A1C test inaccurate — such as if you're pregnant or you have an uncommon form of hemoglobin — your health care provider may use other tests to check for diabetes.

Random blood glucose test

This test may be a part of the routine blood work done during a physical exam. From a needle inserted into a vein, blood is drawn for a variety of laboratory tests. This is done without any special preparation on your part, such as an overnight fast.

Even if you've recently eaten before the test and your blood glucose is at its peak, the level shouldn't be above 200 milligrams of glucose per deciliter of blood

WHAT THE RESULTS MEAN

An international committee of diabetes experts recommends the A1C test for prediabetes and diabetes testing. If the A1C test isn't available, the fasting blood glucose test is another option.

A1C test result	Indicates	Fasting blood glucose test result	Indicates
Less than 5.7%	Standard range	Under 100 mg/dL*	Standard range
Between 5.7% and 6.4%	Prediabetes[†]	100-125 mg/dL on 2 separate tests	Prediabetes[†]
6.5% or higher on 2 separate tests	Diabetes	126 mg/dL or higher on 2 separate tests	Diabetes

* Milligrams of glucose per deciliter of blood.

† Prediabetes means that you're at high risk of developing diabetes.

Based on American Diabetes Association, 2021.

(mg/dL). If it is, and if you're experiencing signs and symptoms of diabetes, it's likely you'll receive a diagnosis of diabetes.

Fasting blood glucose test

The amount of glucose in your blood naturally fluctuates, but within a fairly narrow range. Your blood glucose level is typically highest after a meal and lowest after an overnight fast.

The preferred way to test your blood glucose is after you've fasted overnight or for at least eight hours.

To do the test, blood is drawn from a vein and sent to a laboratory for evaluation. A fasting blood sugar level between 70 and 99 mg/dL is within the standard range.

If the results on two separate tests show a level between 100 and 125 mg/dL, you have what's known as prediabetes. Prediabetes shouldn't be taken lightly. It's a sign that you're at high risk of developing diabetes and that you should see your health care provider regularly and take steps to control your glucose.

Readings of 126 mg/dL or higher on two separate tests indicate diabetes. If your blood glucose is above 200 mg/dL and you have symptoms of diabetes, a second test may not be necessary to reach the diagnosis.

Oral glucose tolerance test

This test is rarely used today because other tests are less expensive and easier to administer.

CAN YOU MISS THE EARLY WARNING SIGNS OF HYPOGLYCEMIA?

Some people who have had diabetes for many years don't experience early signs and symptoms of low blood glucose, such as shakiness or nervousness. That's because chemical changes from long-standing diabetes may mask the symptoms or keep them from occurring. With this condition, called hypoglycemia unawareness, you may not realize your blood glucose is low until later signs and symptoms, such as confusion or slurred speech, set in.

If you're concerned about hypoglycemia unawareness, work with your health care team to identify circumstances that put you at risk of hypoglycemia and discuss ways to help prevent it. For example, most continuous glucose monitoring systems these days have built-in alarms that warn you when your blood sugar is getting low. This allows you to take measures, such as drinking fruit juice or taking a glucose tablet, to prevent a hypoglycemic episode.

An oral glucose tolerance test requires that you visit a lab or your health care provider's office after at least an eight-hour fast. There you drink about 8 ounces of a sweet liquid that contains a lot of sugar — about 75 grams. Your blood glucose is measured before you drink the liquid, after one hour and again after two hours. Health care providers often use a modified version of this test to check pregnant women for gestational diabetes.

MEDICAL EMERGENCIES

Blood sugar that is too low or too high can quickly become a medical emergency that requires immediate attention. (For a quick overview, see "Handling medical emergencies" on pages 298 and 299.)

Low blood sugar (hypoglycemia)

Low blood glucose — a level below 70 mg/dL — is called hypoglycemia (hi-poe-glie-SEE-me-uh). This condition basically results from too much insulin and too little glucose in your blood. If your blood glucose level drops too low — for example, below 50 mg/dL — this could result in confusion, seizures or a loss of consciousness, a condition sometimes called insulin shock or diabetic coma.

Hypoglycemia, also called an insulin reaction, is most common among people taking insulin. It can also occur in people taking oral medications that enhance the release of insulin. See page 125 for more on low blood sugar, including symptoms and what to do if you experience it.

IF I LOSE CONSCIOUSNESS AND NO ONE IS AROUND TO HELP ME, WILL I EVENTUALLY COME OUT OF IT?

A comatose condition can result from dangerously high or low blood glucose. Whether consciousness is regained without assistance depends on many factors, including how high or low your blood glucose level is and how long it has been since you last ate or last received an insulin injection.

If you live alone or are by yourself for much of the day, recruit family members or friends to give you a call if you don't show up for work or to check on you periodically. It may feel like you're imposing, but these people are often happy to help, and they may even save your life.

Also ask your diabetes care team about using a continuous glucose monitor (CGM) with an alarm that can be set to alert you when your blood sugar is dropping too fast. Then you can treat it immediately and prevent a serious hypoglycemic reaction.

High blood sugar (hyperglycemia)

There are two high blood sugar emergencies that are important to know about: hyperglycemic hyperosmolar (hi-pur-oz-MOE-lur) state (HHS) and high ketones (diabetic ketoacidosis). Both can be life-threatening if not treated quickly. For more information on symptoms and treatment of these two conditions, see page 123.

Hyperglycemic hyperosmolar state (HHS)

When your blood glucose reaches a dangerously high level, your blood becomes thick and syrupy. This condition, called hyperglycemic hyperosmolar state, may occur when your blood glucose level rises over 600 mg/dL.

Your cells can't absorb this much glucose, so the glucose passes from your blood into your urine. This triggers a filtering process that draws tremendous amounts of fluid from your body and results in dehydration, a condition caused by too much water loss.

HHS is most common in people with type 2 diabetes, especially people who don't monitor their blood glucose or who don't know they have diabetes. It can occur in people with diabetes who are taking high-dose steroids or drugs that increase urination.

It may also be brought on by an infection (such as a urinary tract infection or pneumonia), illness, stress, drinking too much alcohol or drug misuse. Older adults with diabetes who don't get enough fluids also are at risk of HHS.

Check your blood glucose level. If it's more than 350 mg/dL, call your diabetes care team for advice. If it's 500 mg/dL or higher, seek medical help immediately. This is an emergency situation. Have someone else drive you to the emergency department. Don't drive yourself.

Emergency treatment can correct the problem within hours. You'll likely receive intravenous (IV) fluids to restore water to your tissues and short-acting insulin to help your tissue cells absorb glucose. Without prompt treatment, the condition can be fatal.

High ketones (diabetic ketoacidosis)

When you don't get enough insulin over a period of time, your muscle cells become so starved for energy that your body takes emergency measures and breaks down fat. As your body transforms the fat into energy, it produces blood acids known as ketones. A buildup of ketones in the blood is called ketoacidosis (kee-toe-as-ih-DOE-sis).

Diabetic ketoacidosis (DKA) is a dangerous condition that can be fatal if untreated. DKA is more common in people living with type 1 diabetes. It can be caused by skipping insulin shots or not raising the dose to adjust for a rise in your blood glucose level.

Extreme stress or illness also may cause DKA to occur in people living with either type 1 or type 2 diabetes. When an infection occurs, the body produces certain hormones, such as adrenaline, to help fight off the problem. Unfortunately, these hormones also work against insulin. Sometimes the stress and illness occur together — you get sick and overstressed, and you forget to take your insulin.

In people who are unaware they have diabetes, DKA can be the first sign of diabetes. Early symptoms of DKA can be confused with the flu, which may delay appropriate medical attention.

DKA requires emergency medical treatment, which involves replenishing lost fluids through IV lines and insulin administration. Left untreated, DKA can lead to a coma and possibly death.

LONG-TERM COMPLICATIONS

Diabetes is often easy to ignore, especially in the early stages. You're feeling fine. Your body seems to be working well. No symptoms, no problem. Right? Not really.

The longer you live with diabetes, the greater the damage that occurs. Excess glucose in your blood quietly erodes the very fabric of your body, threatening major organs, including your heart, nerves, eyes and kidneys. You may not feel the effects right away, but eventually you will.

For example, compared with people who don't have diabetes, people living with diabetes are twice as likely to have a heart attack or stroke or die of cardiovascular disease. Diabetes that's left untreated can

also lead to serious problems such as blindness, limb amputation and kidney failure.

Researchers are making great progress in understanding what triggers complications of diabetes and how to manage or prevent them. Several studies show that if you keep your blood glucose close to the standard range, you can dramatically reduce your risks of complications.

And it's never too late to start. As soon as you begin managing your glucose level, you may slow the progression of complications and reduce your chances of developing more health problems.

Heart and blood vessel disease

Heart and blood vessel disease (cardiovascular disease) is the leading cause of death among people living with diabetes. Diabetes can damage your major arteries as well as your small blood vessels, making it easier for fatty deposits (plaques) to form in arteries, a condition called atherosclerosis (ath-ur-o-skluh-ROE-sis). This narrowing of the arteries causes an increased risk of a heart attack, stroke and other disorders from impaired circulation.

Coronary artery disease

Coronary artery disease is caused by atherosclerosis in blood vessels that feed your heart (coronary arteries). Over time, fatty deposits can narrow your coronary arteries, so less oxygen-rich blood flows to your heart muscle. A severe blockage in an artery can leave the heart muscle deprived of oxygen (ischemia), causing a heart attack.

Signs and symptoms of coronary artery disease vary, as does severity, depending on the extent of the disease and the individual. In its early stages, coronary artery disease often produces no signs or symptoms. Later on, however, you may experience signs and symptoms such as shortness of breath, fatigue or rapid or irregular heartbeats (palpitations). Or you may have warning signs of a heart attack.

Heart attack

You could be having a heart attack if you have any of these signs and symptoms:
• Pressure, fullness or squeezing pain in the center of your chest for more than a few minutes

SILENT HEART ATTACKS

If you are living with diabetes, you're at particular risk of silent heart attacks — heart attacks that occur without typical symptoms. Diabetes can damage nerves that transmit chest pain, which typically accompanies a heart attack. Without pain sensations, you may be unaware that a heart attack is occurring.

People living with diabetes also have a greater risk of a fatal heart attack than people who don't have diabetes. Since people living with diabetes are less likely to experience typical symptoms of a heart attack, they may not seek medical attention as quickly. In addition, people living with diabetes are more likely to have high blood pressure and high cholesterol, which increase damage to the arteries that supply oxygen to the heart (coronary arteries), causing a more severe attack.

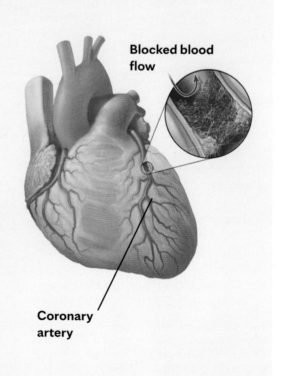

Blocked blood flow

Coronary artery

- Pain extending beyond your chest to your shoulder, arm, back or jaw
- More-frequent or prolonged episodes of chest pain
- Prolonged pain in your upper abdomen
- Shortness of breath
- Sweating
- Impending sense of doom
- Lightheadedness
- Fainting
- Nausea and vomiting

If you think you're having a heart attack, immediately call 911 in the U.S. or a local emergency number.

Damage to your heart from a heart attack increases your risk of developing heart failure.

Stroke

A stroke occurs when the blood supply to a part of your brain is interrupted or severely reduced and brain tissue is deprived of essential oxygen and nutrients. Within a few minutes to a few hours, brain cells begin to die. The interruption can be from a clogged or blocked artery (ischemic stroke) or from a leaking or ruptured artery (hemorrhagic stroke). Ischemic stroke is much more common.

The most common signs and symptoms include:
- Sudden numbness, weakness or paralysis of the face, arm or leg — usually on one side of the body
- Slurred speech or loss of speech

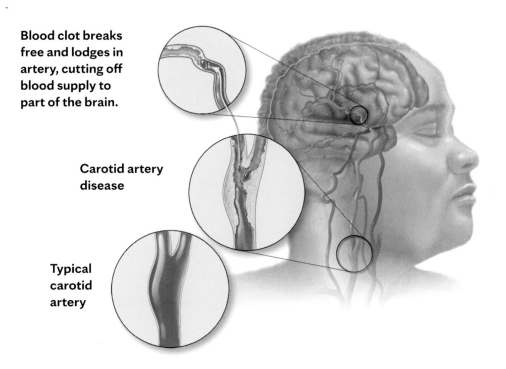

Blood clot breaks free and lodges in artery, cutting off blood supply to part of the brain.

Carotid artery disease

Typical carotid artery

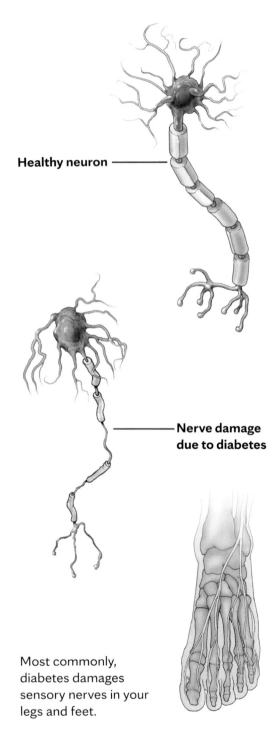

Healthy neuron

Nerve damage due to diabetes

Most commonly, diabetes damages sensory nerves in your legs and feet.

- Sudden blurred, double or decreased vision
- Dizziness, loss of balance or loss of coordination
- A sudden, severe or unusual headache, possibly with a stiff neck, facial pain, pain between the eyes, vomiting or altered consciousness
- Confusion, or problems with memory, spatial orientation or perception.

If you think you're having a stroke, immediately call 911 in the U.S. or a local emergency number.

Nerve damage (neuropathy)

Nerve damage, also called neuropathy (noo-ROP-uh-thee), is a common long-term complication of diabetes. Within your body is a complex network of nerves connecting your brain to muscles, skin and other organs. Through these nerves, your brain senses pain, controls your muscles, and performs automatic tasks such as breathing and digestion.

High blood glucose levels can damage delicate nerves. Excess glucose is thought to weaken the walls of tiny blood vessels (capillaries) that nourish your nerves. Diabetic neuropathy affects about half of all people living with diabetes. Sometimes the results can be painful and disabling. More often the symptoms are mild.

There are many kinds of nerve damage:
- Damage to your sensory nerves may leave you unable to detect sensations such as pain, warmth, coolness and texture.

- Damage to your autonomic nerves can increase your heart rate and perspiration level. In men, such damage can interfere with their ability to have an erection.
- Damage to your gastrointestinal tract can result in diarrhea, constipation or slowed stomach emptying (gastroparesis) leading to a sensation of fullness that can last for hours after you eat.
- Damage to nerves that control your muscles may leave you with weakened muscles and loss of strength.

Most commonly, diabetes damages the sensory nerves in your legs and, less often, your arms. You may experience any of these symptoms, which often begin at the tips of your toes, fingers or both and gradually spread upward:
- A tingling feeling, numbness, pain or a combination of these sensations
- Burning pain that comes and goes
- Stabbing or aching pain that's worse at night
- A crawling sensation

Left untreated, symptoms of decreased sensation can progress, putting you at high risk of injuring your feet without realizing it. Minor injuries, when not recognized early, can lead to bigger problems.

Kidney disease (nephropathy)

Each of your kidneys has about a million nephrons. A nephron is a tiny filtering unit with tiny blood vessels (capillaries). Nephrons remove waste from your blood and send it to your urine. Diabetes can damage this delicate filtering system, often before you notice any symptoms.

Up to 40% of people living with diabetes eventually develop kidney disease, called nephropathy (nuh-FROP-uh-thee). In most cases it is mild, but it can get worse if blood sugar is consistently high. Keeping your blood sugar within a healthy range and managing your blood pressure reduces the risk of nephropathy.

In its early stages, kidney disease produces few symptoms. Generally, kidney damage is extensive before these signs and symptoms occur:
- Swelling of the ankles, feet and hands
- Shortness of breath
- High blood pressure
- Confusion or difficulty concentrating
- Poor appetite
- Metallic taste in the mouth
- Fatigue

Eye damage (retinopathy)

Many tiny blood vessels nourish the light-sensitive tissue at the back part of your eye, called the retina. These blood vessels are often among the first to be damaged by high blood glucose. This damage is called diabetic retinopathy (ret-ih-NOP-uh-thee).

Over time, most people with diabetes develop some form of eye damage. Most have only minor problems, but sometimes eye damage can be severe, resulting in problems such as retinal detachment or glaucoma. There are two types of diabetic retinopathy:

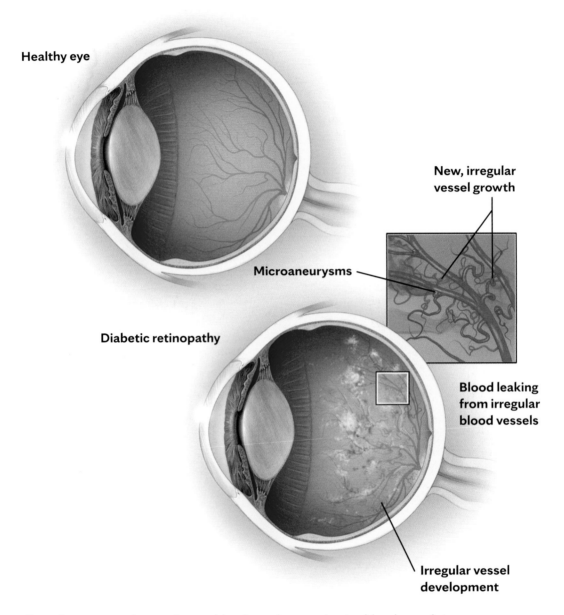

Healthy eye

New, irregular vessel growth

Microaneurysms

Diabetic retinopathy

Blood leaking from irregular blood vessels

Irregular vessel development

Over time, too much sugar in your blood can damage the tiny blood vessels in your retina. They become weak and develop tiny bulges (micronaneuryms). When blood vessels in the retina are damaged, they can leak blood or close off. As a result, the eye attempts to grow new blood vessels. But these new blood vessels don't develop properly and can leak easily.

Nonproliferative

This form is mild and more common. Blood vessels in your retina become weak and may swell or develop bulges or fatty deposits. The condition generally doesn't affect your vision unless swollen vessels form in the tiny portion of your retina called the macula.

Proliferative

When tiny blood vessels in the retina are damaged, they can bleed or close off. New and fragile blood vessels may form and grow (proliferate) in the retina, and they, too, may bleed. If the bleeding is heavy or occurs in certain areas of the eye, it can damage your retina and distort your vision, possibly leading to blindness.

The risk of developing diabetic retinopathy and its progression to more-advanced stages can be greatly reduced by actively managing blood glucose levels.

Early diabetic retinopathy often produces few, if any, visual symptoms. As the damage becomes more severe, these symptoms may develop:
- "Spiders," "cobwebs" or tiny specks floating in your vision
- Blurred vision
- A dark or empty spot in the center of your vision
- Dark streaks or a red film that blocks vision
- Flashes of light
- Poor night vision
- Vision loss
- Increased risk of infection

Other complications

High blood glucose impairs the ability of your immune cells to fight off invading germs and bacteria, putting you at higher risk of infection. Your mouth, gums, lungs, skin, feet, bladder and genital area are common infection sites.

Signs and symptoms of infection vary, depending on its location. A low-grade fever is common with many infections.

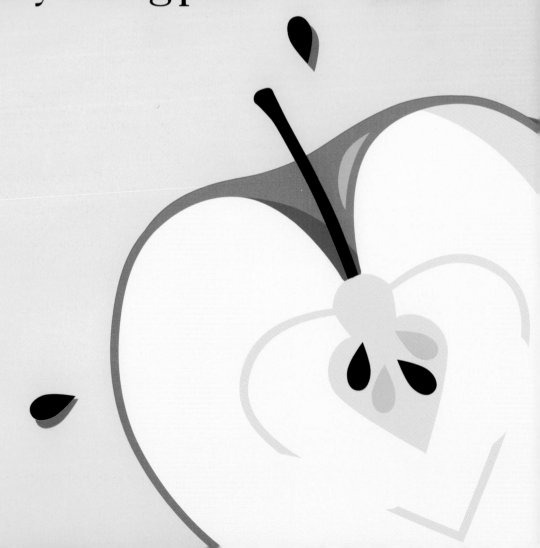

Developing a healthy-eating plan

2

A VISIT WITH GINA R. WIMMER, RDN, LD

"It's important to remember that a healthy-eating plan needs to be sustainable. Meeting with a dietitian annually helps you construct a plan for eating that supports good health and helps you attain lifelong management of diabetes."

A key part of diabetes management is a healthy-eating plan. But does the idea of healthy eating make you cringe just a little? You might think, "Oh no, I'll never get to eat my favorite treats again!" Here's what you need to know. Healthy eating isn't about deprivation or denial. If so, it would be unsustainable. Instead, it means enjoying great nutrition as well as great taste.

Healthy eating can mean learning new ways to cook and prepare meals. It can also mean varying your routine foods with delicious foods you've never tried or adapting favorite recipes to make them tasty and nutritious. And don't forget about consistency. You may choose the healthiest foods in the healthiest amounts, but skipping meals, grazing and other erratic eating patterns can wreak havoc on your blood sugar.

Eating healthy foods in portioned amounts will always be fundamental to good overall health. But diabetes nutrition recommendations are driven by individual nutrition needs and preferences, too.

There are many reasons why nutrition for diabetes may look different from one person to the next. People may have different types of eating plans and patterns that are based on personal preferences, cultural beliefs, as well as daily schedules and other medical issues. If an eating plan seems promising but doesn't really fit your lifestyle, it can be frustrating and difficult to follow. Often, old eating habits return. This is why it's so helpful to work with a dietitian.

A dietitian can help you sort through the plethora of nutrition information out there and develop a healthy-eating pattern that fits with your preferences, schedule and priorities and considers your family's needs too. A dietitian can help you explore the best plan for you right now and in the future.

Visit regularly with your diabetes care team. Because diabetes is a progressive disease, insulin and medications may be added to your care plan or changed to best manage your blood sugar. Changes in medication or insulin may require updates to your nutrition recommendations.

Remember that eating should be a delight, not a chore. The best type of eating plan is the one that you can follow for life — one that allows you to eat healthy, balanced meals that you enjoy.

WHAT'S HEALTHY EATING?

If you think that eating well is all about counting calories or fat grams and depriving yourself of all of your favorite foods, then it's time to think about food in a different way. Eating well means actually enjoying the food that you eat while also getting all of the vitamins, minerals and nutrients that you need to live a long and healthy life.

Because your body is a complex machine, it needs a variety of foods to achieve a balanced mix of energy. An eating plan that emphasizes a variety of vegetables, fruits and whole grains provides a rich supply of nutrients, fiber and other substances associated with better health.

In addition, a variety of foods introduces you to many textures and flavors to increase eating pleasure.

By learning more about how your body uses the nutrients different foods provide, you'll better understand how eating well affects diabetes and your overall health.

Each day you want to eat a variety of foods that help you balance key nutrients. The three main nutrients that your body needs in large quantities (macronutrients) are carbohydrates, protein and fats. These macronutrients, when eaten in the right amounts, form the basis of a healthy-eating plan for anyone, whether living with or without diabetes.

THERE IS NO 'DIABETES DIET'

Contrary to popular belief, living with diabetes doesn't mean that you have to eat special foods or follow a complicated diet. Nor is there a single plan that works for everyone living with diabetes. For most people, eating well when you have diabetes simply means heart-healthy eating in portioned amounts.

This means frequently choosing plant-based foods such as vegetables, fruits and whole grains and opting for smaller servings of lean or low-fat animal foods, such as lean cuts of meat and low-fat and fat-free dairy products. This kind of eating plan is naturally rich in nutrients and low in fat and calories. In fact, it's the kind of eating plan that everyone should aim to follow.

Your dietitian can help you tailor this eating plan to meet your personal needs, taking into account factors such as the type of diabetes you're living with, your blood sugar level, your weight and any other health concerns you may have. Even though the details may differ, the foundation remains the same for all types of diabetes (see opposite page).

HEALTHY EATING FOR ALL TYPES OF DIABETES

The main concepts of healthy eating for diabetes are similar whether you are living with prediabetes, type 1 diabetes or type 2 diabetes. They include these important steps:
- Adopting a heart-healthy eating plan
- Eating in portioned amounts
- Staying consistent with three meals a day at regular times
- Achieving and maintaining a healthy weight
- Limiting your intake of alcohol, sweets and sweetened beverages
- Following up regularly with a dietitian and diabetes care team

However, one size doesn't fit all. The goals and specific nutrition suggestions for the different types of diabetes — as well as for your own individual circumstances — may vary:

Types	Goals	Nutrition suggestions
Prediabetes	Heart-healthy eating, physical activity, and weight loss or maintenance to keep blood sugars within target range and prevent type 2 diabetes	Plate method of eating (see page 45, "Size up your plate") for balanced nutrition in portioned amounts
Type 2 diabetes	Heart-healthy eating, physical activity, weight loss or maintenance, as well as matching your diabetes treatment plan (oral medications, insulin) with your nutrition goals	Any or all: • Plate method of eating for balanced nutrition in portioned amounts • Carbohydrate counting (see page 47) • Exchange system — a meal plan with specific portions of each food group (see page 51)
Type 1 diabetes	Heart-healthy eating and taking insulin to cover carbohydrate-containing foods, physical activity	Carbohydrate counting (see page 47)

Carbohydrates: The foundation

Carbohydrates (carbs) are naturally occurring sugars, starches and fiber found in food. An apple or a slice of bread, for example, consists primarily of carbohydrates. During digestion, carbohydrates break down into a simple sugar called glucose, which is absorbed into the bloodstream and circulates through your body. Your body uses glucose, or blood sugar, to fuel its cells. Your brain, for example, uses glucose as its primary source of energy.

Since carbohydrates are your body's main source of glucose, they can raise your blood sugar levels. But don't be alarmed — carbohydrates are still an important part of your diet, even when living with diabetes. Choosing the healthiest carbohydrates in portioned amounts is the key. Healthy foods rich in carbohydrates include whole grains, vegetables, fruits, milk and yogurt.

Keeping the amount of carbohydrates you eat consistent throughout the day and from day to day is an important way

CARBOHYDRATES: TRUE OR FALSE?

Carbohydrates have gotten a bad reputation over the years. But the truth is, carbohydrates are good for your body when taken in moderation and as part of a healthy, balanced diet. Here's a look at popular beliefs about carbs.

Carbohydrates are bad for you.
False: Carbohydrates are needed to help provide your body, brain and nervous system energy to function. Carbohydrates are the body's main source of energy. They have important vitamins and minerals and are your body's only source of dietary fiber.

Carbohydrates are found in many foods, including fruits, breads and sweets.
True: Carbs are in a of variety foods, such as fruits and fruit juices; milk and yogurt; grains, breads and pasta; starchy vegetables, such as corn and potatoes; and sweets. The key is to choose complex carbohydrates, such as those found in whole foods, over refined carbohydrates, such as those found in ultraprocessed foods — for example, packaged snacks and frozen pizzas.

Carbohydrates make you gain weight.
False: Extra calories make you gain weight. Carbohydrates, just like fat and protein, provide your body with calories. If you eat too many calories, no matter what the food, your body stores the extra calories as fat.

to keep your blood sugar in a healthy range. It's typical for about half of your daily calories to come from carbohydrates. The number of servings of carbohydrate-rich foods you should eat depends on your calorie needs. A dietitian can help you determine your calorie and carbohydrate needs.

Protein: The building blocks

Your body uses protein for the development and maintenance of your muscles and organs. Foods high in protein include meat, poultry, eggs, cheese, fish, legumes, and nuts, seeds and nut butters. If you eat more protein than you need — which many people do — your body stores the extra calories as fat.

Select proteins that are lower in fat, such as fish, poultry without skin, lean meats, and low-fat or fat-free cheese. Whether or not you're a vegetarian, plant sources of protein, such as legumes (beans, dried peas and lentils) and products made from soy (miso, tempeh, tofu, soy milk and soy cheese), can replace meat and dairy products. These foods are also low in fat and cholesterol. Consider this a chance to try something new.

FATS: THE GOOD AND THE BAD

As you read labels, look for products that contain monounsaturated fats with little or no saturated and trans fats. Remember that all fats are high in calories.

Monounsaturated fats ("good" fats) help lower total and low-density lipoprotein (LDL), the "bad" cholesterol. They're found mainly in olive, canola and peanut oils, as well as most nuts and avocados.

Polyunsaturated fats help lower total and LDL cholesterol. They're found mainly in vegetable oils, such as safflower, corn, sunflower, soybean and sesame seed oils.

Saturated fats raise total and LDL cholesterol, increasing your risk of heart disease. They're found mainly in red meats, most whole-fat dairy products (including butter), egg yolks, chocolate (cocoa butter), as well as coconut, palm and other tropical oils.

Trans fats (partially hydrogenated vegetable oil) also raise LDL cholesterol. They're found mainly in stick margarine and shortening and the products made from them — cookies, pastries, candies, snack foods and french fries.

Fats: The calorie heavyweights

Fats are the most concentrated source of food energy. Fat is essential to the life and function of your cells. It's when you eat too much fat — and the wrong kinds — that health problems occur.

Not all fats are created equal. Some are more nutritious than others. Fats are also high in calories, so it's important to limit total fat consumption to help optimize your weight, blood sugar and blood cholesterol.

To limit the amount of fat you eat:
- Eat no more than 6 ounces of cooked lean meat, fish or skinless white meat poultry a day.
- Marinate meats and use herbs and spices to keep meats tender and moist and to give them flavor.
- Avoid fried foods. Instead, bake, steam, grill, broil or roast meat and vegetables.

- Choose fat-free or low-fat dairy products, salad dressings and spreads.
- Use canola or olive oil (in small amounts) for cooking and salads.
- Season vegetables with lemon, lime or herbs rather than butter or oil.

PLAN YOUR MEALS

A meal plan is simply an eating guide with two key roles:
- It helps establish a routine for eating meals at regular times every day.
- It guides you in choosing healthy foods in the right amounts at each meal.

When you're first diagnosed with diabetes, ask your health care provider to refer you to a registered dietitian nutritionist. Eating at irregular times, overeating or making poor food choices can contribute to high blood sugar. A dietitian can help you improve your eating habits.

KEEP AN EYE ON SATURATED FAT AND CHOLESTEROL

Because diabetes puts you at increased risk of heart disease and stroke, it's also important that you limit your intake of saturated fat and cholesterol. Saturated fat elevates your blood cholesterol levels. When there's too much cholesterol in your blood, you may develop fatty deposits in your blood vessels. Eventually, these deposits build up and make it difficult for blood to flow through your arteries. The most concentrated sources of saturated fat and cholesterol include high-fat animal products such as organ meats and processed meats, egg yolks, and high-fat dairy products, including whole milk, cream, ice cream and full-fat cheese. Instead, use lean cuts of meat, egg substitutes, and low-fat or fat-free milk products whenever possible.

DON'T FORGET YOUR OMEGA-3S

Eating foods that are rich in omega-3 fatty acids can help protect against coronary artery disease. Fish is a good source of omega-3s and a good alternative to high-fat meats. Fish high in omega-3s include anchovies, cod, herring, salmon, sardines, freshwater trout and tuna. Eating at least two 4-ounce servings of these types of fish every week is recommended. Omega-3 fatty acids are also found in canola oil, flaxseeds, soybeans and some nuts, especially English walnuts. Of note, nonfish sources will have smaller amounts of omega-3s.

The Food and Drug Administration (FDA) advises pregnant women and nursing mothers to eat between 8 and 12 ounces of fish a week, from choices that are lower in mercury. King mackerel, marlin, orange roughy, shark, swordfish, bigeye tuna and Gulf of Mexico tilefish are some fish that have higher amounts of mercury. Limit albacore tuna and tuna steaks to no more than 4 ounces a week. Check the FDA's website for the latest recommendations.

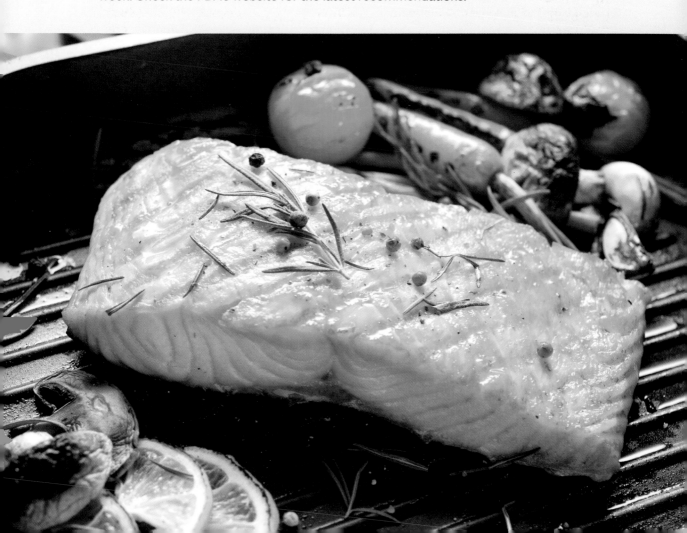

Some people may need to follow a more deliberate meal plan, eating only the recommended number of servings from each food group every day, based on their individual calorie needs. A registered dietitian nutritionist can help you with a plan to improve eating habits and better manage your diabetes.

Working with a dietitian

Understanding the healthiest food choices, how much to eat and how those food choices affect your blood sugar level can be a complex task. A registered dietitian nutritionist can help you make sense of it all and put together a plan that fits your health goals, food tastes, family or cultural traditions, and lifestyle.

The general recommendation is to meet with a dietitian at diagnosis. Then meet annually or whenever you're having trouble meeting your target goals, when complicating factors develop, or when transitions in life and care occur.

At the first meeting, your dietitian will likely ask you about your weight history and your eating habits — what you like to eat and drink, how much you generally eat and drink, as well as when and what time of day you have meals and snacks.

You'll also likely discuss your diabetes treatment goals, what medications you take for diabetes and otherwise, any special health considerations, your physical activity level, your work schedule, your calorie needs, and whether you're trying to lose weight.

When meeting with the dietitian, consider bringing others in your household who are involved in grocery shopping, meal planning or cooking to the appointment. They will benefit from hearing about healthy choices and how they can support you in caring for your health.

Together you and your dietitian will figure out what's practical and achievable for you, and what's not. Then you'll both decide on the best meal-planning tool to help you manage your diabetes. The most common tools for planning meals are the plate method, carbohydrate counting and exchange lists.

Consistency is key

If you're consistent in your eating habits, it can help you manage your blood glucose levels. Every day try to eat:
- At about the same time
- The same number of meals
- About the same amount of food at each meal

Stick to your routine. It's more difficult to manage your blood glucose if you have a small breakfast, skip lunch and eat a large evening meal on the same day. In addition, the more you vary the amount of carbohydrates that you eat from meal to meal or day to day, the harder it is to manage your blood glucose.

Eating at regularly spaced intervals — meals spaced about 4 to 5 hours apart — reduces large variations in blood glucose and allows for adequate digestion and metabolism of your food.

Look for variety

Aim for a wide mix of foods to help you meet your nutritional goals. Your dietitian can help you plan a program that includes a healthy variety of foods.

This doesn't mean that you have to seek out unusual "diet foods." Instead focus on eating more vegetables, fruits, whole grains, lean meats and low-fat dairy products. And it doesn't mean preparing dishes that are complicated or expensive.

Some of the world's most tempting dishes are built around the season's best produce, prepared simply to bring out the fullest flavors. People who regularly enjoy meals made with a variety of healthy ingredients reduce their risk of developing diabetes or complications from the disease. What's more, they also reduce their risk of developing many other diseases, including heart disease, many kinds of cancer, dementia, digestive disorders, age-related vision loss and osteoporosis.

DIETITIAN MYTHS

Some people are scared to talk to a dietitian because of commonly held assumptions. It's time to set the record straight.

Myth: Dietitians just give out meal plans to follow.
Truth: Preset meal plans don't have that great of a track record in real life. If a meal plan doesn't match your schedule, preferences or budget, you likely won't follow it. A dietitian does more than just give you a list of foods to eat. A dietitian asks what your meals look like now, is ready to give you tips and expert advice on how to tweak those meals, and helps you set realistic goals.

Myth: Dietitians will suggest eating foods that are not in my budget.
Truth: Dietitians are aware of potential limitations many people have, especially financial ones. There are many ways to meet healthy goals without breaking the bank. Whether it be grocery shopping advice or resources for public services, a dietitian can help you find your way.

Myth: Dietitians will judge me if I don't eat healthy.
Truth: Dietitians love to help people make the next step toward a healthy life. They know that time, money and long-standing habits can make healthy choices difficult. A dietitian's goal is to help you overcome your hurdles. Be honest about what you eat and what questions you have. That way you'll make your time with your dietitian the best and most useful it can be.

SIZING UP A SERVING

An important part of healthy eating is understanding how much of a particular food makes up a serving. Many people envision servings to be larger than they are, and they eat more than they should. This page provides some visual clues to help you gauge general serving sizes.

Vegetables	Visual cue	
1 cup broccoli	1 baseball	
2 cups raw leafy greens	2 baseballs	

Fruits*	Visual cue	
½ cup sliced fruit	Tennis ball	
1 small apple or medium orange		

Starch (carbohydrates)	Visual cue	
½ cup pasta, rice or dried cereal	Hockey puck	
½ bagel		
1 slice whole-grain bread		

Protein and dairy*†	Visual cue	
2½ ounces chicken or fish	Deck of cards	
1½ ounces beef	½ deck of cards	
1½ ounces beef	4 dice	

Fats	Visual cue	
1½ teaspoons peanut butter	2 dice	
1 teaspoon butter or margarine	1 die	

*Fruits, milk and yogurt contain carbohydrates that can affect blood sugar.

†There are many types of meal-planning tools. The Mayo Clinic Healthy Weight Pyramid groups meats and milk products together, whereas the American Diabetes Association and the Academy of Nutrition and Dietetics separate meats and milk products in their diabetes exchange lists. Work with your health care provider to determine which type of plan will be most effective for you.

WATCH YOUR SERVING SIZES

A serving isn't the amount of food you choose to eat or the amount that's put on your plate. That's called a portion. Rather, a serving is a specific amount of food, defined by standard measurements, such as cups, ounces or pieces.

With the trend toward supersizing, mega-buffets and huge portions in restaurants, it can be difficult to get an accurate idea of what a regular serving size is.

Compared with what's typically served when you're eating out, standard serving sizes may seem small. For example, 3 cups of popcorn (low-fat microwave or popped with no fat added) is one serving. This amount may hardly make a dent in the large bucket you're used to getting at the movies.

Monitoring the number of servings you eat at meals can help you meet your daily nutritional goals and track your carbohydrate intake. Keeping all of the food groups and measurements straight may seem overwhelming. But don't panic. Serving sizes aren't as complex as they may seem. You don't need to have the entire list memorized in your head. Start with the foods that you eat most frequently. Although this approach does take some practice, you'll be surprised at how quickly you'll retain the knowledge you gain.

Sometimes just being aware of the serving size on a nutrition label will help guide you in the right amount to eat.

SIZE UP YOUR PLATE

Consistent, balanced meals are an important aspect of blood sugar control. But this doesn't have to require constant careful calculations.

Another way to approach meals is to use the plate method — a simple but effective way to help you know how much to eat at mealtime. Follow these steps to help you choose the right portions.

1. Fill half your plate with nonstarchy vegetables. These include all vegetables except potatoes, beans and lentils, corn, peas, or winter squash. Enjoy nonstarchy vegetables often and make them the largest part of your plate. Try flavoring vegetables with herbs and spices rather than with salt, fats or other condiments.

2. Keep the portion of protein to no more than one-quarter of your plate (about the size of a deck of cards). Meat includes beef, pork, fish, poultry and other animal proteins, such as eggs. Meat substitutes include cheese, peanut butter, nuts, seeds and tofu. Bake, broil, boil or grill these foods. Avoid adding extra fats or frying. These are high-fat sources of protein, so limit your portions.

3. Use the remainder of your plate for a carbohydrate. Remember that carbohydrate choices can be starches, fruits, or milk and yogurt.

In addition, try to limit the amount of fat you add to your cooking and to your meal. Choose healthier fat options, such as olive, canola and peanut oils.

READ FOOD LABELS

Food labels can be an essential tool for diabetes meal planning. Here are some tips for comparing food labels.

Do the math

The serving sizes listed on food labels may be different from the amounts you're used to eating. If you eat twice the serving size as listed on the label, you also double the calories, fat, carbohydrate and sodium.

Control calories

Calories can add up fast. It's important to be aware of the amount of calories you're eating, especially if you're trying to lose weight. Although some foods may be fat-free or low carb, this doesn't mean they're calorie-free. Think of calories like a daily allowance of money. If the goal is to maintain your weight, it's best to stay within your budgeted amount of calories most of the time. A dietitian can help you determine the right amount of calories for your personal goal, whether it's weight loss or weight maintenance.

Consider carbs in context

Look at the grams of total carbohydrate — which includes sugar, complex carbohydrate and fiber — rather than only the grams of sugar. If you zero in on only the sugar content, you could miss out on nutritious foods that contain natural sugar, such as fruit, yogurt and milk. And you might overdo foods with no natural or added sugar but plenty of carbohydrate, such as certain cereals and grains.

The goal is not to eat as few carbohydrates as you can, but rather to choose the healthiest carbohydrates in consistent amounts from meal to meal.

Put sugar-free products in their place

Products labeled "sugar-free" are often touted as the best choice for people with diabetes. However, sugar-free doesn't mean carbohydrate-free. When choosing between standard products and their sugar-free counterparts, don't assume sugar-free is better. Compare the food labels side by side.

If the sugar-free product has noticeably fewer carbohydrates, it might be the better choice. But if there's little difference in carbohydrates, fat and calories between the two foods, let taste — or price — be your guide.

The same caveat applies to products with a "no sugar added" label. Although these foods don't contain high-sugar ingredients and no sugar is added during processing or packaging, foods without added sugar may still be high in carbs.

Scan the list of ingredients

Keep an eye out for heart-healthy ingredients such as whole-wheat flour, soy and oats. Monounsaturated fats — such as olive, canola or peanut oils — promote heart health, too. Likewise, use food labels to detect unhealthy ingredients, such as hydrogenated or partially hydrogenated oil.

Keep in mind that ingredients are listed in descending order by weight. The main ingredient is listed first, followed by other ingredients used in lesser amounts. For example, if you're looking for a whole-grain product, make sure a whole grain is listed as the first ingredient.

CONSIDER CARB COUNTING

Carbohydrate counting is a method of controlling the amount of carbohydrates you eat at meals and snacks. This is because carbohydrates have the greatest impact on your blood glucose.

It's the balance between the carbohydrates you eat and the insulin available in your body that determines how much your blood glucose levels rise after you eat. With the right balance of carbs and insulin, your blood glucose level will usually come back into goal range.

Carb counting and diabetes

Some people with diabetes — especially those who take diabetes medications or insulin — use carbohydrate counting as a meal-planning tool. They count the amount of carbohydrates in each meal or

IS THE GLYCEMIC INDEX ANOTHER GOOD TOOL FOR PLANNING MEALS?

The glycemic index (GI) ranks carb-containing foods based on their effect on blood sugar levels. High-index foods are associated with greater increases in blood sugar than are low-index foods. But low-index foods aren't necessarily healthier. Foods that are high in fat tend to have lower GI values than do some healthy foods.

Using the glycemic index for meal planning is a fairly complicated process. Many factors affect the GI value of a specific food, such as how the food was prepared and what you eat with it. Another meal-planning tool is the glycemic load, which multiplies the GI of a food by the amount of total carbohydrates in a serving. For example, eating small amounts of a food with a high glycemic load may have less impact on blood glucose.

Talk with a registered dietitian nutritionist if you have questions. Currently there isn't enough evidence of benefits to recommend using GI diets as your main strategy in meal planning.

snack. This helps keep their blood glucose from going too high or too low throughout the day.

However, carbohydrate counting doesn't mean that you can go overboard on foods that are low in or free of carbohydrates, such as meat and fats. These foods are high in calories. Too many calories and too much fat and cholesterol over the long term increase your risk of weight gain, heart disease, stroke and other diseases, as well as make it difficult to control your blood sugar.

Understand the terms

If you're counting carbs, be aware that the term *net carbohydrates* or *net carbs* on product labels can be misleading. These marketing terms aren't approved by the Food and Drug Administration (FDA). So if you use the net carb number on the label, you may not accurately be counting your carbohydrates. And if you're on insulin, you could underestimate how much you need. Work with your dietitian to learn how to count carbs properly to meet your specific needs.

Be consistent

With carb counting, and diabetes in general, consistency is important — it plays a key role in glucose management. Large variations in your carbohydrate intake throughout the day — such as skipping meals and then eating a huge meal — can cause blood glucose levels to go too high or too low.

Also, it's important not to confuse carb counting with popular-diet terminology. Following a low-carb diet or a ketogenic diet is not the same as carb counting.

How to count carbs

You may be thinking that carb counting sounds like a lot of work. But it's not as much as you might think. Your dietitian will help you determine how many carbs you should aim for at meals.

You also don't have to memorize how many carbs are in a cookie or a piece of fruit. Instead, you can purchase books or search online resources or apps that list carb counts for thousands of foods. Most packaged foods are required to list their carbs on the label.

What about homemade foods? How do you count the carbs in dishes with multiple ingredients? Do you have to add together the carbohydrate amounts for each separate ingredient?

For some foods, that may be the easiest way to do it. Take a tuna salad sandwich, for example. It includes two slices of bread, half a can of tuna and a couple of tablespoons of mayonnaise. Check the serving sizes and carb counts for the bread, tuna and mayonnaise. In this case, the tuna and mayo have minimal carbs, so you only need to count the bread.

At first, you may have to measure your foods to get a sense of how much you use. But after a while, you'll be able to eyeball the serving sizes pretty well.

There are also different apps and software that will help you track your carb intake. Some will calculate nutrition facts for you after you add or subtract ingredients from recipes, or even enter your own recipes.

Here are a few tips to get you started:
- Start with the serving size. For example, one serving of chili con carne equals 1 cup, and 1 cup of this type of chili contains 22 grams of carbs.
- Next, guess how much you'll probably eat. Is it about 1 cup, or more like 2 cups? Then do the math. Two cups have 44 grams of carbohydrates.
- Now think about the other foods you're going to eat with your chili. Crackers and a piece of fruit? There are carbs in these foods, too. About how much will you eat, and what's the total carb count?

THE REAL SCOOP ON SUGAR

For years, people with diabetes were warned to avoid sweets and sugars. But what researchers understand about diabetes nutrition has changed — and so has the advice on sweets.

It was once assumed that honey, candy and other sweets would raise your blood sugar level faster and higher than fruits, vegetables or foods containing complex carbohydrates. But many studies have shown this isn't true, as long as the sweets are eaten with a meal and balanced with other foods. Although different types of sweets can affect your blood sugar level differently, it's the total amount of carbohydrate that counts the most.

Of course, it's still best to consider sweets only a small part of your overall diet.

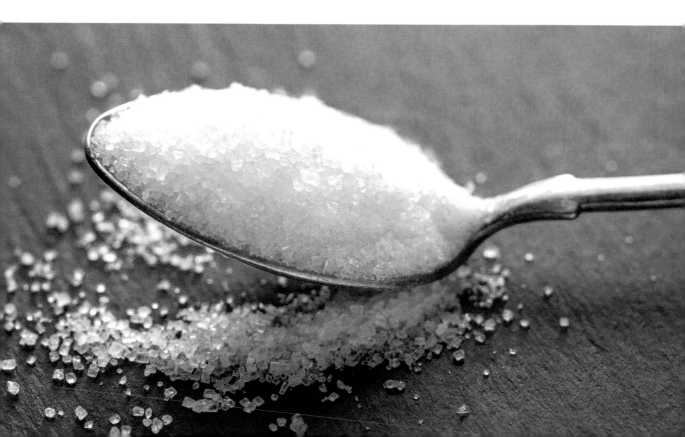

Candy, cookies and other sweets have little nutritional value and are often high in fat and calories.

'Have your cake and eat it too'

Sweets count as carbohydrates in your meal plan. The trick is substituting small portions of sweets for other carbohydrates — such as bread, tortillas, rice, crackers, cereal, fruit, milk or yogurt — in your meals. To allow room for sweets as part of a meal, you have two options:
- Replace some of the carbohydrates in your meal with a sweet.
- Swap a carb-containing food in your meal for something with fewer carbohydrates.

Let's say your typical lunch is a turkey sandwich with a glass of skim milk and a piece of fresh fruit. If you'd like a cookie with your meal, look for ways to keep the total carb count in the meal the same. Trade your usual bread for low-calorie bread with fewer carbs or eat an open-faced sandwich with only one slice of bread. Then when you add a cookie, the total carb count stays the same.

To make sure you're making even trades, read food labels carefully. Look for the total carbohydrate in each food, which tells you how much carbohydrate is in one serving.

Consider sugar substitutes

Artificial sweeteners offer the sweetness of sugar without the calories. Artificial sweeteners may help you reduce calories and total carbohydrates and stick to a healthy plan — especially when used instead of sugar in coffee and tea, on cereal, or in baked goods.

In fact, artificial sweeteners, by themselves, are considered "free foods" because they contain very few calories and don't increase blood sugar significantly.

Examples of artificial sweeteners include:
- Acesulfame potassium, also called Ace-K (Sweet One, Sunett)
- Advantame
- Aspartame (Equal, Sugar Twin)
- Neotame
- Saccharin (Sweet'N Low, Necta Sweet)
- Sucralose (Splenda)

But artificial sweeteners don't necessarily offer a free pass for sweets. Many products made with artificial sweeteners, such as baked goods and artificially sweetened yogurt, still contain calories and carbohydrates that affect your blood sugar level.

The same goes for sugar alcohols, another type of reduced-calorie sweetener often used in sugar-free candies and desserts. Check product labels for ingredients such as sorbitol, maltitol, mannitol, xylitol, lactitol, isomalt and hydrogenated starch hydrolysates (HSH).

Although sugar alcohols are lower in calories than is regular sugar, sugar-free foods containing sugar alcohols still have calories. And in some people, sugar alcohols can cause side effects such as diarrhea, gas and bloating.

ARTIFICIAL SWEETENERS: HEALTHY OR UNHEALTHY?

Artificial sweeteners, also known as high-intensity sweeteners, are synthetic sugar substitutes. They may be made from naturally occurring substances, such as herbs or sugar itself. Artificial sweeteners can be an appealing alternative to sugar, since they contain minimal calories and only a small amount is needed to provide the same sweetness as sugar. The decrease in calories as well as carbohydrates could contribute to better blood sugars and weight loss. However, it's important to remember that many food items that use artificial sweeteners often contain calories and carbohydrates from other ingredients. Read nutrition labels carefully to understand how many calories along with grams of carbohydrates are in these foods.

The FDA regulates artificial sweeteners and has approved the following artificial sweeteners: Ace-K, advantame, aspartame, neotame, saccharin and sucralose. Also, the sweeteners lou han guo (monk fruit) and stevia are generally recognized as safe. The FDA sets acceptable daily intake for each artificial sweetener at very conservative levels.

While artificial sweeteners aren't considered carbohydrates and don't contain calories, there's no clear-cut evidence that using them will help blood sugar, weight-loss efforts or heart health. Choosing an item sweetened with an artificial sweetener doesn't make an unhealthy choice healthy. It simply means it's less unhealthy than one with sugar. Artificial sweeteners can be great alternatives to sugar for some individuals, but it is a personal decision. Remember that just because a product is sweetened with an artificial sweetener, it isn't necessarily calorie-free. When it comes to beverages, water is always your best choice, since it's naturally free of calories and carbohydrates.

A change in taste

Don't be surprised if your tastes change as you adopt healthier eating habits. As your taste buds adapt, food that you once loved may seem too sweet — and healthy substitutes may become your new idea of delicious.

USING EXCHANGE LISTS

Meal plans that include exchanges are one type of tool you might consider using to control your blood sugar and weight while striving to get balanced nutrients. In the exchange system, foods are grouped into basic types — carbohydrates such as starches, fruits, milk and yogurt; protein; and fats. The foods within each group contain about the same amount of carbohydrates and protein, although the amount of calories and fat can vary.

That means you can exchange, or trade, foods within a group because they're similar in nutrient content and the manner in which they affect your blood sugar.

An exchange is basically one serving within a group. One starch exchange, for instance, might be half of a medium baked potato (3 ounces) or ⅓ cup of baked beans or ½ cup of corn.

Your dietitian may recommend a certain number of daily exchanges from each food group based on your personal needs and preferences. Together you'll decide the best way to spread the exchanges throughout the day.

Exchange lists, which are developed by the American Diabetes Association and the Academy of Nutrition and Dietetics, help ensure variety and balance in your meal plan as well as the proper serving sizes to help keep your blood sugar level within your target range.

Food categories

In the exchange system, foods are grouped into these main categories:
- Carbohydrates (starches, fruits, milk and yogurt)
- Nonstarchy vegetables
- Protein
- Fats

TO SNACK OR NOT TO SNACK: IT DEPENDS

When you're considering a snack, one of the first questions to ask yourself is why are you snacking. Are you truly hungry? Or maybe just bored?

Living with diabetes doesn't mean that you need to snack or that you shouldn't snack. What's important is to understand how snacking affects your blood sugar. Healthy snacks don't raise your blood sugar or cause you to gain weight. Snacking on carbohydrate-rich foods might be encouraged during pregnancy. It might also be appropriate for children, people trying to gain weight, and people taking insulin or medication. Talk with your diabetes care provider or dietitian about your snack and carbohydrate needs.

Low-carbohydrate snacks include nonstarchy vegetables and small amounts of low-fat cheese, nuts and seeds. Healthy snacks that contain carbohydrates include fruit, yogurt, whole-wheat crackers and popcorn.

DIABETES AND ALCOHOL: DO THEY MIX?

Many people with diabetes wonder if it's OK to drink alcohol. The best advice is to ask your doctor about appropriate alcohol intake for your specific situation. If you're having trouble controlling your blood glucose or if you have high levels of triglycerides — a type of blood fat — you may be advised to avoid alcohol. But a light to moderate amount may be fine if your diabetes is well managed and it doesn't interfere with your medication.

If you choose to drink alcohol, do so in moderation. For healthy adults, that means up to one drink a day for women, and up to two drinks a day for men. One drink equals one 12-ounce can of regular beer (about 150 calories), one 5-ounce glass of wine (about 100 calories) or one 1.5-ounce shot glass of hard liquor (about 100 calories). Always drink alcohol with a meal or with food. Never drink on an empty stomach because of the risk of low blood glucose. Remember, high-calorie beverages — especially mixed drinks that include sugary sodas and juices — can raise blood glucose and contribute to weight gain.

The exchange system also includes information on determining exchanges when eating or drinking:
- Combination foods
- Restaurant foods
- Sweets and other carbs

Talk to your dietitian about how using exchange lists might help you improve your eating habits, lose weight and better manage diabetes.

STAYING MOTIVATED

Sticking to a healthy eating plan is one of the most challenging aspects of living with diabetes. The key is to find ways to keep motivated and overcome obstacles.

Common hurdles

Common hurdles to following a healthy-eating plan include:

Financial concerns

Buying lots of fresh fruits and vegetables can get expensive. But keep in mind that you're probably buying fewer foods that aren't as nutritious, such as chips and sweets, which also can be costly.

You also save money if you buy less meat. And frozen and canned fruits (without added sugar) and vegetables (without added salt and fat) are less expensive, healthy options that don't spoil as quickly as fresh produce.

Cultural traditions

Food is an expression of culture. But all cuisine can be prepared in healthier ways. You can find cookbooks for people with diabetes that focus on foods from various cultures, with plenty of ideas for making recipes healthier.

Family and social situations

Sometimes family members and friends may not understand why you're making changes to your meals — and to theirs. Discuss your diabetes treatment goals with family and friends and ask them for their support. The changes you're making will help keep you and your family healthy.

If family and friends seem offended if you say no to their special dishes, enlist their aid to help make that special recipe a healthy option. Ask your dietitian for recipe suggestions so that you can include family favorites in your meal plan. If you're going to attend a special gathering where you don't know the people well, before you arrive think through what you'll eat and drink once you get there. You might also consider bringing along your own healthy snacks to nibble on and share with others.

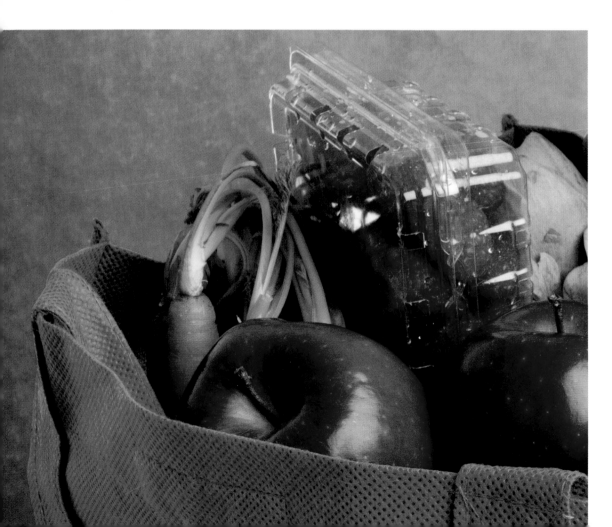

Rewards of staying on plan

Motivation to stick with your healthy-eating plan will improve as you begin to experience the benefits of your hard work:

- You'll experience fewer episodes of high and low blood glucose.
- You'll be better able to manage your weight.
- You'll feel better and have more energy.
- You'll have a greater impact on your diabetes.

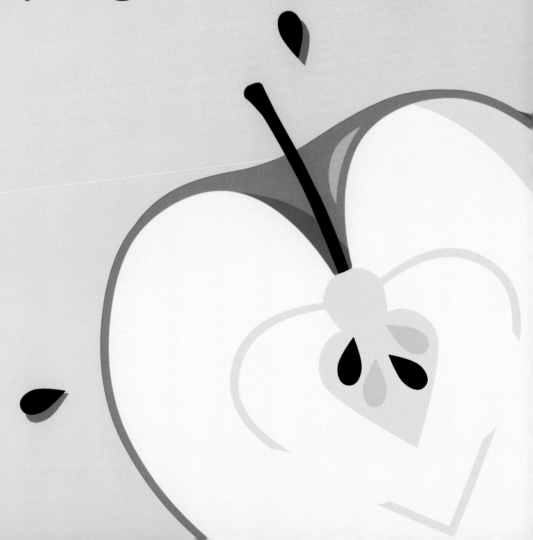

CHAPTER 3

Achieving a healthy weight

A VISIT WITH DONALD D. HENSRUD, M.D., M.S.

"The good news is that weight loss can reverse insulin resistance, and the effect can be immediate. Within a couple of days of losing weight, blood glucose values improve, sometimes dramatically."

The main risk factors for type 2 diabetes — the most common form of diabetes — are a family history of diabetes, excess body weight (particularly around the abdomen), a sedentary lifestyle and poor diet. Of these, the most important risk factor you can control is body weight. As you well may know, the main reason the prevalence of diabetes is increasing in the United States is that the number of people who are overweight or obese is increasing.

When it comes to diabetes, the hormone insulin is a key factor — it helps lower blood sugar (glucose) by helping transport glucose into cells. The way excess weight increases your risk of diabetes is that as you gain weight, your body becomes resistant to insulin's effects because of excess body fat. Initially, your body produces more insulin to overcome this resistance. But as time goes by, your body becomes even more resistant to insulin and it can't keep increasing production. Finally, blood glucose values start to rise and you develop diabetes.

The good news is that weight loss can rapidly reverse this process. Within a few days of losing weight, blood glucose values improve, sometimes dramatically, particularly in younger people. Every plan to lose weight should include lifestyle changes — changing what and how much you eat and being more physically active. In some cases, diabetes can be completely reversed and blood glucose values can return to standard range or close to it.

Positive lifestyle changes that produce weight loss will decrease your risk of diabetes and related complications such as eye disease, kidney disease, nerve damage and particularly heart disease.

In addition, weight loss can help improve other health conditions related to being overweight, including high blood pressure, abnormal blood fats (lipids), obstructive sleep apnea and more.

Finally, eating better and getting more exercise will simply help you feel better, and this can happen soon after starting to make changes in these areas.

Healthy-lifestyle habits can give you the best chance to manage your diabetes and prevent health complications. Yes, losing weight takes work — or more correctly, planning — but the rewards are great. With the right attitude, you can have fun and feel great while adding years to your life!

Being overweight is by far the greatest risk factor for type 2 diabetes. An overwhelming majority of people who develop this type of diabetes are overweight. By contrast, most people with type 1 diabetes are at or below their ideal weights.

Why is weight such an important factor in type 2 diabetes? Fat alters how your body's cells respond to the hormone insulin — it causes them to become resistant to insulin's effects, reducing the amount of blood sugar (glucose) that's transported into your cells. As a result, more glucose remains in your bloodstream, increasing your blood glucose level.

The good news is that you can reverse these processes in type 2 diabetes. As you lose weight, your cells become more responsive to insulin, allowing the hormone to do its job. For some people living with type 2 diabetes, losing weight is all that's necessary to control their diabetes and return their blood glucose to their target range.

And the amount of weight you need to lose to see benefits doesn't have to be extreme. A modest weight loss of 5% to 10% of your weight can lower your blood glucose level, as well as provide many other health benefits, such as reducing your blood pressure and adjusting blood cholesterol levels.

Losing weight can be a challenge — as you well may know. However, with a positive attitude and the right advice, it's a challenge you can meet. As you develop healthier habits, the pounds will gradually begin to come off.

DO YOU NEED TO LOSE WEIGHT?

Before figuring out if you're overweight by medical standards, keep in mind that many fashion models and celebrities are unrealistically thin, and you shouldn't expect to look like them. Your goal is to achieve a healthy weight — one that improves your blood glucose control and reduces your risk of other medical problems.

To see if you could benefit from weight loss, consider these three factors — your body mass index (BMI), your waist circumference, and your personal and family medical history.

Body mass index

Body mass index is a measurement based on a formula that takes into account your weight and height in determining whether you have a healthy or unhealthy percentage of body fat. To estimate your BMI, use the chart on the opposite page.

A BMI under 19 indicates that you're underweight, 19 to 24 is considered a healthy range, 25 to 29 indicates overweight, and 30 or greater means you're obese.

BMI provides a reasonable estimate of body fat for most people. However, it has limitations. For example, BMI may:
- Underestimate body fat for older adults or people with low muscle mass
- Overestimate body fat for people who are very muscular and physically fit

WHAT'S YOUR BMI?

To determine your body mass index (BMI), find your height in the left column. Follow that row across until you reach the column with the weight nearest yours. Look at the top of the column for your approximate BMI.

	Healthy		Overweight					Obese				
BMI	**19**	**24**	**25**	**26**	**27**	**28**	**29**	**30**	**35**	**40**	**45**	**50**
Height	**Weight in pounds**											
4'10"	91	115	119	124	129	134	138	143	167	191	215	239
4'11"	94	119	124	128	133	138	143	148	173	198	222	247
5'0"	97	123	128	133	138	143	148	153	179	204	230	255
5'1"	100	127	132	137	143	148	153	158	185	211	238	264
5'2"	104	131	136	142	147	153	158	164	191	218	246	273
5'3"	107	135	141	146	152	158	163	169	197	225	254	282
5'4"	110	140	145	151	157	163	169	174	204	232	262	291
5'5"	114	144	150	156	162	168	174	180	210	240	270	300
5'6"	118	148	155	161	167	173	179	186	216	247	278	309
5'7"	121	153	159	166	172	178	185	191	223	255	287	319
5'8"	125	158	164	171	177	184	190	197	230	262	295	328
5'9"	128	162	169	176	182	189	196	203	236	270	304	338
5'10"	132	167	174	181	188	195	202	209	243	278	313	348
5'11"	136	172	179	186	193	200	208	215	250	286	322	358
6'0"	140	177	184	191	199	206	213	221	258	294	331	368
6'1"	144	182	189	197	204	212	219	227	265	302	340	378
6'2"	148	186	194	202	210	218	225	233	272	311	350	389
6'3"	152	192	200	208	216	224	232	240	279	319	359	399
6'4"	156	197	205	213	221	230	238	246	287	328	369	410

Asians with a BMI of 23 or higher may have an increased risk of health problems.

Based on *Circulation.* 2015;129(suppl 2):S102 and NHLBI Obesity Expert Panel, 2013.

In addition, BMI may underestimate risk for people of Asian descent, in part because it doesn't factor in the risk conferred by excess abdominal fat.

Therefore, it's useful to look at waist size (measured slightly above the hipbones in adults) in addition to BMI. Health risks go up with increasing waist size, regardless of BMI.

Waist circumference

Another way of determining if you're at a healthy weight is to measure your waist circumference. This gives you an idea of how much weight you carry around your abdomen.

If you carry most of your weight around your waist or upper body, you have an apple shape. If you carry most of your weight around your hips and thighs, you have a pear shape. Generally, it's better to have a pear shape than an apple shape. That's because excess fat around your abdomen is linked with greater risk of weight-related diseases such as type 2 diabetes and heart disease.

To determine whether you're carrying too much weight around your abdomen, measure your waist circumference horizontally at the top of your hip bones. Men with a waist more than 40 inches or women with a waist more than 35 inches are at higher risk of health problems.

In general, the greater the waist measurement, the greater the health risks.

Personal history

An evaluation of your medical history is equally important in determining if your weight is healthy.

- Do you have a health condition that would benefit from weight loss? For most people living with type 2 diabetes, the answer to this question is yes. This is especially important if you also have another condition that would benefit from weight loss, such as hypertension.
- Have you gained much weight since high school? Weight gain in adulthood is associated with increased health risks.
- Do you smoke cigarettes, have more than two alcoholic drinks a day or live with too much stress? Combined with these behaviors, excess weight has greater health implications.

Your results

If your BMI indicates that you aren't overweight and you're not carrying too much weight around your abdomen, there's probably no health advantage to changing your weight. Your weight is healthy.

If your BMI is 25 to 29 and your waist circumference exceeds healthy guidelines, you could probably benefit from losing a few pounds, especially if you answered yes to at least one personal health question above.

Discuss your weight with your health care provider during your next checkup. If

ARE YOU READY?

1. How motivated are you to lose weight?
   a. Highly motivated
   b. Moderately motivated
   c. Somewhat motivated
   d. Slightly motivated or not at all

2. Considering the amount of stress affecting your life right now, to what extent can you focus on weight loss and on making lifestyle changes?
   a. Can focus easily
   b. Can focus relatively well
   c. Can focus somewhat or not at all
   d. Uncertain

3. In the long run, it's best to lose weight at a steady rate of 1 to 2 pounds a week. How realistic are your expectations about how much you'd like to lose and how fast you want to lose it?
   a. Very realistic
   b. Moderately realistic
   c. Somewhat realistic
   d. Slightly or very unrealistic

4. Aside from special celebrations, do you ever eat a lot of food rapidly while feeling that your eating is out of control?
   a. No
   b. Yes

5. If you answered yes to the previous question, how often have you eaten like this during the last year?
   a. About once a month or less
   b. A few times a month
   c. About once a week
   d. About three times a week or more

6. Do you eat for emotional reasons, for example, when you feel anxious, depressed, angry or lonely?
   a. Never or rarely
   b. Occasionally
   c. Frequently
   d. Always

7. How confident are you that you can make changes in your eating habits and maintain them?
   a. Completely confident
   b. Moderately confident
   c. Somewhat confident
   d. Slightly confident or not at all

8. How confident are you that you can exercise several times a week?
   a. Completely confident
   b. Moderately confident
   c. Somewhat confident
   d. Slightly confident or not at all

If most of your responses are:
- a and b, you're probably ready to start a weight-loss program.
- b and c, consider if you're ready or if you should wait and take action to prepare yourself.
- d, you may want to hold off on your start date and take steps to prepare yourself. Reassess your readiness again soon.

Note: If your answer to question 5 was b, c or d, discuss this with your doctor. If you might have an eating disorder, it's crucial that you get appropriate treatment.

your BMI is 30 or more, losing weight can improve your overall health and reduce your risk of serious weight-related diseases, including complications of diabetes.

ASSESS YOUR READINESS

You need to decide whether now is the right time to start a weight-loss program. It's OK if it's not. Starting before you're ready can set you up for failure. But you don't want to put off your start date any longer than necessary, especially if your health is at risk. The questions on page 61 may help you make your decision.

Why readiness is important

If you're going to lose weight because you want to — and not because you think it's expected of you — you'll quickly appreciate the benefits that come from weight loss. If you feel positive about most of your responses to the readiness assessment on page 61, start your weight-loss program now.

The fewer obstacles you have, the more likely you are to succeed in establishing healthy eating and fitness habits in place of unhealthy habits.

If you're not ready to start

If you're uncertain about many of the questions on page 61, consider waiting for a better time. If you're not ready to start a weight-loss program, talk with your health care provider. Together you can come up with ideas on how to prepare yourself. For example:

- If you're under a lot of stress, would you benefit from a stress management course?
- If this is an emotional time for you, for whatever reason, where can you get support?
- If a hectic schedule is an issue, how can you prioritize, trim your task list and make time for yourself?

Looking ahead

Set a date to reassess your readiness. Even if you're not ready to move ahead full force with a weight-loss program, consider taking a few simple steps first (see the table on page 64).

SET REALISTIC GOALS

Goal setting puts your thoughts into action. But your ability to reach weight goals is closely tied to how realistic your expectations are. Goals that are unrealistic or too long term just set you up for frustration and disappointment. When planning, include both process goals and outcome goals.

- A process goal measures specific activities. For example, rather than vowing to lose 20 pounds, commit to walking for 30 minutes a day, five days a week.
- An outcome goal is generally longer term and measures the end result but not how you achieve the result — for example, a goal to lose 20 pounds.

YOU HAVE THE POWER!

Don't sell yourself — and your efforts — short.

Recognize your success. When you do well and meet your goals, congratulate yourself on your effort and self-control. Don't give your weight program the credit. *You* did it. The program just guided you.

Reward yourself. Celebrate reaching short-term as well as long-term goals. Consider what you've already accomplished — whether it's changing your diet, getting more physically active, going down one size in clothing or walking a flight of stairs without getting winded. Reward yourself with a fun day trip or a new CD, or simply take time to relax.

Cheer yourself on. If you get discouraged about continuing, write down why you feel better as a result of your weight loss up to this point. Look at how you've succeeded in changing your eating and activity habits. Focus on your successes, not what you have left to do. You may reap benefits that you never anticipated.

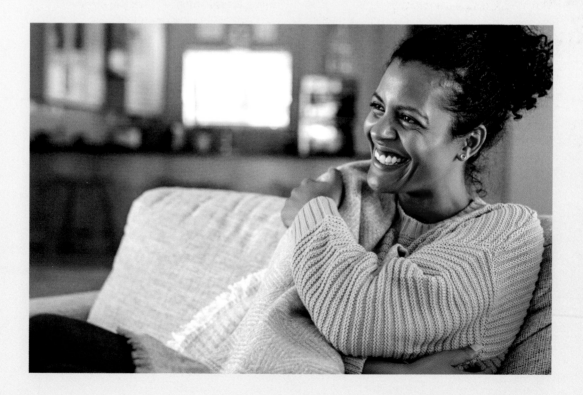

What I'll do	How I'll do it
I'll eat more fruit each day instead of sweets.	• I'll put out a bowl of fruit at home so that it's easy to grab. • I'll eat low-fat fruit yogurt. • I'll eat fruit at the beginning or end of meals.
I'll eat more vegetables each day, and I'll eat less meat.	• I'll buy ready-to-eat, snack-size veggies, such as cherry tomatoes or baby carrots. • I'll eat a salad with a variety of colorful veggies at lunch or supper. • I'll put more veggies and less meat on my plate.
I'll increase my physical activity on most days of the week.	• I'll take the stairs instead of the elevator. • I'll park farther away from my destination. • I'll ride my bike instead of driving my car. • I'll walk first thing in the morning or as soon as I get home. • I'll walk at lunchtime with a co-worker.

Be SMART about your goals

Set goals that are SMART: specific, measurable, attainable, relevant and time-limited.

- *Specific.* State exactly what you want to achieve, how you're going to do it and when you want to achieve it.
- *Measurable.* Track your progress. For example, if your goal is to eat more servings of vegetables and fruits, track the number of servings you eat each day in a food record or food diary. If your goal is to walk for 30 minutes a day or jog 3 miles a day five days a week, track this in an exercise log. Review your progress each week.
- *Attainable.* Ask yourself whether a goal is reasonable before you set it. Tailor your expectations to your personal situation. Are you allowing enough time and resources? Start slowly and work your way up to larger goals.
- *Relevant.* Pick a goal that's relevant for you at the stage you're at in life. Think about what's most important to you and what will truly benefit your life.
- *Time-limited.* It's helpful to plan a series of small goals that build on each other instead of one major long-term goal. Setting and achieving short-term goals helps keep you motivated. Choose a definite start date.

Once you've developed your SMART goals, make a commitment to sticking with them. Try not to look too far ahead. Focus on what can you do today or even right now to make this weight-loss plan work for you.

Write down your goals

Work with your diabetes care provider, registered dietitian or certified diabetes care and education specialist to develop your process and outcome goals. Talk about what worked and what didn't work well in the past and why. Were your goals SMART? What can you do differently to increase your chance of success?

Write down your initial goals and review them often. But remember that your goals may change over time. If so, add your new ones.

Reassess and adjust

If you have difficulty with your weight program, be willing to reassess and adjust your goals — or your plan to achieve them. You may need to change your goals so that they're a better fit for your needs. Review your goals with your diabetes care team. Make sure all of the goals are yours and not someone else's. Keep them realistic.

Remember, you will lose weight. And your life will change. But it takes time and commitment.

SIMPLE FIRST STEPS

You're eager to start losing weight. But you don't have time to read the details about another new approach. Or you're overwhelmed by the thought of another new approach, and you just want some simple first steps. What can you do now?

DAILY CALORIE GOAL FOR HEALTHY WEIGHT LOSS

To lose weight, the following daily calorie goals often work well.

Weight	Starting calorie goal	
Pounds	Men	Women
250 or less	1,200	1,400
251 to 300	1,400	1,600
301 or more	1,600	1,800

Choose one or more of the steps outlined in the table on page 64 to get started toward developing a healthier you. While simple, they are significant measures you can take to begin dropping pounds. After two weeks, if you're ready, move on to the full program described in the next section and start reaping the benefits of getting to a healthy weight.

THE MAYO CLINIC HEALTHY WEIGHT APPROACH

The same healthy-eating plan for managing your blood glucose can also help you lose weight, as long as you pay attention to the total amount of calories you consume each day.

For many people, simply replacing a few servings of fats, meat and processed food with lower calorie vegetables, fruits and whole grains is enough to reach their calorie goals.

Small changes also add up. For example, by switching from whole milk to fat-free milk, you save 60 calories a cup. If you drink a cup of milk each day, that's 420 calories a week. Over time, simple steps can save a lot of calories.

Mayo Clinic has developed a common-sense approach to weight control that encourages smart decisions and healthy behaviors grounded on the fundamentals of the Mayo Clinic Healthy Weight Pyramid (page 272). Instead of a diet that you go on and off, it's a lifestyle program to better your health.

The Mayo Clinic approach recognizes that for successful, long-term weight loss, you need to focus on more than just the food you eat and the pounds you lose. You need to focus on your overall health and well-being. A key element of the Mayo Clinic Healthy Weight Pyramid — shown in the center of the pyramid — is incorporating physical activity into your daily routine. You'll read more about physical activity in the next chapter.

Food groups: Your best food choices

Here's a look at the food groups that make up the Mayo Clinic Healthy Weight Pyramid. Keep in mind that serving sizes are important.

Vegetables

As nutritional powerhouses, most vegetables are low in calories and fat and high in fiber. Focus on fresh vegetables, but frozen or canned without added fat or salt are OK. Go for variety. Note: Starchy, higher calorie vegetables (such as corn, potatoes and winter squash) are counted as carbohydrates.

Fruits

Practically all types of fruit fit into a healthy diet. But fresh, frozen and canned fruits without added sugar are better choices. They're filling and packed with nutrients and fiber. Different colors have different nutrients, so eat a variety. Limit fruit juices and dried fruits — they have more calories and are less filling than whole fruits.

Carbohydrates

Most foods in this group are grains or are made from grains. Whole grains are best because they're higher in fiber and other important nutrients. Examples include whole-grain cereals, breads and pastas, and oatmeal and brown rice. When shopping, look for specific terms such as whole wheat or whole oats as a first ingredient on the label.

Protein and dairy

The best protein and dairy choices are those that are high in protein but low in saturated fat and calories, such as legumes — beans, peas and lentils, which are also good sources of fiber — fish, skinless white meat poultry, fat-free dairy products and egg whites.

DAILY SERVING RECOMMENDATIONS FOR DIFFERENT CALORIE LEVELS

Food group	Starting calorie goal				
	1,200	1,400	1,600	1,800	2,000
Vegetables*	4 or more	4 or more	5 or more	5 or more	5 or more
Fruits*	3 or more	4 or more	5 or more	5 or more	5 or more
Carbohydrates	4	5	6	7	8
Protein/dairy†	3	4	5	6	7
Fats†	3	3	3	4	5
Sweets†	75 calories a day				

*The recommended servings for fruits and vegetables are minimums — eat as much as you like.

†The recommended servings for carbohydrates, protein/dairy, fats and sweets are maximums.

Fats

Your body needs certain types of fat to function properly, but saturated fats and trans fats increase your risk of heart disease. Focus on including healthier fats in your diet, such as olive oil, nut butters and avocados.

Sweets

This group includes candies, cakes, cookies, pies, doughnuts and other desserts, as well as table sugar. Most of these foods are high in calories and fat without many nutrients. When it comes to sweets, less is more. You don't need to cut sweet treats out of your life entirely, but save them for special occasions and keep portions small.

Tailor the pyramid to meet your needs

Use the Mayo Clinic Healthy Weight Pyramid in the way that works best for your needs. Here's how to get started:

- **Determine your calorie goal.** To lose weight, follow the daily calorie goals shown on page 65, unless your health care provider advises otherwise. If you feel exceptionally hungry at this calorie level — despite eating lots of vegetables and fruits — or you're losing weight faster than desired, move up to the next calorie level. Fewer than 1,200 calories a day for women and 1,400 calories a day for men generally isn't recommended — you may not get enough nutrients. But don't become so focused on calories that you lose sight of the big picture — adopting a healthier lifestyle.

ENERGY DENSITY: EAT MORE AND LOSE WEIGHT

The Mayo Clinic Healthy Weight Pyramid is based on the concept of energy density. Here's how it works. Feeling full is determined by the volume and weight of food eaten — not by the number of calories. If you choose foods with low energy density — few calories for their bulk — you can eat more volume but consume fewer calories because of two key factors:

- *Water.* Most vegetables and fruits contain a lot of water, which provides volume and weight but few calories. Half a large grapefruit, for example, is about 90% water and just 50 calories.
- *Fiber.* The high fiber content in foods such as vegetables, fruits and whole grains provides bulk to your diet, so you feel full sooner. Fiber also takes

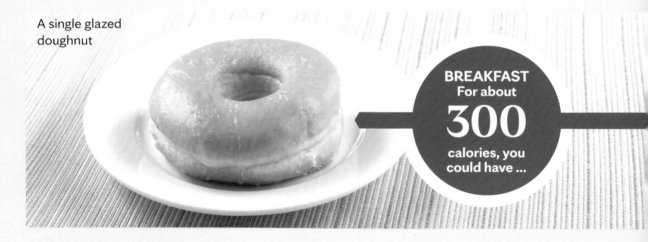

A single glazed doughnut

BREAKFAST
For about
300
calories, you could have ...

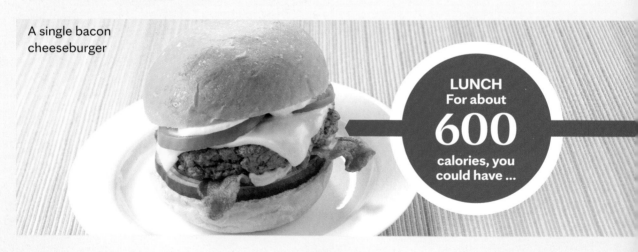

A single bacon cheeseburger

LUNCH
For about
600
calories, you could have ...

longer to digest, making you feel full longer. Adults need about 25 to 35 grams of fiber a day, but on average, most adults consume much less. Increase your fiber gradually while increasing the fluids in your diet.

High vs. low density

Most high-fat foods, desserts, candies and processed foods are high in energy density — so a small volume of these foods contains a lot of calories. If you choose your foods wisely, you can eat more volume but with fewer calories, as shown in the comparisons below.

A bowl of bran flakes with fat-free milk, blueberries and a slice of whole-wheat toast with peanut butter

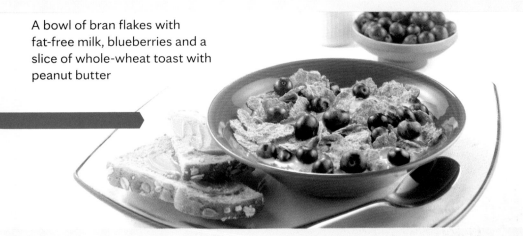

A sandwich with soup, fresh fruits and veggies, and a few crackers

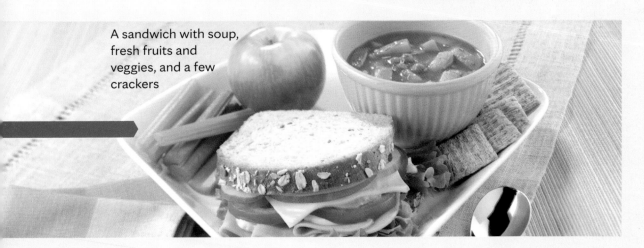

- *Determine the number of servings.* Use the table on page 67 to determine the number of servings to eat each day. Eat as many fresh or frozen vegetables and fruits as you like — they're low in calories and packed with nutrition. Adjust your goals as necessary. If, for example, you don't reach your vegetable goal on Monday, eat extra vegetables on Tuesday.
- *Learn serving sizes.* Many people regularly eat more than they should because they don't know how to estimate a serving size. Use the visual cues on page 44 to help you gauge what equates to a serving.
- *Keep a daily food record.* This has helped many people to successfully lose unwanted pounds. Throughout the day, record what foods you eat, the amount, the number of servings of each and the food groups to which they belong. Or track this data using your computer or smartphone. Too much information? Write a short summary each day in a food journal. Consider including your thoughts and feelings.
- *Include physical activity in your day.* Whether it's informal, such as brisk walking, or structured exercise, move as much as you can during the day. The key to keeping physically active is making it convenient.

WHAT ARE YOUR EATING TRIGGERS?

Does your food record reveal any consistent patterns? Maybe the challenge is your love of particular foods, such as ice cream or salty snacks. Or perhaps you feel compelled to clean your plate.

To help you be successful in losing weight, identify the factors that lead to your unhealthy habits. Take a few minutes to think about eating triggers and check those that apply to you:

- *Time of day.* Are there certain times of the day when you're more inclined to eat?
- *Activities.* When you watch TV or read, do you always have food in your hand? Do you eat fast at your desk while you work?
- *Foods.* What and how much do you eat? Do you find that the sight or smell of certain foods tempts you to overeat?
- *Physical factors.* When you're tired, do you turn to junk food for energy? If you have chronic pain, do you use food to distract you from the pain?
- *Emotions.* Do certain feelings, such as stress, cause you to snack endlessly? How do you feel before and after you eat? Do you eat more when you're with certain people? When you're alone?

Addressing your triggers

As you explore solutions, keep these tips in mind:

- Avoid keeping unhealthy food in the house or at work. So when you get the urge to eat, you'll grab something healthy.
- Limit your time in front of the TV. Keep a glass of water nearby to sip from when you're watching TV or reading. If you get hungry, munch on fruits or veggies. Exercise while watching TV.
- Take every opportunity to move around and stay physically active to increase your energy. Get adequate rest.

KEEPING A FOOD RECORD

Most people underestimate the amount of food they eat by at least 20%. When you first begin your weight-loss program, a daily food record can help you see how much you actually eat in a day and where you need to make improvements. Research shows that people who record what they eat each day are often more successful at losing weight.

Food*	Amount	Servings	Food group
Breakfast			
Whole-wheat flake cereal, dry	1 cup	2	Carbohydrates
Fat-free milk	1 cup	1	Protein/dairy
Banana	1 small	1	Fruits
Snack			
Orange	1 medium	1	Fruits
Lunch			
Greek salad			
Spinach	2 cups	1	Vegetables
Tomato	1 medium	1	Vegetables
Green pepper	½	1	Vegetables
Cucumber	½	1	Vegetables
Olive oil	2 tsp	2	Fats
Bread, whole-grain	1 slice	1	Carbohydrates
Snack			
Apple	1 small	1	Fruits
Dinner			
Fish (cod, salmon, tuna)	3 ounces	1	Protein/dairy
Pasta, whole-grain	½ cup	1	Carbohydrates
Tomato sauce	¼ cup	1	Vegetables
Salad			
Lettuce	2 cups	1	Vegetables
Cherry tomatoes	8	1	Vegetables
Dressing	2 tbsp.	1	Fats
Snack			
Strawberries	1½ cups	1	Fruits

*Calorie-free beverages, such as black coffee, unsweetened iced tea or sparkling water, don't count.

- If coping with pain is an issue, talk with your doctor about pain management strategies.
- Do something to distract yourself. Take a walk, listen to music or call a friend.

Adapting recipes

Many recipes can be modified so that they're healthier. Experiment with some of your favorite recipes using these tips:
- Reduce the amount of sugar. You can reduce the amount of sugar in most recipes by one-third to one-half of the original amount without significantly affecting the flavor. Follow the general guideline of a quarter cup of sweetener (sugar, honey or molasses) for every cup of flour.
- Use less fat. Fat in many baked products and casseroles can be reduced by one-third to one-half. In baked goods, substitute half the shortening with applesauce or puréed fruit. Look for the words *fat-free* or *low-fat* in products such as milk, yogurt, cheese and spreads.
- Make substitutions. In casseroles, cut the amount of meat in half or replace the meat with carrots, onions, lentils or beans. Replace half the flour in baked goods with whole-grain flour. Replace butter with olive oil when sautéing food.
- Delete an ingredient. Eliminate ingredients that are used primarily for appearance or included by habit, such as coconut, frosting or cheese, as well as high-fat or high-sodium condiments such as ketchup, mayonnaise or jam.
- Reduce your serving size. Determining a true serving size is half the battle. But sometimes you don't need to eat an

WHAT ABOUT ALL THOSE FAD DIETS?

In general, fad diets can be risky to your health. And most people stick with fad diets for only a short while before they go off them and eventually gain their weight back. If a diet sounds too good to be true, it probably is. The reason why there are so many fad diets is that none of them has led to lasting weight loss and improved health.

Whether a diet is low carb, low fat or somewhere in between, here are a few points to keep in mind:
- Calories count. To lose weight, the number of calories you consume needs to be less than the calories you expend.
- To keep weight off, your diet needs to be practical, enjoyable and sustainable.
- Both low-carb and low-fat diets can be made healthier with good food choices, such as emphasized in the Mayo Clinic Healthy Weight Pyramid.

entire serving to enjoy a food. By eating half a serving, you consume only half the calories, sugar and fat.

- Change the method of preparation. Instead of frying, use low-fat cooking methods, such as baking, broiling, grilling, poaching or steaming.
- Invest in a good cookbook. Visit the American Diabetes Association (ADA) website at www.diabetes.org to view cookbook titles that are especially helpful for people with diabetes. Also search for healthy recipes on www.MayoClinic.org.

BE A SMART SHOPPER

These simple strategies will help ensure that you have the right foods available to follow your healthy-eating plan.

Plan ahead

Decide how many main meals you'll be shopping for. Then consider the number of food items you'll need for breakfasts, lunches and snacks. Take an inventory of your staples, such as fresh fruits, frozen vegetables, healthy proteins and whole grains.

Make a list

A list makes your shopping trip more efficient and helps you avoid impulse purchases, saving both your eating plan and your budget. But don't let your list prevent you from looking for or trying new healthy foods. When making your list, use your weight-loss menus as your guide. Make sure your list includes healthy and convenient snack foods.

Shop the perimeter of the store

Chances are that the produce, dairy case, and meat and seafood sections of your grocery store are all located on the perimeter. That's where to focus your shopping when using the Mayo Clinic Healthy Weight Pyramid. Whole, unprocessed foods are generally better than ready-to-eat foods because they don't contain added sugar, sodium or artificial ingredients, and you can control any ingredients that you add while cooking. Whole foods also tend to be higher in vitamins, minerals and fiber. Flash-frozen fruits and vegetables are as nutritious as fresh, and may be less expensive.

Don't shop when hungry

It's harder to resist buying high-fat, high-calorie snack items when you're hungry. So set yourself up for success and shop after you've eaten a good meal. If you do find yourself shopping on an empty stomach, drink some water or buy a piece of fruit to munch on to avoid unhealthy impulse buys.

Read nutrition labels

If you're buying processed foods, check nutrition labels. Remember, even foods advertised as low fat or fat-free can pack a lot of calories. Don't be fooled. The label

WHAT'S YOUR MEAL ROUTINE?

As you examine your eating behaviors and try to identify unhealthy habits, it's important to reflect on your mealtimes. Answer these questions to help assess if your meal routine is helping or hurting your efforts to lose weight. (Snacking isn't considered a meal.)

1. How many meals do you eat in a day?
    A. Two or less
    B. Three
    C. Four
    D. Five or more

Having just one or two meals a day generally isn't the best approach to eating, especially if you're skipping breakfast or snacking throughout the day. When snacking, you probably don't pay attention to how much you eat, and chances are that you'll overeat. Aim for three planned, balanced meals each day.

2. How many between-meal snacks do you have each day?
    A. One or none
    B. Two
    C. Three
    D. Four or more

Snacking between meals to relieve hunger is OK, as long as you're nibbling on something healthy. Remember, you can eat unlimited amounts of vegetables and fruits. However, snacks shouldn't take the place of healthy, balanced meals.

3. Where do you most often eat your meals?
   A. At the kitchen or dining room table
   B. At the kitchen counter
   C. In another room in the house
   D. On the go, such as in your car or office

Get into the habit of eating meals at the kitchen or dining room table. Mealtime should be a time to relax and not be rushed or distracted.

4. What else are you doing while you're eating?
   A. Watching a movie or TV
   B. Reading
   C. Preparing food
   D. Sitting at the table and focusing on eating

Eating while you do other things can be distracting and lead to eating more calories than you intended to. You may even begin to feel the need to eat whenever you do these activities. Break the link — enjoy your food without distraction.

5. How long does it generally take you to eat a meal?
   A. Less than five minutes
   B. Five to 10 minutes
   C. 10 to 20 minutes
   D. 20 minutes or more

The longer it takes you to eat a meal, the more time your brain has to register that you're full. Eating too fast creates a time lag: You overeat before you begin to feel full. Slow down. You'll likely eat less and enjoy the experience more.

will list the calories, fat, cholesterol, sodium and added sugars for one serving — but keep in mind that you might eat more than one serving at a time. Compare similar products so that you can choose the healthiest.

BUMPS IN THE ROAD: OVERCOMING SETBACKS

It's inevitable that you'll have setbacks, and that's OK. But don't use your setbacks as an excuse to dump your eating goals. Instead, renew your determination and simply continue on with your plan. For example, if you ate a rich dessert that you hadn't planned on, think about what triggered you to do so and try to learn from it.

Getting back on track

Use the following tips to help you get back on track after a setback.

Take charge

Accept responsibility for your own behavior. Remember that ultimately only you can help yourself lose weight. Along with your efforts will come success that's ultimately yours as well.

Avoid risky situations

If restaurant buffets are just too tempting, avoid them — at least until you feel more in control of your new eating habits.

Think it through

If you're tempted to indulge in an old favorite food, first ask yourself if you're really hungry. Chances are, your craving is more from habit than hunger. Wait a few minutes and see if the desire passes. Or try distracting yourself from your urge to eat — call a friend or take the dog for a walk.

Let your brain catch up

If you're having trouble limiting your portions, eat a healthy amount slowly. Then stand up for a bit before having a second helping. It takes a few minutes for your stomach to let your brain know that you're full. By the time you sit down again, you may not be as hungry as you thought.

Be gentle with yourself

Practice self-forgiveness. Don't let negative self-talk ("I've blown it now!") get in your way of getting back on track with your eating goals. Try not to think of your slip-up as a catastrophe. Remember that mistakes happen and that each day is a chance to start anew.

Ask for and accept support

Accepting support from others isn't a sign of weakness, nor does it mean that you're failing. Asking for support is a sign of good judgment. Positive support from others helps keep you on track.

WILLPOWER VS. SELF-CONTROL

You may think that you can reach a healthy weight if you exert enough willpower. You just won't eat those foods that cause you to gain weight. Unfortunately, this can set you up to fail as your willpower inevitably cracks. This is when many people give up. "I already broke the rules, so I might as well keep eating."

Don't be too hard on yourself. Be realistic — make healthy behavior choices easier through planning so you can rely on self-control instead of willpower. These examples show the difference:

Willpower	Self-control
I'll make a cheesecake for the family, but I won't eat any of it.	I won't make a cheesecake, but I can have an occasional slice when I dine out.
We'll go to the buffet, but I'll just have salad.	We'll go to a restaurant that offers small portions and low-fat or vegetarian items.
I'll bring my favorite chocolate dessert for my co-workers, but I won't have any of it.	I'll bring a tasty healthy dessert for my co-workers so that I can have some, too.

Find healthy ways to deal with stress

Everyone experiences stress differently. Yet some sources of stress are common, such as too much to do and too little time. Perhaps you can take a fresh look at your schedule or learn to say no to extraneous requests. You might benefit from learning a few relaxation techniques, such as deep breathing or meditation.

Make sure you get enough sleep and set aside at least one night each week for recreation. Go for a quiet walk in a park or play a game of pickleball with friends. You might also consider taking a stress management class. Don't be afraid to seek professional help if needed.

Plan your strategy

Clearly identify the problem, and then create a list of possible solutions. Try a solution. If it works, you've got a strategy for preventing another lapse. If it doesn't, try the next solution and keep trying until you find one that works.

Reevaluate your goals

Your weight-loss goals may change over time. Review them periodically and make certain they're still realistic. Change them as needed. Remember, healthy weight loss comes gradually — 1 or 2 pounds a week.

IS IT OK TO HAVE MEAL REPLACEMENT SHAKES AND PRODUCTS IN PLACE OF MEALS IF I DON'T HAVE TIME TO EAT?

Focusing the bulk of your diet on whole grains, fruits, vegetables and lean proteins is best. But a meal replacement product on occasion is a convenient alternative when eating a healthy meal isn't possible.

Most meal replacement products, such as shakes or meal bars, provide fewer than 400 calories a meal and are fortified with vitamins and minerals. Ask your doctor or dietitian if meal replacement products fit into your specific meal planning.

When you do need to replace a meal with a bar or shake, ignore the packaging claims and read the nutrition label. Look for whole-grain ingredients or whole-food ingredients, such as nuts or seeds. An ingredient like nuts can boost the protein in a bar and can contribute to the product's fiber content, which will help you feel fuller longer. Also, try to avoid added sugars, which are sugars and syrups added to foods during processing. They contribute calories but not nutrients.

Although setbacks are disappointing, they can help you learn to keep your goals realistic, know what high-risk situations to avoid and determine what strategies don't work for you.

Above all, realize that you're not a failure. Reverting to old behaviors doesn't mean that all hope is lost. It just means that you need to recharge your motivation, recommit to your program and return to healthy behaviors.

Habits for a lifetime

It takes time and regular reinforcement for your new healthy behaviors to become habits. Eventually you'll know how to identify healthy foods, determine a serving and calculate how many servings you need. Also strive to make physical activity and exercise a daily routine. Once these become habits, you're on your way to maintaining a healthy weight for life.

Remember to use whatever works for you. If you favor computers, tablets or mobile apps, or other technical tools, use them to your advantage. Use whatever devices or functions — trackers, reminders or alarms — that can help you meet your goals.

BEVERAGES: HOW MANY CALORIES ARE YOU DRINKING?

Although some beverages, such as juice and milk, have important nutrients, they also contain a lot of calories. Drinking reduced-calorie ("light") juices or diluting juices with plain or sparkling water can help lower calories. But whole fruit, packed with fiber and nutrients, is a much better choice and more filling. To help cut calories in milk yet still get calcium, switch to low-fat or fat-free milk. Water is still the best choice when it comes to satisfying thirst and cutting the urge to snack. Try sparkling water if you don't like plain water.

Beverage	Serving size*	Average calories*
Water	8 oz.	0
Coffee	8 oz.	2
Tea, hot or cold, brewed with water (unsweetened)	8 oz.	0-2
Tea, iced (pre-sweetened with sugar), ready to drink	8 oz.	125-240
Milk, whole	8 oz.	150-160
Milk, 2%	8 oz.	120-140
Milk, 1%	8 oz.	100-120
Milk, fat-free	8 oz.	90-100
Fruit juice (100%, no added sugar), ready to drink	8 oz.	100-180
Fruit drinks	8 oz.	100-150
Soda, regular	16 oz.	130-250
Soda, diet (artificially sweetened)	16 oz.	0-10
Beer, regular (light in color)[†‡]	12 oz.	150-190
Beer, light (reduced in calories)[†]	12 oz.	100-145
Wine	5 oz.	120-130
Liquor, 80-proof (gin, rum, whiskey, vodka)	1½ oz.	95-110

*Serving sizes vary. [†]Calories may vary by brand. [‡]Dark beer may have up to 220 calories in 12 oz.

Based on USDA National Nutrient Database for Standard Reference, Release 28, and product labels.

Getting more active

CHAPTER 4

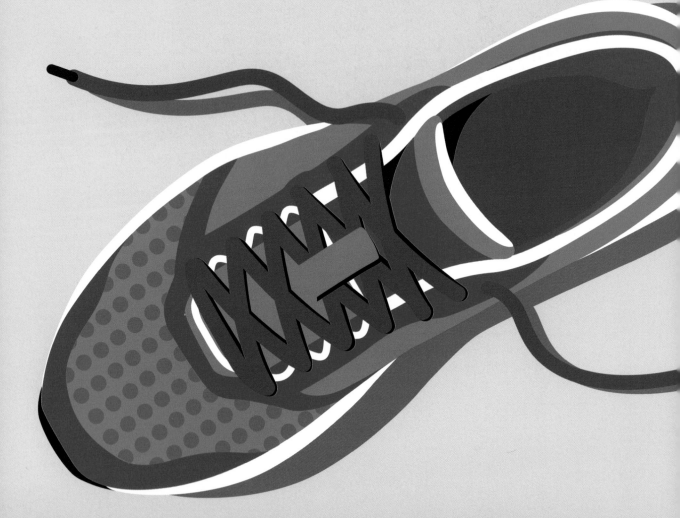

A VISIT WITH CARMEN TERZIC, M.D., PH.D.

"Research shows that being active is important when it comes to management of diabetes. Physical activity and exercise improve blood glucose control, reduce cardiovascular risk factors, contribute to weight loss and improve well-being."

You may have heard it before, and it's true. Being active is key to good health and to diabetes management. Physical activity improves your body's ability to use insulin and lowers your blood sugar (glucose). There are many other benefits, too, such as help with weight loss, better control of blood pressure and cholesterol, reduction in stress levels, a lower risk of heart disease and stroke, and much more.

If you're thinking, "That sounds great, but I don't have time to be active," you're not alone. Time is the No. 1 barrier to being physically active. But being fit doesn't have to mean hours of gym time each day; it simply means moving more — finding simple ways to build activity into your day, being creative in combining exercise with other social or leisure activities, and doing what works for you.

In combination with daily physical activity, work toward engaging in aerobic activity. Aerobic activity is the kind that gets your heart rate up. Examples include walking, biking or swimming. Your goal is to work up to 30 to 40 minutes of physical activity at least five days a week. You can break it up, too. Bouts of activity spaced throughout your day can give you the same benefit.

The first step is the hardest, and if you're reading this, you've already started to take that first step. Good for you. Next, ask yourself these two questions: What can I do to be physically active today? What am I ready for? Answer these questions and then fill in the blank: Today I will _____ to be active. No one can tell you what's best for you; only you can determine that. Start slow and go one day at a time.

Talk with your diabetes care team before starting a regular physical activity program. Ask if there's a need to change any medicines, how often to check your blood glucose and if there are exercises to not do based on your past health history. Once you've met with your team, you are ready to move forward.

In this chapter you can learn more about the benefits of being physically active in managing diabetes, how to get started with an activity program as well as other tips to help you increase your personal success. Remember, being physically active and taking care of yourself are for you. Taking time to be healthy is not selfish; it's simply a must. Your body will thank you for it.

DIABETES AND EXERCISE

Our bodies are designed to move, even if modern society makes it easy to do anything but that. You may sit at a desk all day and then come home and watch TV or put your feet up and read. It can take a special effort to incorporate exercise and other physical activity into your day. But that effort brings a bounty of health benefits — especially if you are living with diabetes.

Benefits

Staying active and fit is important for everybody. Keeping your body in regular motion extends your life and reduces your risk of disease, whether you have diabetes or not. If you live with diabetes, regular activity helps you to:
• Better control your blood glucose
• Lower your risk of heart disease
• Improve your blood pressure and cholesterol
• Stay at a healthy weight
• Increase your overall fitness
• Feel more energetic
• Improve your flexibility
• Improve your sense of well-being

The information in this chapter can help you get started on the road to a more active life. You don't have to knock yourself out to reap the benefits. Limiting time spent sitting is in itself a tool that helps you to be active. Moving more throughout the day and adding a moderate amount of exercise to your daily routine can improve your fitness and help you manage your diabetes.

Risks

For people living with type 2 diabetes, the risks of engaging in low- to moderate-intensity activities are low. If you don't have any symptoms or complications and are receiving appropriate diabetes care, you don't need medical clearance to start a low- to moderate-intensity exercise program. As a rule of thumb, this includes anything not exceeding the demands of a brisk walk. As you become more fit, you can likely engage in higher intensity activities.

If you're living with type 1 diabetes, the only common concern with exercise is the possibility of your blood sugar dropping too low (hypoglycemia). In some cases, blood sugar may rise too high but this is less common. Monitoring your blood sugar, adjusting carbohydrate intake and other strategies (see page 103) before, during and after an exercise session can help to counteract the risk of hypoglycemia.

If you're older, you have multiple chronic conditions, or you haven't been very active recently, talk to your primary care doctor or diabetes care team before you start exercising.

REDUCE THE TIME YOU SIT

Compared with the early half of the last century, people today move less. At work, where many of us sit at our desks for hours, we're burning an average of 130 fewer calories a day. We're less active at home as well, where it's all too tempting to park ourselves in front of the TV for the evening. And with conveniences such as online shopping, banking and socializing, we hardly need to leave the comfort of our chairs.

All that inactivity adds up. On average we spend half our days sitting, and it's taking a toll. Prolonged periods of sitting are associated with an increased risk of health problems, including diabetes, heart disease and some cancers — not to mention weight gain and obesity.

And while regular exercise is important, unfortunately it doesn't seem to overcome the long-term health effects of too much sitting. As an example, people who sit for eight hours or more a day have an increased risk of heart disease even if they exercise an hour daily.

The American Diabetes Association recommends that you get up and move about every 30 minutes or so to maximize blood glucose benefits, especially if you have type 2 diabetes.

Moving more at work

You don't need to overhaul your entire workday to move more; you just need to be more proactive. If your job involves a lot of sitting, make a point of breaking up your day by walking around or stretching for a minute before you sit back down. Another strategy is to attach small movements to simple tasks. On the phone a lot? Walk while you're talking. Stand up when you're reading emails or stretch whenever you hit send.

Changing your office setup also can increase your amount of physical activity. If you trade in your chair for a stability ball, you'll activate your core muscles and use more energy by lightly bouncing. If you have access to a treadmill desk or workstation, try to spend at least part of your day working there.

Moving more at home

At the end of a long day, most of us look forward to some downtime, whether it's watching TV, browsing the internet or playing video games. Like anything, though, moderation is key.

Before seeking out that recliner, do something to get yourself moving. Go for a walk around your neighborhood, clean up the garage, or sweep up the house. See if you can get the whole family moving with a game of tag or beanbag.

When doing chores around the house or in the garage, put an extra spring in your step by turning on some lively music. And when it's time to enjoy that downtime, consider incorporating some physical activity. Stretch, walk on a treadmill or use a stationary bike for an hour while streaming a movie or watching TV. Or get up and move during commercials.

GET MORE FIT

In addition to moving more, regularly exercising your body with intentional structured movements can help you get fit and strong, improve your metabolism,

and burn more calories. Typically, there are four aspects of a well-rounded fitness program:
- Aerobic exercise
- Strength (resistance) training
- Flexibility exercise
- Stability and balance exercise

Aerobic exercise

Aerobic activities are those that involve repeated and continuous movement of your large muscle groups. They get your heart rate up, make you breathe a little harder and make you sweat — such as dancing or playing basketball. Even a brisk walk can get your heart pumping.

Aerobic activities wake up your body and set in motion a lot of beneficial biological processes. For example, aerobic activities increase the density of mitochondria in your cells. Mitochondria are like tiny energy factories that power your cell functions. Aerobic exercise makes them bigger and better. Aerobic exercise increases your cells' sensitivity to insulin and uptake of blood sugar. It improves the flexibility and responsiveness of your blood vessels, makes your lungs stronger, boosts your immune function, and increases the strength and function of your heart.

An aerobic workout generally includes:
- ***Warm-up phase.*** Before your activity, warm up for 5 to 10 minutes to gradually rev up your cardiovascular system and increase blood flow to your muscles. Try a low-intensity version of your planned activity. If you plan to walk, warm up by walking slowly.

START WITH WALKING

A simple walking program, such as the example below, may be the best aerobic activity to start with, especially if you haven't been particularly active. Begin with slow, short walks and gradually increase your frequency, time and intensity.

Once you can walk a distance without much strain, you can vary the intensity by walking hills, increasing your pace or swinging your arms more. Also consider including other types of physical activity.

When walking or doing other activities that involve being on your feet, make sure you wear comfortable athletic shoes that fit well and provide support (see opposite page).

Week	Minutes/day	Comments
1	15	4 days this week
2	20	5 days this week
3	25	Begin 7 days this week
4	30	
5	35	
6	40	Increase intensity
7	45	
8	50	
9	55	
10	60	Increase intensity

WALKING SHOES: FEATURES AND FIT

Purchase walking shoes that are comfortable and fit properly to help prevent blisters, calluses and other injuries. Use this checklist to help you choose:

- Consider buying shoes at an athletic store with professional shoe fitters. Shoes that provide motion control (arch and heel support) are preferable.
- Wear the same socks you'll wear when walking.
- Ask the salesperson to measure both feet and help determine your foot type (typical, flat or high arches).
- If one foot is larger than the other is, buy shoes to fit your larger foot.
- Wiggle your toes to be sure you have at least a quarter-inch space after your longest toe.
- Be sure the shoe is wide enough. The width and heel should be snug, but not tight.
- If you can detect the outline of your toes in the top or on the side of the shoe, try a larger size or wider shoe.
- Walk in the shoes before buying them. They should feel comfortable right away.

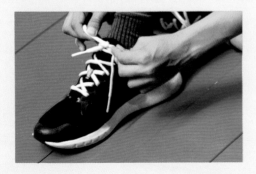

- *Conditioning.* Perform your planned aerobic activity.
- *Cool-down phase.* After conditioning, cool down for 5 to 10 minutes. Stretch your calf muscles, upper thighs, hamstrings, lower back and chest. After-workout stretching improves muscle flexibility and allows your heart rate to return to usual.

It may sound simplistic, but 30 minutes of exercise a day most days of the week can do a world of good. Even if you do 10 minutes of aerobic activity three times a day, you'll still get health benefits. Having a fitness buddy can increase your motivation to be active and make it more fun.

Also, use new technologies to your advantage. There are many new and innovative ways to work out from the comfort of your own home. Use a fitness app or join a virtual fitness group. You can find almost any kind of workout on your smart phone, tablet or TV, including cycling, yoga, kickboxing, tai chi, weightlifting and more. New apps and programs are always popping up.

The best exercise is the one you enjoy doing!

Resistance training

In addition to aerobic exercise, strength or resistance training also helps improve life with diabetes.

For people living with type 2 diabetes, strengthening or resistance exercises decrease insulin resistance, body fat and

MONITORING YOUR PROGRESS: ACTIVITY TRACKERS

You're moving more during the day and getting more steps in. But are you doing enough to see results? Using activity-tracking devices and apps can help you set and reach your fitness goals.

Activity trackers, also known as activity monitors or fitness trackers, are the modern equivalent of pedometers. But they do more than count steps. Activity trackers can determine how far you've traveled and what type of movement you were doing, such as walking or jogging. And many measure sleep quality and length, compute calorie intake and the number of calories burned, monitor your heart rate, and serve as alarm clocks or watches. Some display your progress in real time; all can show it later on a smartphone, tablet or computer. They can even provide social support through apps or websites. And activity trackers can assist with your goal setting by giving cues and rewards to encourage healthy behaviors.

Many activity trackers are made to be worn on your wrist, like a watch or bracelet, although some can be clipped to your clothing. Most can be worn for 24 hours. Accuracy can be hit or miss but most are accurate enough to provide some helpful information. Some popular examples of activity trackers include ones from Amazon, Apple Watch, Fitbit, Garmin and others.

When choosing an activity tracker consider whether the tracker:
- Is affordable
- Is simple to use and easy to read
- Can be used in indoor and outdoor lighting
- Has a decent battery life
- Is lightweight and convenient to wear
- Has the features you prefer, such as GPS, heart rate monitoring, automatic workout tracking, sleep tracking, water resistance, notifications, companion apps or social features
- Helps you stay motivated to be more active

Even if you don't have a wearable device, an activity tracker app on your smartphone may help you quantify your daily activity, such as the number of steps taken, the flights of stairs climbed, the distance walked or ran, the amount of calories burned, and how much time you spent being physically active in general. Many apps also have social connection aspects, where you can share goals and successes.

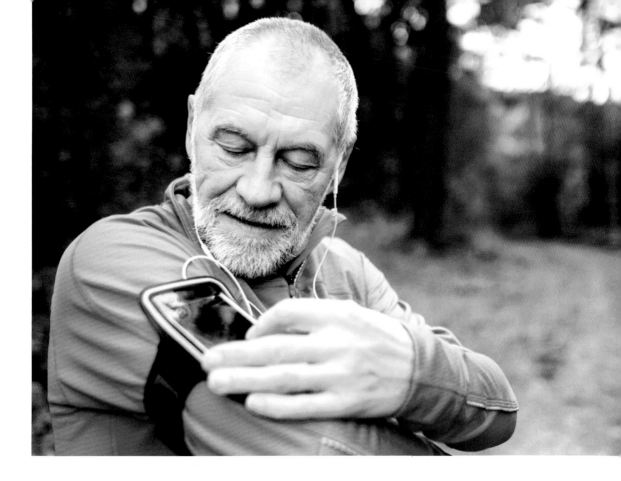

blood pressure, and increase strength and lean muscle. Combining aerobic and resistance training is better for optimal blood sugar management than just doing one or the other.

For people living with type 1 diabetes, resistance training can also help minimize the risk of hypoglycemia. If you do both resistance and aerobic exercises in one session, doing resistance training first results in less risk of hypoglycemia than if you do aerobic training first.

Resistance training slightly increases your rate of metabolism (the number of calories your body uses while just sitting), which can help keep your weight in check. Increased lean muscle mass provides you with a bigger "engine" to burn calories. Because muscle tissue burns more calories than does fat tissue, the more muscle mass you have, the more calories you burn, even at rest.

Resistance training involves working your muscles against some form of resistance. This is typically done with free weights, weight machines or resistance bands.

You can also exercise using the weight of your own body as the resistance. You can

STRENGTHENING EXERCISES

Strengthening exercises can be performed at home, using your own body weight or elastic bands, or in a fitness facility. It doesn't take much time to complete a strengthening exercise program that includes all of your major muscle groups.

Here are four strengthening exercises that you can perform at home using your own body weight. Start with about 1 to 3 sets of 8 to 15 repetitions of each. Use slow and controlled motions when lifting.

Squat

To start, stand with your feet slightly more than shoulder-width apart. Put your hands on your waist or on a table or counter. Maintaining a comfortable back arch, slowly bend through the hips, knees and ankles as shown. Bend your knees as far as is comfortable, but no more than 90 degrees. Keep your knees in line with your feet and not ahead of your toes. Pause, then return to the starting position.

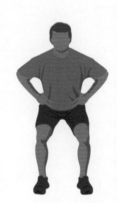

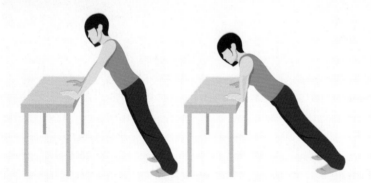

Wall or table pushups

Lean on a wall or table as shown. Slowly bend your elbows and lean your upper body toward the wall or table, supporting your weight with your arms and keeping your heels on the floor. Straighten your arms and return to the starting position.

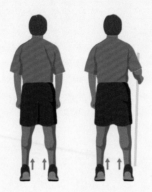

Calf strengthening

Stand with your feet shoulder-width apart. If necessary for balance, hold on to the back of a sturdy chair or another sturdy object. Slowly raise your heels from the floor and stand on your tiptoes. Hold. Slowly return to the starting position.

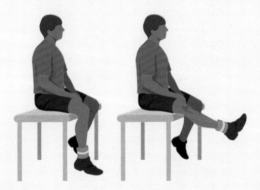

Knee extension*

Start as shown at left, with an ankle weight* on your right leg. Spine is in a neutral position. Maintaining alignment, slowly straighten your right knee as shown at right, pause, then return to the starting position. Do both legs.

*If you have a history of knee or back pain, don't use an ankle weight until you improve your strength. People with back problems or older adults may want to use a chair with lumbar support.

see this occur with exercises such as pushups, lunges and standing squats.

Regardless of the method you choose, begin slowly. If you start with too much resistance or too many repetitions, you may damage muscles and joints. A single set of 12 repetitions (reps) can help you gain strength just as effectively as doing multiple sets.

If you're otherwise healthy, begin with a weight you can lift comfortably eight times, and build up to 12 reps. The weight should be heavy enough so that the last 3 to 4 reps are difficult to complete. After you can easily do 12 reps, increase the weight by up to 10%.

Before each session, take a 5- to 10-minute walk to warm up your muscles. You can work your whole body during each session, or you can focus on your upper body during one session and your lower body during the next.

To allow time for your muscles to recover, take at least one day off before working the same muscle group again.

If you're new to resistance training, consider working with a certified professional at a fitness center to learn proper technique. Or look for a class offered through a community education program.

Try to do resistance training 2 to 3 days a week. Here are some guidelines to follow:
- *Use good form.* Complete all movements slowly and with control. If you're not able to maintain good form, decrease the weight or number of reps.
- *Breathe freely.* Exhale as you lift a weight and inhale as you lower it.
- *Stop if you feel pain.* The intensity level should be somewhat hard, but you shouldn't feel pain.
- *Mix it up.* Change your routine frequently. Do this to avoid injury and prevent boredom.

IS IT OK TO EXERCISE IF I'M PREGNANT OR HAVE GESTATIONAL DIABETES?

If you're pregnant, you can still exercise even if you have diabetes. In fact, regular physical activity — say, a daily 20- to 30-minute brisk walk — before and during your pregnancy is good for you and your baby. It improves your heart health and overall fitness and decreases the risk of complications such as preeclampsia or cesarean delivery. If you use insulin, follow the guidelines for safe exercise on page 103. The same benefits apply if you're at risk of gestational diabetes. A daily brisk walk before and during your pregnancy can help reduce your risk. If you have gestational diabetes, either aerobic exercise or resistance training can improve insulin action and blood sugar control.

CAN I STILL EXERCISE IF I HAVE COMPLICATIONS FROM DIABETES?

Yes. Daily light to moderate low-impact activities such as walking or pedaling a stationary bike can improve blood sugar and benefit your heart, lungs, brain and muscles even if you have complications. The American Diabetes Association recommends caution with certain activities depending on your condition.

If you have ...	Take caution with ...
Heart or lung disease	• Very strenuous activity • Heavy lifting or straining • Holding strength training positions such as a plank or wall sit • Exercising in extreme heat or cold
High blood pressure	• Very strenuous activity • Heavy lifting or straining • Holding strength training positions such as a plank or wall sit
Kidney disease	• Strenuous activity
Peripheral neuropathy	• High-impact, strenuous or prolonged weight-bearing activities (walking long distances, running, jumping or hopping) • Standing or weight bearing when you have a foot injury, open sore or ulcer
Autonomic neuropathy	• Exercising in extreme heat • Rapid movement changes that increase your risk of fainting
Retinopathy	• Strenuous exercise • Heavy lifting or straining • Holding your breath while lifting or pushing • Jarring, high-impact head-down activities
Peripheral vascular disease, osteoporosis or arthritis	• High-impact activities

WANT A MORE EFFICIENT WORKOUT? TRY HIIT

If you're interested in a quicker workout that still increases your fitness, and you're physically capable of stepping up your program, a form of exercise called high-intensity interval training (HIIT) may be for you.

Scientists have discovered that short, repeated bursts of high-intensity exercise separated by periods of resting or low-intensity exercise can help you achieve the same (and even better) aerobic fitness as a prolonged period of moderate-intensity exercise.

In addition, for people living with type 2 diabetes, HIIT promotes rapid improvement of cardiorespiratory fitness, insulin sensitivity and blood glucose control. Some evidence suggests it may be even more beneficial in these ways than a traditional aerobic exercise program.

HIIT is also safe for people with type 1 diabetes. In fact, high-intensity bouts of exercise — either before, after or during moderate aerobic exercise — can help protect against a rapid decline in blood sugar.

HIIT can help with weight loss. When you exercise, the increase in activity boosts the number of calories you burn, not just during the activity but for a while afterward as well. With low-intensity activities, the afterburn tails off fairly quickly. But with higher intensity activities, the afterburn is longer.

Intervals are one example of incorporating higher intensity activity into your workout. You can do interval training with just about any activity. This can be as simple as walking fast for a while, then slower, and repeating. Or you could alternate between walking and climbing stairs or hiking up a hill. Pedaling a bike, swimming or dancing faster then slower repeatedly — these work too! A sport such as basketball is inherently high-intensity.

You don't have to do intervals. Afterburn can also be extended without the short bursts, simply by increasing the intensity of activity throughout. For example, you could walk more briskly for the duration of your usual walk.

Before increasing the intensity, make sure you're ready — that you've built a good foundation. Remember — frequency first, then duration, then intensity. And check with your doctor if you're uncertain about your health.

GAUGING EXERCISE INTENSITY

When you're doing physical activity, exercise intensity correlates with how hard the activity feels to you. It's also reflected in how hard your heart is working. Here are some clues to help you judge your exercise intensity:

Light exercise intensity
• You have no noticeable changes in your breathing pattern.
• You don't break a sweat (unless it's very hot or humid).
• You can easily carry on a full conversation or even sing.

Moderate exercise intensity
• Your breathing quickens, but you're not out of breath.
• You develop a light sweat after about 10 minutes of activity.
• You can carry on a conversation, but you can't sing.

Vigorous exercise intensity
• Your breathing is deep and rapid.
• You develop a sweat after a few minutes of activity.
• You can't say more than a few words without pausing for breath.

• *Listen to your body.* Mild muscle soreness for a few days after starting resistance training is typical. Sharp pain and sore or swollen joints can mean that you've overdone it.
• *Stretch your muscles afterward.* Before your workout, simply warm up your muscles by slowly easing into your chosen activity.

Stretching and flexibility

Most aerobic and resistance training programs cause your muscles to tighten. Stretching doesn't affect blood sugar, but it can increase flexibility and range of motion, helping you in your day-to-day activities and in the other components of your exercise program. When stretching, follow these steps:
• *Warm up first.* Stretching muscles when they're cold increases your risk of injury, including pulled muscles. Warm up by walking while gently pumping your arms, or do a favorite exercise at low intensity for five minutes. You want to stretch your muscles after exercise — when your muscles are warm.
• *Target major muscle groups.* Focus on your calves, thighs, hips, lower back, neck and shoulders. Also stretch muscles and joints that you routinely use at work or play.

STRETCHING EXERCISES

Stretching before and after aerobic activity helps increase the range of motion around your joints and helps prevent joint pain and injury.

But don't stretch a "cold" muscle: If you stretch before you exercise, do a short 3- to 5-minute warmup first, such as low-intensity walking. If you only have time to stretch once, stretch after you exercise, when your muscles are warmed up. Stretch slowly and gently, only until you feel slight tension in your muscles.

Here are four stretches. Stretch each muscle group once. Try to do them 3 to 5 days a week and after physical activity.

Seated hamstring stretch

Sit on a sturdy chair as shown. Maintain a comfortable back arch. Slowly straighten your left knee until you feel a stretch in the back of your thigh (hamstring). You may apply gentle downward pressure with your hands. Hold for 30 seconds. Relax. Repeat with the other leg.

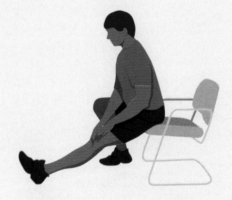

Chest stretch

Stand with arms at your sides. Then move your arms backward while rotating your palms forward as shown at right. Squeeze your shoulder blades together, breathe deeply, and lift your chest upward. Hold for 30 seconds while breathing freely, then relax. Return to starting position. Repeat.

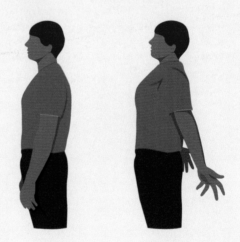

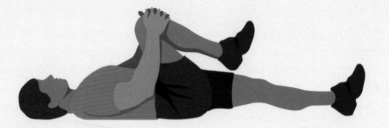

Knee-to-chest stretch*

Lie on a firm surface with your right knee bent (heel flat on the surface) and your left leg straight — or keep both knees bent if that's more comfortable. Gently pull the right knee toward your right shoulder with both hands as shown to stretch your lower back. Hold for 30 seconds. Relax. Repeat with the other leg.

*If you have osteoporosis, don't do this stretch because it can increase the risk of a compression fracture in your spine.

Calf stretch with straight knee

Stand an arm's length from the wall as shown. While maintaining a straight right knee (right heel on the floor), bend your left knee as if to move it toward the wall. This stretches your right calf. Hold for 30 seconds. Relax. Repeat with the other leg.

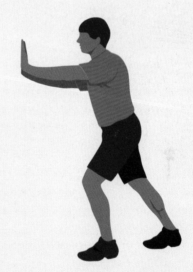

- *Hold each stretch for at least 30 seconds.* It takes time to lengthen tissues safely. Try to hold your stretches for 30 to 60 seconds, if possible. Then repeat the stretch on the other side. For most muscle groups, a single stretch is usually sufficient.
- *Don't bounce.* Bouncing as you stretch can cause small tears in the muscle. These tears leave scar tissue as the muscle heals, which tightens the muscle even further — making you less flexible and more prone to pain.
- *Focus on pain-free stretching.* You may feel tension while you're stretching, but it shouldn't hurt. Back off to the point where you don't feel pain, and hold the stretch.
- *Relax and breathe freely.* Don't hold your breath.

As a general rule, stretch whenever you exercise. If you're particularly tight, you might want to stretch every day or even twice a day.

Another option to consider is signing up for a yoga or tai chi class (see next sections). These activities help promote flexibility. Plus, it may be easier to stick with a stretching program if you're in a class.

Balance

Diabetes may affect your balance. It is important to include balance training into your overall physical activity. Balance exercises improve your stability and gait, even if you have peripheral neuropathy.

If you're an older adult, balance exercises are especially important because they can help you prevent falls and maintain your independence. It's a good idea to include balance training along with physical activity and strength training in your regular activity.

Nearly any activity that keeps you on your feet and moving, such as walking, can help you maintain good balance. But specific exercises designed to enhance your balance are beneficial to include in your daily routine and can help improve your stability.

For example, balance on one foot while you're standing for a period of time at home or when you're out and about. Or, stand up from a seated position without using your hands. Or try walking in a line, heel to toe, for a short distance. For some examples of balance exercises, see pages 98 and 99.

You can also try forms of movement training such as tai chi or yoga that may improve balance and stability and reduce the incidence of falls.

Tai chi

Tai chi is an ancient Chinese form of martial art, that comprises a series of slow and gentle movements.

When performed on a regular basis, tai chi has been shown to improve balance, posture, strength, flexibility and stability, while reducing the incidence of falls. Studies have shown that tai chi also

WHEN'S THE BEST TIME TO EXERCISE?

The best time to exercise depends on your diabetes treatment. If you take insulin, avoid exercising for the three hours after injecting rapid- or short-acting insulin because of the potential risk of low blood sugar. Both insulin and exercise lower your blood glucose. Ask your doctor whether you need to adjust your insulin dose before exercising and how long to wait to exercise after injecting insulin.

Don't exercise for more than an hour unless you've discussed your insulin needs with your doctor. If you are living with type 1 diabetes and you exercise for more than an hour or do strenuous activities, you may benefit from a snack before you begin or while exercising.

For most people living with type 2 diabetes, a snack before exercise generally isn't necessary. If you don't take medications to control your diabetes, it also may be OK to exercise after you eat, when your blood glucose level is generally highest.

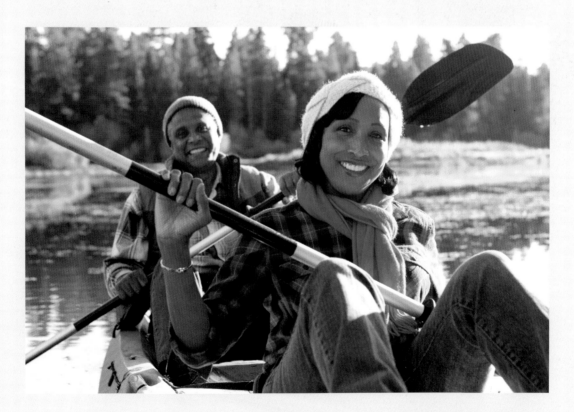

BALANCE EXERCISES

Balance exercises are important for stability and strength, and to help prevent falls and fractures. Here are a few exercises to get you started.

Shifting weight side to side

When you're ready to try balance exercises, start with weight shifts:

A 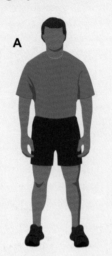 B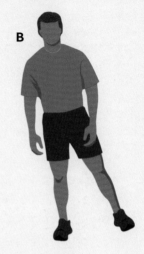

- Stand with your feet hip-width apart and your weight equally distributed on both legs (A).
- Shift your weight to your right side, then lift your left foot off the floor (B).
- Hold the position as long as you can maintain good form, up to 30 seconds.
- Return to the starting position and repeat on the other side. As your balance improves, increase the number of repetitions.

Balance on one foot

Standing on one leg is another common balance exercise:

A 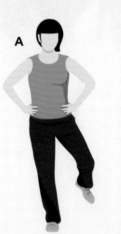 B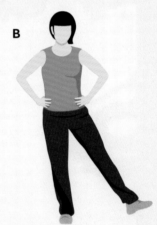

- Stand with your feet hip-width apart and your weight equally distributed on both legs. Place your hands on your hips. Lift your left leg off the floor and bend it back at the knee (A).
- Hold the position as long as you can maintain good form, up to 30 seconds.
- Return to the starting position and repeat on the other side. As your balance improves, increase the number of repetitions.
- For variety, reach out with your foot as far as possible without touching the floor (B).
- For added challenge, balance on one leg while standing on a pillow or other unstable surface.

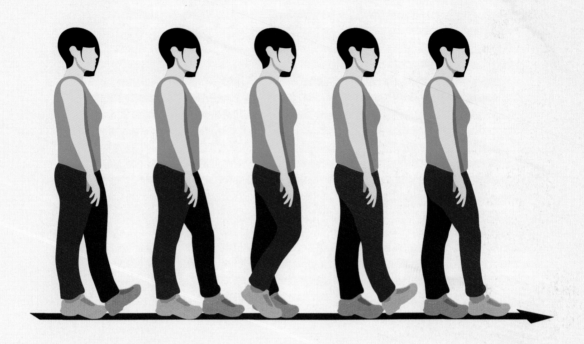

Walking in a line, heel to toe

Walk forward for 20 steps in a straight line. Put your heel down first, then your toes. This is called walking heel to toe.

RAINY DAY WORKOUT

For those days when it's too icky to go outside, or you don't have the time or the energy to leave the house, you can still get a workout in right at home:

- Grab your TV remote control or set up your tablet or other digital device. Pick a favorite half-hour show.
- Before you hit play, do one pushup and two squats. Think of hitting play as your reward for doing those two things.
- Hit play, then march in place. Or if you have one, ride a stationary bike, walk on a treadmill, or use a rowing machine. (Tip: You can purchase relatively inexpensive bike stands that transform a regular bike into a stationary bike.)
- If a commercial comes on, use that as your cue to do another pushup or a few squats. (Or do a few bicep curls or resistance band exercises.)
- Keep this up for the duration of the show. (Or stop when you can't go any longer. Next time, you can do a little more.)
- Workout done!

If you do this workout often, your fitness will improve. You can add in variations to your routine, such as more pushups and squats, marching with high knees or doing jumping jacks for a minute or two, or pedaling faster. Find creative ways to challenge yourself just a little each time.

decreases blood sugar levels in individuals living with type 2 diabetes. You can learn tai chi either by signing up for classes near your home or through many videos and classes available online.

Yoga

Yoga is another gentle form of exercise that has been shown to lower blood sugar levels. In addition, it improves strength, flexibility and balance, and it can decrease anxiety and stress and lower blood pressure. There are different forms and intensities of yoga, but most combine physical poses, controlled breathing, and meditation or relaxation.

Yoga can be performed in your home space or in a group class. If you have any orthopedic conditions or history of osteoporosis, talk with your doctor before enrolling in a yoga class.

AVOIDING INJURY

As you get more active, you'll start to feel better all around and more confident in your movements. But don't forget about safety. Follow these tips.

Wear proper clothing and shoes

Select clothes that are right for the weather and your activity. Physical activity increases your body temperature, so it's better to underdress than overdress. In cool weather, dress in layers so that you can remove or replace layers as you warm up or cool down.

In warm weather, wear lightweight, light-colored clothes. Sweating more won't help you lose fat, just water, which increases your risk of overheating and becoming dehydrated. Use sunscreen and wear a hat.

Make sure your shoes fit well and they aren't too tight. Replace them when they begin to show signs of wear. Always put on clean, smooth-fitting socks.

Examine your feet

Check your feet before you exercise. If you see any signs of irritation, cushion the area to avoid injury. If you have cuts, wash them with soap and water, use an antibiotic ointment, and bandage them.

After exercise, check your feet again. Look for blisters, warm areas or redness. If you have an open sore that doesn't heal, see a doctor.

Drink plenty of fluids

You lose fluid when you sweat, and it's important to replace this fluid. Water is the best choice. But if you're exercising for a long period, you may want the

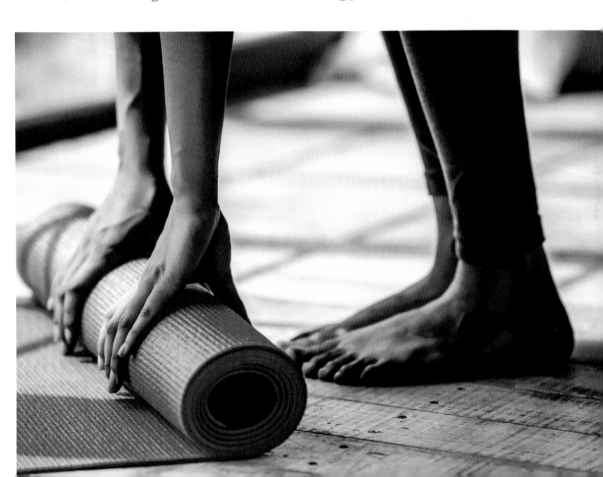

STAYING HYDRATED

When you exercise, you need extra water to maintain your normal body temperature and to replace fluid lost through perspiration. Drink water before and after physical activity. If you take a brisk walk for more than 45 minutes, drink water every 15 to 20 minutes, especially in hot weather. An easy way to tell if you're well-hydrated is if the color of your urine is clear or light. But if your urine is a dark yellow or amber color, you may not be getting enough water. Drinking plenty of water is essential to good health. It:

- Regulates body temperature
- Moistens tissues such as those in the mouth, eyes and nose
- Lubricates joints
- Protects body organs and tissues
- Helps prevent constipation
- Carries nutrients and oxygen to the cells of your body
- Lessens the burden on the kidneys and liver by flushing out waste products
- Helps dissolve minerals and other nutrients to make them accessible

What about energy and sports drinks?

Some energy and sports drinks may be useful in certain circumstances — but others may actually be harmful. Here's a brief summary:

- *Energy drinks.* These drinks typically contain a lot of carbohydrates, caffeine and other stimulants. Carbohydrates can boost energy, but too much caffeine or other stimulants can make your heart beat faster, raise your blood pressure, and cause nervousness, irritability and insomnia.
- *Sports drinks.* These products, such as All Sport, Gatorade and Powerade, typically contain carbohydrates and electrolytes, which can increase energy and replace minerals lost during sweat. Sports drinks may help if you've exercised for 90 minutes, or for 60 minutes if your activity is particularly intense or it's very hot. Beware of products that offer extra ingredients to improve performance — they can be risky.
- *Fitness water.* This water has some vitamins, minerals, carbohydrates, flavoring and sometimes caffeine. There's little, if any, added value of nutrients in the amounts supplied. But if you like them, just avoid the products with caffeine.

calories and electrolytes found in sports drinks. Drink fluids before, during and after exercise. The hotter the weather, the more important it is to keep your body hydrated.

Pay attention to your environment

Extreme temperatures can stress your body. On hot days, exercise indoors, or early in the morning, or late in the evening. In general, don't exercise outside if the temperature is higher than 80 F, especially if the humidity or the heat index is high. The heat index is based on a formula that uses both heat and humidity. Also avoid extremely cold temperatures.

EXERCISING SAFELY WITH DIABETES

Exercise is a key step to improving your health when you have diabetes. But exercise does affect your body's insulin production and blood sugar levels — something to take into account if you're on insulin therapy. Both insulin and exercise lower your blood glucose. To exercise safely, you'll need to track your blood sugar before, during and after an exercise session. This shows you how your body responds to exercise. Knowing this helps you prevent potentially dangerous blood sugar fluctuations with only a few simple steps.

If you don't take medications for your diabetes or you don't use medications commonly linked to low blood sugar levels, you probably won't need to take any special precautions before exercising.

If you're uncertain about an activity or have questions, check with your primary care provider.

Before your workout

Before starting a fitness program, get your doctor's OK to exercise — especially if you've been inactive. Ask your doctor how activities you're contemplating might affect your blood sugar. Your doctor can also suggest the best time to exercise and explain the potential impact of medications on your blood sugar as you become more active.

If you're taking insulin or other medications that can cause low blood sugar (hypoglycemia), test your blood sugar 15 to 30 minutes before exercising.

Below are some general guidelines for preexercise blood sugar levels. The measurements are expressed in milligrams per deciliter (mg/dL) and millimoles per liter (mmol/L).

- *Lower than 100 mg/dL (5.6 mmol/L).* Your blood sugar may be too low to exercise safely. Eat a small snack containing 15 to 30 grams of carbohydrates, such as fruit juice, fruit, crackers or even glucose tablets before you begin your workout.
- *100 to 250 mg/dL (5.6 to 13.9 mmol/L).* You're good to go. For most people, this is a safe preexercise blood sugar range.
- *250 mg/dL (13.9 mmol/L) or higher.* This is a caution zone — your blood sugar may be too high to exercise safely. Before exercising, test your urine for ketones — substances made when

your body breaks down fat for energy. The presence of ketones indicates that your body doesn't have enough insulin to control your blood sugar.

If you exercise when you have a high level of ketones, you risk ketoacidosis — a serious complication of diabetes that needs immediate treatment. Instead of exercising immediately, take measures to correct the high blood sugar levels and wait to exercise until your ketone test indicates an absence of ketones in your urine.

During exercise

Watch for symptoms of low blood sugar.

When you exercise, low blood sugar is sometimes a concern. If you're planning a long workout, check your blood sugar every 30 minutes — especially if you're trying a new activity or increasing the intensity or duration of your workout. Checking every half-hour lets you know if your blood sugar level is stable, rising or falling, and whether it's safe to keep exercising.

This can get cumbersome if you're participating in outdoor activities or sports. Still, this precaution is necessary until you know how your blood sugar responds to changes in your exercise habits.

Using a continuous glucose monitor (CGM) can be helpful, but at first be sure to confirm your blood sugar levels with fingerstick checks until your routine is stable.

The following steps also can help stabilize your blood sugar levels:
- Interspersing high-intensity activities with moderate-intensity activities (for example, sprinting with jogging, or speed walking with brisk walking).
- Combining resistance training (such as squats and pushups) with aerobic exercising (riding a stationary bike). Do resistance training first followed by aerobic exercising right after.

Stop exercising if:
- Your blood sugar is 70 mg/dL (3.9 mmol/L) or lower
- You feel shaky, weak or confused

Eat or drink something that contains approximately 15 grams of fast-acting carbohydrate to raise your blood sugar level, such as:
- Glucose tablets or gel (check the label to see how many grams of carbohydrate these contain)
- ½ cup (4 ounces) of fruit juice
- ½ cup (4 ounces) of a regular (nondiet) soft drink
- Hard candy, jelly beans or candy corn (check the label to see how many grams of carbohydrate these contain)

Recheck your blood sugar 15 minutes later. If it's still too low, have another 15-gram carbohydrate serving and test again 15 minutes later.

Repeat as needed until your blood sugar reaches at least 70 mg/dL (3.9 mmol/L). If you haven't finished your workout and want to keep exercising , you can continue once your blood sugar returns to a safe range.

After your workout

Check your blood sugar as soon as you finish exercising and again several times during the next few hours. Exercise draws on reserve sugar stored in your muscles and liver. As your body rebuilds these stores, it takes sugar from your blood, causing your blood sugar to go down.

The more strenuous your workout, the longer your blood sugar is affected. Low blood sugar is possible even 4 to 8 hours after exercise. Having a snack with slower acting carbohydrates, such as a granola bar or trail mix, after your workout can help prevent a drop in your blood sugar.

If you do have low blood sugar after exercise, eat a small carbohydrate-containing snack, such as fruit, crackers or glucose tablets, or drink a half-cup (4 ounces) of fruit juice.

CHAPTER 5

Monitoring
your blood sugar

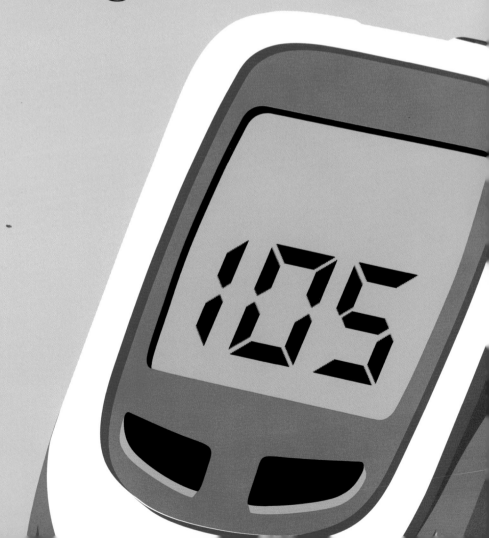

A VISIT WITH ANNA KASPER, R.N., CDCES

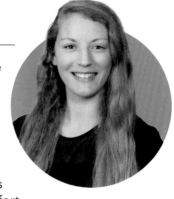

"A lack of education and empowerment can lead to a lot of concerns regarding monitoring blood sugar. Meeting with a certified diabetes care and education specialist (CDCES) can ensure your success and comfort in this routine of self-care when you live with diabetes."

"My doctor just told me that I have diabetes, and that I need to test my blood sugar regularly. Does that mean I have to prick my finger with a needle? I've heard that it can hurt. Isn't there some other way to test my blood sugar? Besides, my diabetes isn't that bad. And I feel fine. If I was on insulin, my diabetes would be more serious. Then I would have to test my blood sugar, right?"

As a certified diabetes care and education specialist, I frequently hear many of these comments when people who've just been diagnosed with diabetes find out that they need to begin blood sugar monitoring.

Fear, misconceptions and past negative experiences are often why people respond to monitoring in the way that they do. Certainly, it's understandable to be afraid of something new — particularly for a procedure that may cause some discomfort, such as monitoring your blood sugar. However, most people find the procedure isn't nearly as difficult or painful as they imagined, and after a while it simply becomes a new self-care routine.

When I'm working with someone who's fearful about blood sugar testing, I often suggest doing the test at the beginning of the education session. The person usually finds out that the procedure causes only mild discomfort. And testing right away means that the person won't have to sit through the session anticipating the fingerstick.

I explain that the needles (lancets) are very fine, which reduces the discomfort associated with a fingerstick. Then we talk about how there are fewer nerve endings on the sides of the finger pads than on the fingertips. We discuss how all lancing devices are customizable to allow for personalized comfort. There also are many new diabetes technology tools that can help lessen the need for daily fingersticks. (You can read more on diabetes technology in Chapter 7.)

People with newly diagnosed diabetes often want to know why it's so important to monitor their blood sugar. The answer is that monitoring provides valuable, real-time information about how exercise, food, medications, stress and many other factors affect blood sugar. It provides important data not just to the diabetes care team but to the person with diabetes. A blood sugar check can provide an instant snapshot of current blood sugar levels.

Monitoring your blood sugar (glucose) can be a hugely valuable tool in your diabetes self-management plan. At the same time, keep in mind that your blood sugar will likely go up and down and that there's no such thing as perfectly controlled blood sugar. There are many elements that impact your blood sugar, and it would be impossible to control all of them. Instead of thinking of your blood sugar in terms of control, think about managing it in the setting of many factors that can dynamically impact your blood sugar.

If you have days when your blood sugar doesn't fall within your desired range, it doesn't mean that you've failed. Everyone has hard days now and then. The goal is for you to do the best you can, with the tools that you have, so that you can thrive while living with diabetes.

If you have diabetes, managing your blood sugar level so that it stays within a healthy range is one of the most important things you can do to feel your best and prevent long-term complications.

But how do you do this? Managing diabetes includes six basic steps:
- Monitoring your blood glucose as prescribed
- Eating a varied and healthy diet
- Staying active
- Maintaining a healthy weight for you
- Using medications as prescribed
- Maintaining your emotional well-being and seeking support as needed

This chapter focuses on the first of these six self-care routines. Blood sugar monitoring is essential — it's the main way to know whether you're reaching your treatment goals day in and day out.

If you've just been diagnosed with diabetes, or your treatment has changed, monitoring can seem overwhelming at first. You might feel angry, upset or fearful about having diabetes. You may be anxious about testing — afraid that it will take over your life, that it will be painful or disruptive. These feelings are common.

But as you learn how to measure your blood glucose and understand how regular testing can help you, you'll likely feel more comfortable with the procedure and be able to live mindfully with your diabetes.

Work with your primary diabetes care provider, certified diabetes care and education specialist (CDCES), and other members of your diabetes care team to determine a monitoring schedule that's right for your needs. Also know that these monitoring needs may change throughout your life with diabetes.

HOW OFTEN AND WHEN TO TEST

How often you need to test your blood glucose and at what time of day depends on the type of diabetes you have and your treatment plan. If you take insulin, you'll test your blood glucose frequently, at least twice a day. Your diabetes care provider may advise testing three or four times a day or even more often based on activity and needs.

WHAT YOU'LL NEED

Testing your blood glucose is a quick and easy process that generally takes less than two minutes. Some tools you'll need include:

Lancet and lancing device

A lancet is a small needle that pricks the skin on your finger so that you can draw a drop of blood. A lancing device holds the lancet. Because people differ in skin thickness, lancing devices can be customized for different depths.

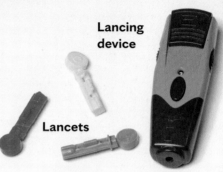

Lancing device

Lancets

Test strip

Test strip vial

Control solution

Test strips

Test strips are small strips that interpret your blood glucose. Typically, you insert the test strip into the blood glucose meter before drawing blood. Most blood glucose meters require small amounts of blood compared with earlier meters.

Note that test strips need to be kept in their container (test strip vial) and protected from moisture. They also should not be exposed to temperatures outside of the range listed on their label to ensure accurate readings. These strips also should not be used beyond their expiration date. You can use the control solution (reagent) to test the validity of your test strips (see page 118).

Blood glucose meter

A blood glucose meter, also called a blood glucose monitor, is a small computerized device that measures and displays your blood glucose level. These meters come in many forms (see page 112).

Blood glucose meter

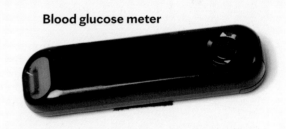

ALTERNATE SITE TESTING

Glucose meters may offer what's called alternate site testing. That means you can test your blood from sites other than the fingertip — such as the palm, forearm, upper arm and thigh. But the Food and Drug Administration (FDA) points out that blood from your fingertips shows changes in blood glucose levels (after a meal or exercise, for example) more accurately than does blood from other sites. This is why the fingertip is preferred for your safety and for accuracy of results. Use blood from your finger rather than other sites if:

- You think your blood glucose is low
- Your blood glucose is rapidly changing because of food or medication
- You've just finished exercising
- You suspect that the results from the alternate site is unreliable

When using an alternate site, you'll need to massage the puncture site to stimulate the flow of blood before you use the lancing device. Check the instructions that come with the glucose meter to see which sites the FDA approved for the product you're using. Ask your diabetes care team if it's acceptable to use sites other than your fingertips.

Testing is commonly done before meals and at bedtime — in other words, when you haven't eaten for four or more hours. This allows for a clear picture of your blood glucose, apart from your food intake. Your diabetes care provider may also advise you to check your blood glucose level 1 to 2 hours after a meal. Ask your provider what testing times might provide the best glucose information to help you live safely with your diabetes and treatment plan.

A change in your regular routine may be another reason to test your blood glucose, especially if you live with type 1 diabetes. These changes may include increasing your physical activity, eating less than usual or traveling. Special circumstances, including pregnancy or illness, also may warrant increased testing.

If you live with type 2 diabetes and you don't currently need insulin, test your blood glucose as often as directed by your diabetes care provider to make sure it's within your goal range. For some people this may mean daily testing, while for others it might be twice a week.

In general, if you're able to manage your blood glucose with diet and exercise and without using medication, you probably won't need to test your blood glucose as often. If you and your diabetes care provider decide you need to test more frequently, talk to your provider or CDCES about the best way to incorporate additional blood glucose testing into your management plan.

PERFORMING THE TEST

Once you have the right equipment, you're ready to start testing your blood glucose on the schedule recommended by your diabetes care provider.

Testing basics

It's important to follow the instructions that come with your particular blood glucose meter. In general, here's how the process works:

1. Before pricking your finger, wash your hands with soap and warm water. Then dry them well.
2. Remove a test strip from the container and replace the cap immediately to prevent damage to the strips.
3. Insert the test strip into the meter.

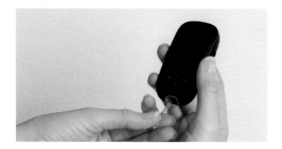

4. Place the tip of the lancing device on your finger. Stick the side of your

finger pad, not the tip or way out by the edge of your fingernail. This way you'll be less likely to have sore spots. If needed, hold your hand down to encourage a drop of blood to form.

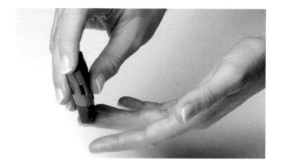

5. When you have a drop of blood, carefully touch the test strip to the blood droplet. The test strip pulls in the sample. You don't need to assist with the uptake of the droplet. Wait to see confirmation on your meter screen that you've provided enough blood.

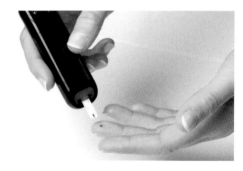

6. Warm hands allow for easier droplet creation than do cold hands. To help the blood flow, gently squeeze your finger from the base toward the site

CHOOSING THE RIGHT METER

Blood glucose meters come in many forms with a variety of features. So how do you know which device is right for you? Your diabetes care team may recommend a meter or help you select one. Keep in mind that some health insurance plans require their participants to use a specific meter. When choosing a meter, consider these factors:

Cost

Most insurance plans, including Medicare and Medicaid, cover the cost of a blood glucose meter and test strips after you pay your deductible and any coinsurance. Find out what your insurance covers before you buy. Some plans limit the total number of test strips allowed. Meters vary widely in price, so shop around before you buy. The test strips are the most expensive part of a monitoring system. Figure out which type of strip is most cost-effective for you. Make sure the test strips are the right ones for your meter.

Ease of use and maintenance

Some meters are easier to use than are others. Are the meter and strips comfortable to hold? Can you easily see the numbers on the screen? How easy is it to get blood onto the strips? Most meters use cell batteries, which last a long time. A battery symbol shows up on the screen when the battery is low and needs to be changed.

Special features

Ask about the meter's features to see what might fit your specific needs. For example, some meters are large with strips that are easier to handle. Some are compact and easier to carry. Others have a backlight or audio capability. People with impaired vision can buy a meter with a large screen or a "talking"

you poked. Be careful not to squeeze too hard as this can skew the reading. If you have trouble obtaining a droplet, adjust the lancing device depth or contact your diabetes care team for help.

7. Within a few seconds of transferring blood to the test strip, the meter will display your blood glucose level.

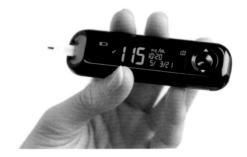

meter that announces the results. For children, there are even colorful meters or stickers made to fit around the display screen.

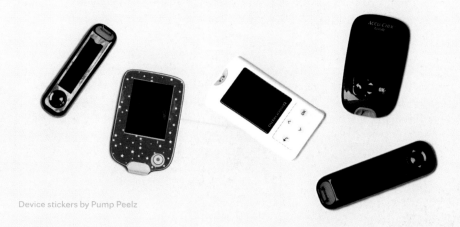

Device stickers by Pump Peelz

Some meters include USB rechargeable batteries that work with a wall or computer charger. This allows for quick and easy recharging, much like recharging a cellphone.

Also consider how the meter stores and retrieves information. Many track the time and date of a test, the result, and trends over time. Some track high and low blood glucose patterns within preset or customizable target ranges. For most meters available, you can download the meter information to an app or software program for your review. You can send this information to your diabetes care team, or the team can download the data during your office visit.

More expert tips

Your fingertips contain a lot of nerve endings, so make sure to rotate the sites where you stick your fingers to minimize any discomfort. You can use all fingers.

You may have the option to test your blood glucose from other sites, such as your forearm or palm. But check with your diabetes care team first to find out if alternate site testing is appropriate in your case. Read more about alternate site testing on page 110.

Although finger pricks remain the gold standard for blood sugar monitoring, other products are being developed to

WHOLE-BLOOD GLUCOSE LEVELS VS. PLASMA GLUCOSE LEVELS?

Home glucose meters use whole blood to measure glucose levels. But when blood is drawn at your medical appointment and sent to a lab, the red blood cells are removed, leaving only plasma, before glucose is measured.

Because of this difference, results from labs and home meters aren't exactly the same. Plasma tests tend to be more accurate, and the results are 10% to 15% higher than are whole-blood test results. But most home meters, especially new ones, are calibrated to give a plasma test result, even though they use whole blood for the test. Your home meter's results are considered accurate if they fall within 15% of the lab test result.

minimize the discomfort with the process as well as make meter use accessible for all. You might ask your diabetes care provider or CDCES about these potential alternatives and if they would be an option for you.

For more on advances in monitoring tools and diabetes technology, see Chapter 7.

RECORDING YOUR RESULTS

Blood sugar monitoring can provide more than just an immediate measurement of your blood glucose. It can help you assess your progress in managing your diabetes.

Each time you check your glucose, log your results. This information helps you see how food, physical activity, medication and other factors affect your blood glucose. As patterns occur, you can begin to understand how your daily activities cause your blood glucose level to go up or

down. This puts you in a better position to manage your diabetes day by day and even hour by hour.

Your life is often not the same from one day to the next. Some days you exercise more or eat less. Maybe you're sick or you're having trouble at work or at home. Changes such as these can affect your blood glucose level.

By keeping an accurate record of both day-to-day events and your blood glucose levels, you may identify some problem areas for you. By addressing these areas you'll be better able to manage your blood sugar as well as celebrate your successes.

With the information you gain, you can even learn how to anticipate problems before they occur. You can plan ahead for changes in your routine that you know will affect your blood glucose levels. This may include activities such as traveling, eating out or exercising harder than usual.

Date	Medication dose	Blood glucose test results				Comments*
		Before morning meal	Before noon meal	Before evening meal	Bedtime	

*Record relevant factors such as changes in diet and activity, weight, insulin reactions, illness, urine ketones and stress levels.

What to track

Your diabetes care team may have given you a record book for tracking your test results. If not, you can use any type of notebook. You can also log your results digitally, using a computer or a smartphone. Many software programs are available for recording and tracking blood glucose levels — ask your diabetes care team for a recommendation.

Every time you check your blood glucose, do your best to record:
- The date and time
- The test result
- The type and dosage of medication you're taking

Also include room for notes, where you can record any other information that might help explain a change from your usual blood glucose level. Examples of

---

BE MINDFUL OF THE NUMBERS GAME

When you're testing and recording your blood glucose frequently, it's easy to get caught up in a numbers game. The "right" numbers equal your success, while the "wrong" numbers represent your failure. At times, you may end up feeling upset, confused, angry, frustrated or discouraged about your blood glucose results. It's also easy to become overly focused on testing and test results.

Living with diabetes, you can sometimes feel burned out with all the numbers and record-keeping involved in monitoring your blood glucose.

Try to remember that these numbers are not tied to your self-worth. They're simply data to help you track how well your treatment plan is working for you. There may be times when your results indicate that you need to make changes in your treatment, but not always. Your glucose results shouldn't be seen as representations of your perceived successes or failures.

No matter how focused you are with your plan or how hard you try, your blood glucose readings won't be "perfect" every time. And that's OK. Sometimes out-of-range readings happen for no obvious reason. Give yourself some grace and use your data as a learning tool. Try to stay curious and open about finding the best ways to care for you.

If you find that these numbers are impacting you emotionally or your ability to care for yourself, reach out to your diabetes care team for support and guidance.

different circumstances or factors that might affect your blood glucose include:

- A change in your diet (such as having a birthday dinner, eating at a restaurant or eating more than usual)
- A change in exercise or activity level
- Going on a trip
- Unusual excitement or stress
- An illness

Take your records and blood glucose meter with you when you see your diabetes care team. The team reviews your records and uses the information to help you interpret the results. The team may recommend changes in your medication and ask to discuss your diet, level of physical activity and other lifestyle considerations. The more complete your records are, the more useful they'll be.

Record-keeping is often more intense when you start tracking your blood glucose. The more information you collect, the more familiar you'll become with your body's unique patterns and trends. This important data also allows your diabetes care team to quickly make any needed adjustments to your treatment plan. Over time, however, you'll likely find a comfortable pace of record-keeping that will keep you safe but not burn you out.

Remember, these records are for your information and self-empowerment. When you bring them to your diabetes care team, you won't get graded on your performance. Your records are used as a starting point for a joint discussion on what's helping or not helping with your diabetes management plan. Your diabetes care team is there to assist you, not to judge you.

STAYING WITHIN YOUR RANGE

As you check and record your blood glucose levels, you want your glucose to stay within a healthy range — not too high or too low. This range is individualized and often referred to as your target range or your goal range.

In people without diabetes, the typical range for a fasting blood glucose level is 70 to 100 milligrams of glucose per deciliter of blood (mg/dL). But that's not realistic, or always safe, for most people living with diabetes. Instead, your focus will be on a fasting blood glucose level that's in your goal range. You and your diabetes care team will determine your blood glucose goals together.

Because blood glucose naturally rises after eating, your goal after meals will be different from that before meals. Your goal before bed also may be different from your goal during the day.

In determining what blood glucose goals to recommend for you, your diabetes care team takes into account several factors, including your age, whether you have any diabetes-related complications or other medical conditions, and whether you can recognize when your blood glucose is low.

Recognizing the signs and symptoms of low blood glucose (hypoglycemia) is important because if your blood glucose drops too low, you may lose consciousness or have a seizure. See page 125 for more information on the warning signs of hypoglycemia.

These are the blood glucose goals that adults living with diabetes generally aim to meet:
- Before meals — 80 to 130 mg/dL
- About 2 hours after a meal — under 180 mg/dL
- Before bedtime — customized, if needed

Your goals may differ, especially if you have complications, you're pregnant or you're older — so always follow the advice of your diabetes care team.

TROUBLESHOOTING PROBLEMS

Blood glucose meters are generally accurate and precise. Human error rather than a nonfunctioning machine is more likely to produce an inaccurate meter reading.

If you think something's not right with your readings, start with the basics.

Check the test strips

Throw out damaged or outdated strips.

Check the meter

Make sure the meter is at room temperature, and the strip guide and the test window are clean. Replace the batteries in the meter if needed.

To check your meter and your testing skills, take the device along with you when you visit your diabetes care team or have an appointment for lab work. Members of your team can help you check your blood glucose at the same time that blood is drawn for lab tests. That way, you can compare the reading you get with the lab results.

Check the system measurement scale (calibration)

This is becoming very rare, but some meters must be calibrated to each container of test strips. If your meter requires it, be sure the code number in the device matches the code number on the container of test strips.

Do a quality control test

You can do a quality control test to ensure your meter and strips are working properly together. It's a good idea to do a quality control test when:
- You suspect your results are higher or lower than your current blood sugar levels
- Your meter or strips have been exposed to environmental elements, such as heat, cold, humidity or water, according to your meter manufacturer's instructions
- The meter has been dropped or damaged

To do a quality control test, follow your usual blood-testing procedure, but use a liquid control solution supplied by the meter manufacturer instead of a blood sample. Follow the manufacturer's instructions for doing the control test. The resulting blood glucose value displayed on your meter should be within the control solution range listed on the test strip container. If the reading isn't within the specified range, then there may be a problem with the test strip, control solution or meter. See the manufacturer's instructions for trouble-shooting steps.

Control solutions are available at most drugstores and pharmacies and need to match your meter and strips. If you have questions about this procedure, such as which solution to use or what to do if the results are outside of the listed range, ask your diabetes care team for help.

Check your technique

Wash your hands with soap and water before pricking your finger. Allow your hands to dry. If you use an alcohol wipe to clean your finger, wait to prick your finger until the alcohol has dried completely. Apply a generous drop of blood to the test strip. Don't add more blood to the test strip after the first drop was applied.

Check for other possible problems

Other factors that can lead to an inaccurate reading include:
- Not enough blood applied to the test strip
- More blood added to the test strip after the first drop was applied

- Alcohol, lotion, hand sanitizer, food, dirt or other substances on your finger or alternative site
- A meter or control solution that's not at room temperature
- A damaged meter

After troubleshooting, do another control test. If the results are still not in range, talk to your diabetes care team or call the meter manufacturer for help.

FACTORS AFFECTING BLOOD GLUCOSE

The amount of glucose in your blood continuously varies. That's because many factors affect how your body metabolizes food into glucose and how it uses this glucose. Self-monitoring helps you learn what makes your blood sugar level rise and fall so that you can make adjustments in your treatment. It can also help you understand why your blood glucose level may be different from day to day or hour to hour.

Food

The food you eat raises your blood glucose level. About 1 to 2 hours after a meal, your blood glucose is typically at its highest level. Then it starts to fall. What you eat, how much you eat and at what time of day you eat all affect your blood glucose level.

These patterns can look different depending on the type of diabetes you have and at what stage. As you work to learn about your personal responses, strive for

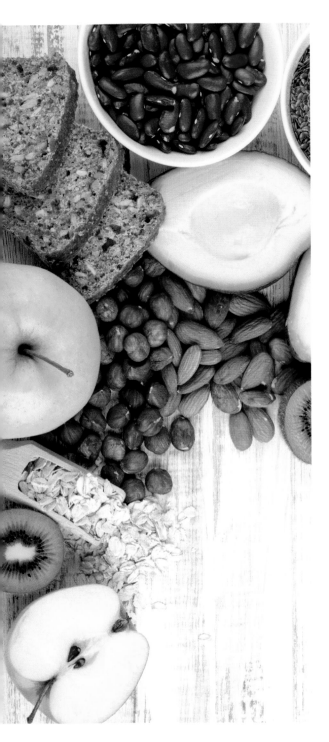

consistency from day to day in the time you eat and the amount of food you eat. Doing so will help you better identify patterns in the beginning. Work with a registered dietitian nutritionist to ensure you follow a meal plan that works for you.

By understanding when and how much you eat, you may be able to manage the times your blood glucose is higher, such as after meals. You can also better manage how much your blood glucose goes up after a meal.

Depending on your medication regimen, if you eat too much, your blood glucose will likely be higher than usual. Too little food may result in lower than usual blood glucose. If you take insulin, eating too little with some insulin types could put you at risk of very low blood glucose (hypoglycemia). It's also important to understand that different foods have different effects on your blood glucose.

Food is made up of carbohydrates, protein and fat. All can increase blood glucose, but carbohydrates have the most noticeable and immediate effect. Within the carbohydrate group, different types have varying effects. See Chapter 2 for more on food and how it affects your blood glucose.

Your liver

As mentioned in Chapter 1, glucose is stored in your liver in the form of glycogen. Your liver also makes new glucose from other substances, such as protein and fat.

WHAT ABOUT STRESS?

Stress can affect blood glucose in two ways. When you're under a lot of stress, it can be easy to lose your usual routine. You may exercise less, eat less healthy foods and not test your blood sugar as often. As a result, stress indirectly may cause your blood glucose to rise or be more irregular.

Occasionally, stress can have a direct effect on your blood glucose level. Physical and psychological stress may cause your body to produce hormones that prevent insulin from working properly, increasing blood glucose levels.

If you want to explore how your blood glucose reacts to stress, log your stress level on a scale of 1 to 10 every time you log your blood glucose level. After a couple of weeks, look for a pattern. Do high glucose levels often occur with high stress levels and low glucose levels with low stress? Do your current stressors impact your ability to practice your self-care routines? If so, stress may be affecting your blood glucose management, something you can discuss with your diabetes care team.

When your glucose level falls, your liver breaks down glycogen and releases it into your bloodstream. This generally happens when you haven't eaten for a while.

The process of storing and releasing glucose causes natural variations in blood glucose levels, but it's more pronounced when you live with diabetes and can be impacted by the type and stage of diabetes you are living with.

Exercise and physical activity

Typically, exercise and physical activity lower your glucose level. With help from insulin, exercise and physical activity promote the transfer of glucose from your blood to your cells, where the glucose is used for energy. The more you exercise, the more glucose you use and the faster it's transported to cells, lowering the amount of glucose in your blood. Exercise makes your cells more responsive to insulin, so it works more efficiently.

Although fairly uncommon, sometimes exercise has the opposite effect — it raises your blood glucose. This usually happens if your blood glucose is very high to begin with or when you're engaging in short bursts of intense physical activity (anaerobic exercise), such as weightlifting or sprinting. Until you know how your body responds to exercise, test your blood glucose before and after exercising and again several hours later.

Medications

Insulin and noninsulin injectable and oral diabetes medications can lower your blood glucose level. The time of day you take your medication and how much you take affect how much your blood glucose level drops. If your medication is causing your blood glucose to drop too much, or not enough, your diabetes care provider may need to make adjustments to your dosage.

Medications taken for other conditions can affect blood glucose. Whenever you're prescribed a new medication for another health condition, remind your health care provider that you live with diabetes and ask if the medication may alter your blood glucose level.

By being aware of a medication's effects and following simple precautions, such as increased glucose monitoring, you may keep it from causing significant changes in your blood glucose levels. If the drug does make it harder for you to manage your blood glucose, talk with your diabetes care team about it.

Illness

The physical stress of a cold, the flu or another illness, especially a bacterial infection, causes your body to produce hormones that can increase blood glucose. Injury or a serious health problem such as a heart attack also can increase your blood glucose level.

The additional glucose is meant to help promote healing. But in people with diabetes, more glucose can be a problem. When you're sick it's important to monitor your blood glucose frequently and be in contact with your diabetes care team for guidance and support.

Alcohol

Alcohol consumption prevents your liver from releasing glucose and can increase the risk of your blood glucose falling too low. If you take insulin or certain oral or noninsulin injectable diabetes medications and you drink alcohol, you risk experiencing hypoglycemia. This is true even with as little as 2 ounces of alcohol. If you choose to drink alcohol, work with your diabetes care team to create a safe, realistic plan for you.

To prevent your blood glucose from dropping too low, never drink on an empty stomach or if your blood glucose is already low. (See "Diabetes and alcohol: Do they mix?" on page 53.)

Depending on the drink ingredients, however, an alcoholic beverage can do the opposite of lowering your blood glucose — it can cause your blood glucose to rise. This could happen, for example, with the sugary sodas or juices used in mixed drinks. Monitor your blood glucose before and after drinking alcohol to see how your body responds to its use.

Be aware that even if a drink raises your glucose now, it can place you at risk of low blood sugar later. Alcohol can also mask the signs and symptoms of hypoglycemia, so make sure those around you know to assist you in monitoring your blood sugar levels as needed. And don't forget to reach out to your diabetes care team for support in learning how to enjoy an alcoholic beverage safely.

WHEN TEST RESULTS SIGNAL AN ISSUE

Watch for patterns that show that your blood glucose readings are persistently above or below your goals. This might indicate that your medication needs to be adjusted. If you're not taking medication and your glucose levels are above your goals, it may indicate that your diet and exercise efforts aren't enough and medication is warranted. This doesn't mean that you've failed in managing your diabetes. Diabetes can be progressive despite your best efforts.

Persistently high or low blood glucose readings put you at risk of complications of diabetes (see Chapter 1). Experiencing high or low blood glucose levels once in a while — especially if you can identify the reason — isn't cause for immediate alarm. However, frequent, unexplained high or low readings need attention.

It's important to call your diabetes care team if:
- Your blood glucose is persistently higher than 300 mg/dL
- Your blood glucose readings are persistently above or below your goals
- Your blood glucose is greater than 250 mg/dL for more than 24 hours during an illness
- You frequently have signs and symptoms of low blood glucose (hypoglycemia)

AVOIDING THE HIGHS AND LOWS

Blood sugar levels that are consistently out of your target range can cause a problem, especially if the levels are very high or very low. Here's what to watch for and how to react.

High blood sugar (hyperglycemia)

Anyone can have occasional episodes of high blood sugar — what's known as hyperglycemia. Still, hyperglycemia is nothing to take lightly.

If you feel more fatigued than usual, your urination frequency has increased and you've been thirsty all day, check your blood sugar. When you do, you may discover it's a lot higher than your target range.

Some of the most common causes of hyperglycemia include:
- Eating too much food or a lot of high-carb foods
- Exercising too little
- Physical stress, such as an infection or other illness
- Emotional stress, such as family conflict or workplace challenges
- Forgetting to take your diabetes medication
- Problems with your insulin, such as not giving yourself enough insulin at the right time or using expired insulin

What to watch for

Paying attention to the early signs and symptoms of hyperglycemia can help you manage the trend promptly and get your blood glucose back in goal range.

Watch for these common warning signs:
- Frequent urination
- Increased thirst
- Blurred vision
- Fatigue

If your blood sugar level climbs high enough and stays elevated, you may develop diabetic ketoacidosis or hyperglycemic hyperosmolar syndrome.

When you have diabetic ketoacidosis, your body begins to break down fat for energy. This produces toxic acids known as ketones. When you have hyperglycemic hyperosmolar syndrome, your blood becomes thick and syrupy due to extreme dehydration along with extremely high blood sugars. Left untreated, both conditions are life-threatening.

What to do

If you experience any signs or symptoms of hyperglycemia — even if they're subtle — check your blood sugar level. If your blood sugar level is higher than usual, and you've been taught to do so, use a home test kit to check your urine for ketones. It's a good idea to also check your ketone level if you're feeling sick or especially stressed.

Most home kits use chemically treated strips that you dip into your urine. When you have high amounts of ketones in your blood, excess ketones are excreted in your urine.

Test strips in the kit change color according to the level of ketones in your urine — low, moderate or high. If the color on your test strip shows a moderate or a high ketone level, call your diabetes care team right away for advice on how much insulin to take. In addition, drink plenty of water to keep yourself from getting dehydrated. If you have a high ketone level and you can't reach anyone on your diabetes care team, go to the nearest emergency department.

Diabetic ketoacidosis requires emergency medical treatment, which involves replenishing lost fluids through intravenous (IV) lines. Insulin, which may be combined with glucose, is injected into an IV line so that your body will stop making ketones. Gradually, your blood glucose level is brought back to a healthy level.

Adjusting your blood glucose too quickly can produce swelling in your brain. This complication appears to be more common in children, especially those with newly diagnosed diabetes.

If no ketones are in your urine — or you've not been instructed to monitor for ketones — and you're not ill, you may be able to treat hyperglycemia on your own.
- Take your medication as directed. If you have frequent episodes of hyperglycemia, your diabetes care provider may adjust the dosage or timing of your medication.
- Get physical. Gentle exercise, such as walking or biking, is often an effective way to lower blood sugar. But there's a caveat. If you have ketones in your urine, exercise can drive your blood

WEARABLE MEDICAL IDS

It's a good idea to wear a medical ID that identifies you as someone who lives with diabetes. There are seat belt covers, bracelets, necklaces and many more options available for this important identification need.

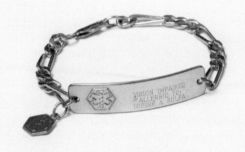
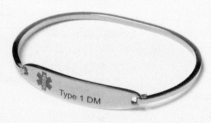

sugar even higher, so avoid strenuous exercise during this time.
- It may help to avoid sugary beverages and eat more well-rounded meals. If you're having trouble sticking to your meal plan, ask your diabetes care provider or dietitian for help.

Prevention steps

Long periods of hyperglycemia aren't good. They can lead to damage in your nerves, blood vessels and many organ systems.

You can prevent these complications by following your diabetes management plan and by treating episodes of high blood sugar quickly. Work with your diabetes care team to make sure your management plan is meeting your needs. Be sure to work with your team to create a plan for hyperglycemia and sick-day management of your blood glucose levels.

Low blood sugar (hypoglycemia)

Hypoglycemia — often defined as blood sugar below 70 milligrams per deciliter (mg/dL) — occurs when there's too much insulin and not enough glucose in the blood. Hypoglycemia is most common among people who take insulin, but it can occur in people taking certain oral or noninsulin injectable diabetes medications. Reasons for low blood sugar may include:
- Taking too much diabetes medication
- Not eating enough to match medication
- Postponing or skipping a meal

- Increasing physical activity (such as housework, exercise or intimacy)
- Drinking alcohol

What to watch for

Paying attention to the early signs and symptoms of hypoglycemia can help you treat the condition promptly. Red flags include:
- Shakiness
- Dizziness
- Weakness
- Sweating
- Hunger
- Irritability or moodiness
- Headache
- Blurry or double vision
- Pounding heartbeat
- Clumsiness
- Confusion

If you develop hypoglycemia during the night, you might wake to sweat-soaked pajamas or a headache.

It's important to take your warning signs seriously. Hypoglycemia can increase the risk of serious — even deadly — accidents. Left untreated, hypoglycemia can lead to seizures and loss of consciousness. Rarely, severe hypoglycemia can be fatal.

What to do

If you think that your blood sugar may be dipping too low, check your blood sugar level. If the results confirm that you're experiencing hypoglycemia, eat or drink something that will raise your blood sugar level quickly. This is something that equals roughly 15 grams of pure, readily absorbable carbohydrates. Examples include:
- Four ounces fruit juice
- Four ounces regular — not diet — soda
- One tablespoon sugar, jelly, honey or syrup
- Fifteen regular-size jelly beans
- Four glucose tablets (available without a prescription at most pharmacies)

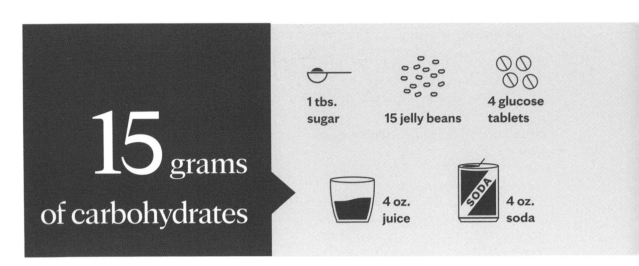

15 grams of carbohydrates

1 tbs. sugar

15 jelly beans

4 glucose tablets

4 oz. juice

4 oz. soda

If you experience symptoms of low blood sugar but can't check your blood sugar level right away, treat yourself as though you have hypoglycemia. In fact, carry at least one item listed above with you at all times, especially if you're on blood glucose-lowering medications. Never treat low blood sugar with foods that contain fat, protein or high amounts of fiber, as these all delay your digestion.

If you check your blood sugar and it is at or below 54 mg/dL, it's recommended that you double the initial treatment to 30 grams of pure carbs, instead of 15 grams. For some people, treatment amounts may vary. Work with your diabetes care team to create a plan that suits your needs.

Check your blood sugar level again 15 minutes later. If it's still below your blood sugar goal range, eat or drink something containing 15 grams of pure carbs again.

Continue to check every 15 minutes and treat again until you're in your goal blood glucose range. When your blood glucose is stable again, be sure to eat meals and snacks as usual.

Emergency hypoglycemia treatment

If you lose consciousness or for some other reason can't swallow, you'll need an injection of glucagon, a fast-acting hormone that stimulates the release of glucose into your blood. Teach your close friends and family members how to give you the medication in case of an emergency. Also tell them to call 911 or a local emergency number if you don't regain consciousness quickly.

A traditional glucagon emergency kit includes the medication and a syringe. The shot is easy to administer and is generally given in the arm, buttock, thigh or abdomen. Newer glucagon administration formats include nasal glucagon powder and a ready-to-use glucagon autoinjector pen.

When you meet with your diabetes care team, mention any episodes of hypoglycemia. They will help you consider what triggered the hypoglycemia. There is

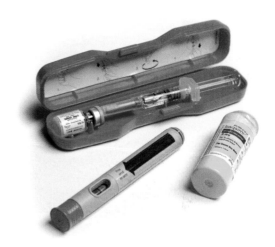

Emergency glucagon administration can rapidly correct very low blood sugar levels. Glucagon is available in different formats. Clockwise from the top: traditional syringe and medication vial, glucagon nasal powder and glucagon autoinjector pen.

nothing to be embarrassed about regarding these levels, but your disclosure of them will help you and your team work to prevent additional episodes. If necessary, your diabetes care team may change your treatment plan to prevent future problems with low blood sugar.

Prevention steps

The best way to manage hypoglycemia is to prevent it from occurring:
- If you live with diabetes, follow the diabetes management plan you and your diabetes care team have developed.
- If you haven't been diagnosed with diabetes but have recurring episodes of

---

HOW TO SAVE MONEY ON DIABETES CARE SUPPLIES

The cost of supplies for diabetes care can add up quickly. But there are ways you can save money. Ask your diabetes care team about these options or others they may know about:
- Patient-assistance programs offered by health care companies, manufacturers or nonprofits
- Free products from drug companies or product manufacturers
- Local or state savings programs
- Veteran or military benefits
- Health insurance, Medicare or Medicaid coverage
- Pharmacy discount cards

---

hypoglycemia, eating frequent small meals throughout the day may keep your blood sugar levels from getting too low. In this case, work closely with your health care team to determine the cause of these episodes.

OVERCOMING BARRIERS

Despite the advantages of blood glucose monitoring, many people living with diabetes don't test their blood glucose as often as recommended — or at all. Here are some common reasons why, along with some suggested solutions.

Cost

Some diabetes care supply companies offer low-cost solutions. In addition, many diabetes drug companies have patient-assistance programs. If cost is a factor for you, ask your diabetes care team if there's a local or nationwide program that can help lower your expenses. Those on your team may also be able to help you find a more affordable option covered by your insurance plan. If you are uninsured or underinsured, work closely with your diabetes care team to find the most affordable option for your needs.

Limited access to health care

If getting to a medical center is a challenge, check with your local, county or state health department about outreach health care and social services. Virtual medicine (telemedicine) is beginning to bridge these gaps, so ask if your diabetes care team can facilitate this for you.

Lack of information and misperceptions

Some people are simply unaware of the benefits of blood glucose monitoring and believe there is nothing they can do to improve their disease. But blood glucose monitoring is one of the most powerful tools available to give you an inside look at your condition. It can help you learn much more about your disease than you would without monitoring. And that knowledge is key to managing the effects of diabetes on your life. Also, remember that your needs for support, empowerment and education will evolve throughout your life.

Fear

If you fear the discomfort of pricking your finger, work closely with a certified diabetes care and education specialist to come up with solutions that will ease your concerns and ensure maximum comfort with this important self-care routine.

Lifestyle issues

Even with a hectic or unpredictable work schedule or lifestyle, you can find ways to build monitoring into your daily routine. With this investment in your self-care, you will likely feel better overall. Your diabetes care team can help with this.

Privacy issues

Testing is quick, and monitors are portable. You may be able to find a private place, such as a bathroom, to do your tests if that's more comfortable for you. Just remember that when you check your blood glucose in public, millions of other people do it every day too, and that this simple act is an important investment in your health. There should be no embarrassment in that.

If any of these barriers or other considerations are stopping you from monitoring your blood glucose as recommended, reach out to your diabetes care team. There are many solutions available. Sometimes all it takes is someone to guide you to a new approach.

CHAPTER 6

Medical treatment

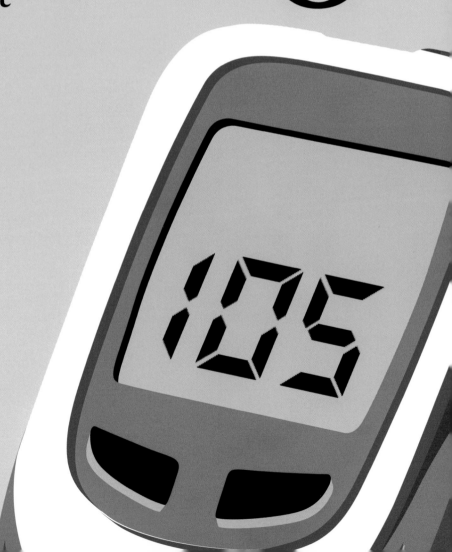

A VISIT WITH PANKAJ SHAH, M.D.

"You and your family are the best advocates for your diabetes. Speak up. Talk to your doctor if your treatment seems overwhelming, is too expensive, or is causing side effects. And remember that you're not alone. Working together with your diabetes care team, you can manage your diabetes and prevent its complications — and do it with minimal disruption of your regular lifestyle."

only glucose management but also management of cholesterol, blood pressure and body weight as well as regular exercise, healthy eating and not using tobacco.

A healthy diet and regular exercise are an essential part of diabetes treatment. And for many people living with type 2 diabetes, they may be the only measures needed — at least early on. In a person living with diabetes, the supply of insulin declines over time. The decline is faster if the need for insulin is high — for example, when factors such as high blood sugar, excessive calorie intake (often because of too much sugar and refined starch), sickness, certain medicines and tobacco use are present.

Managing blood sugar (glucose) levels is key. Very high glucose levels — higher than 300 milligrams per deciliter (mg/dL) — can cause dehydration and life-threatening complications. Glucose levels higher than 180 mg/dL raise the risk of infections and interfere with wound healing. In addition, diabetes increases the risk of serious long-term complications, such as kidney failure, blindness and amputations. It almost doubles the risk of heart attack and stroke. All of these complications are largely preventable through optimal management of diabetes. This includes not

When diet and exercise aren't enough to maintain acceptable blood sugar levels in people with type 2 diabetes, oral or sometimes injectable medications may be prescribed. Many times, people need a combination of oral medications and injections.

For people living with type 1 diabetes who have little insulin to begin with, insulin injections are necessary. You may need to take insulin injections several times a day or use an insulin pump. The amount of insulin needed will depend on your blood sugar levels and the foods you eat. Work closely with your diabetes care team to learn how to manage your insulin doses. Regular follow-up with your team to assess the adequacy of your treatment is important.

Effective diabetes management can reduce the risks of complications down to the risks seen in people without diabetes. If you already have some complications of diabetes, proper management can prevent further damage.

DIABETES MEDICATIONS OTHER THAN INSULIN

Noninsulin medicines are meant for people living with type 2 diabetes. They're usually not recommended for people living with type 1 diabetes.

When diet and exercise aren't sufficient to maintain acceptable blood sugar (glucose) levels, medications in the form of tablets, injections or a combination of the two can help keep blood sugar within the target range.

Some medicines trigger release of insulin from your pancreas. Other medicines reduce the need for insulin by making your body more sensitive to its effects, slowing digestion of carbohydrates, or causing loss of sugar in urine.

Talk with your diabetes care team about the pros and cons of each drug. The team can help you find an option that suits your specific needs and desires. The table on page 300 in the appendix lists several classes of noninsulin diabetes drugs, with examples of their main advantages and disadvantages.

Your diabetes care team will want to know if you have any of the following conditions, because certain medicines are preferred in these situations:
- Atherosclerotic cardiovascular disease, such as coronary artery disease, stroke or peripheral artery disease
- Heart failure
- Kidney disease

Other factors that influence the choice of medicine include:
- High risk of developing cardiovascular disease, heart failure or kidney disease
- High blood pressure
- Desirability of weight loss
- Not being able to take certain drugs

HOW TO HELP YOUR DIABETES CARE TEAM CHOOSE THE BEST TREATMENT FOR YOU

Sharing in the decision-making process can help your diabetes care team make treatment decisions that best fit your life.
- Tell your diabetes care team about other problems, conditions or illnesses you're experiencing.
- Tell your team how you're feeling about all of your daily diabetes-related tasks. Do these tasks feel manageable? Are you feeling overwhelmed? Is it difficult to remember everything you need to do?
- Let your team know if the cost of caring for your diabetes is affecting you. Your diabetes care team can take that into account when considering your options.

- Side effects
- Cost
- Need for blood tests and frequency of testing
- Complexity of self-management

Metformin

Metformin improves your body's response to insulin, decreasing insulin resistance. It also reduces the amount of glucose your liver releases. As a result, you need less insulin to lower your blood glucose.

Metformin is also available in extended-release pills (Glumetza, Fortamet) and in liquid form (Riomet). It is usually inexpensive, doesn't cause weight gain and may even promote slight weight loss (possibly 1 to 2 pounds).

Precautions

Metformin isn't toxic to your kidneys. However, it's not recommended when you have advanced kidney disease with a glomerular filtration rate (GFR) of less than 30 milliliters per minute (ml/min); with a GFR of less than 45 ml/min, it may be prescribed at a lower dose. Metformin usually isn't recommended for people who've had lactic acidosis.

Metformin is often withheld before a big surgery or procedure (such as cardiac, vascular or radiologic procedures using contrast agents) and restarted about two days later if all goes well. If the procedure leads to significant kidney damage, use of metformin or a reduction of its dose needs to be reconsidered.

Possible side effects

In the long run, most people tolerate metformin well. Initially it may cause some nausea. This usually settles down over the next few days to a few weeks. It can also cause diarrhea and vomiting. If you develop diarrhea or vomiting while taking metformin, hold or reduce the very next dose of metformin and let your diabetes care provider know.

Some people take vitamin B-12 supplements while taking metformin because long-term metformin use has been associated with vitamin B-12 deficiency.

Let your diabetes care provider know if you experience any of these side effects:
- Loss of appetite
- Vomiting
- Gas or diarrhea
- Abdominal bloating, discomfort or pain
- Changes in taste, such as an unpleasant metallic taste in your mouth

How it's usually given

You typically take metformin twice a day. Some extended-release formulations can be taken once a day.

Initially, metformin is often started at 500 milligrams (mg) once a day with the biggest meal of the day. After at least one week of making sure that it's not causing any abdominal discomfort, nausea, vomiting or diarrhea, the dose is increased to 500 mg twice a day with the two biggest meals of the day (or if extended release preparation, 1,000 mg with the biggest meal of the day).

The dose may be further increased at increments of no more than 500 mg a day each week, up to a maximum of 1,000 mg twice daily (with the largest meals or 2,000 mg of extended release preparation, also with the biggest meal of the day).

If at any dose, there is nausea or abdominal discomfort, the dose should not be increased. If at any dose, there is vomiting or diarrhea the very next dose should be reduced (or stopped). Follow up with your diabetes care provider.

SGLT-2 inhibitors

Sodium-glucose cotransporter-2 (SGLT-2) inhibitors — such as empagliflozin (Jardiance), canagliflozin (Invokana), dapagliflozin (Farxiga) and ertugliflozin (Steglatro) — lower blood sugar levels by causing urinary loss of glucose and salt. This loss of glucose in the urine (and therefore loss of calories) also causes some weight loss. These are relatively expensive medications. Insurance coverage and copay vary by the insurance plan.

At least some of these drugs have been shown to be helpful in specific ways, as they:
• Reduce the risk of serious kidney disease (as well as dialysis, renal transplant or death) by about 15% to 25%

• Decrease the risk of cardiovascular disease (heart attack, stroke, or death) by about 10% to 20%
• Decrease the risk of acute heart failure by about 25% to 40%
• Reduce liver fat content and reverse fatty liver disease to some extent

Some SGLT-2 inhibitors are added to the treatment plan for people with kidney disease, heart disease or heart failure even when glucose is within the target range.

Precautions

SGLT-2 inhibitors either aren't recommended or are used with great caution if you have or have had:
• Type 1 diabetes
• Diabetic ketoacidosis (DKA)
• Severe or recurrent urinary tract infections (UTIs)
• Severe kidney failure
• Active foot ulcer or infection

These medicines are typically stopped if you develop:
• A UTI
• A genital bacterial or yeast infection
• Persistent dehydration
• High blood ketone levels

In addition, these medicines are usually discontinued 3 to 4 days before any scheduled major surgery to reduce the risks of DKA.

If you're also taking high blood pressure (hypertension) medications — including water pills or diuretics — these may need to be stopped if you develop dehydration or lightheadedness upon standing, which suggests your blood pressure is low. If you're taking other diabetes medicines, their dosages may need to be adjusted.

Possible side effects

Side effects that may occur when you take SGLT-2 inhibitors include:
- Increased thirst
- Increased urination frequency (if this disrupts your sleep or daily routine, talk to your diabetes care team)
- Dehydration (if you're not drinking enough water)
- Elevated ketones and ketoacidosis
- Yeast infection
- Urinary tract infection

How they're usually given

These medicines are started at a small dose. If needed and if tolerated, the dose is increased after a few weeks to months.

GLP-1 agonists

These medicines mimic the action of a normally occurring hormone called glucagon-like peptide 1 (GLP-1). They're also called GLP-1 receptor agonists or GLP-1 analogs.

GLP-1 agonists do a couple of things. One, they increase insulin levels on an as-needed basis. Two, they decrease appetite and increase feelings of fullness, causing significant weight loss (5 to 10 pounds).

While taking these medicines, you can expect to feel hungry less often. When you eat, you'll likely feel full sooner after eating a smaller amount of food. Some of these medicines have been approved for weight loss, even in people without diabetes.

At least some of these drugs have specific benefits, as they may:
- Decrease the risk of cardiovascular disease (including heart attack, stroke, or death) by about 10% to 15%
- Reduce the progression of kidney disease by about 15% to 25%
- Reduce liver fat content and reverse fatty liver disease to some extent

Some GLP-1 agonists are prescribed for these benefits even if glucose is well-managed. GLP-1 agonists aren't recommended in combination with DPP-4 inhibitors (see page 137). If you're taking other diabetes drugs, their dosages will likely need to be adjusted.

GLP-1 agonists are relatively expensive medications, depending on the brand and the dose. Insurance coverage and copay vary by the insurance plan.

Precautions

These medicines shouldn't be used if you develop or have a history of pancreatitis or pancreatic cancer. They're also not recommended if you've had medullary thyroid cancer or multiple endocrine neoplasia tumors (MEN 2), or you have a family history of medullary thyroid cancer or MEN 2.

ARE THERE ANY HERBAL REMEDIES THAT WILL HELP TREAT TYPE 2 DIABETES?

Some people with diabetes take herbal remedies in an effort to ease their symptoms. The effectiveness and side effects of these remedies aren't well understood. These preparations are not regulated by the Food and Drug Administration (FDA).

If you're interested in taking such remedies, try to research what is known about them and buy only the ones that are packaged and sold by a reliable source. Be cautious about using herbal products manufactured or bought outside of the United States. The American Diabetes Association cautions against the use of herbal supplements because little research exists to prove the remedies are safe and effective.

Possible side effects

In the long run, most people tolerate these medicines well, but initially they often cause nausea and abdominal fullness after eating. Nausea usually settles down over the next 3 days to 3 weeks of continued use. About 5% to 10% of people taking GLP-1 agonists won't be able to take a full dose.

These side effects can be minimized by slowly escalating the dose. If you develop diarrhea or vomiting, reduce the very next dose. Let your diabetes care provider know about these side effects and that you've reduced the dose.

GLP-1 agonists don't cause low glucose (hypoglycemia) unless they are used in combination with sulfonylurea agents, such as glipizide, glyburide or glimepiride (see page 139).

How they're usually given

Some GLP-1 agonists are given as injections under the skin, such as daily liraglutide (Victoza) or weekly semaglutide (Ozempic), dulaglutide (Trulicity) and long-acting exenatide (Bydureon BCise). Semaglutide (Rybelsus) is a tablet that you take daily by mouth.

These drugs are started at the smallest dose and increased only when the lower dose is tolerated. If you develop vomiting or diarrhea, reduce the very next dose of the drug and tell your diabetes care provider.

DPP-4 inhibitors

Dipeptidyl-peptidase 4 inhibitors — such as alogliptin (Nesina), linagliptin (Tradjenta), saxagliptin (Onglyza) and sitagliptin

WHAT SHOULD I DO IF I FORGET TO TAKE MY MEDICATION?

You forgot to take your diabetes medication. What should you do? That depends on which drugs you take. For example, if you're on a sulfonylurea (such as glipizide, glyburide or glimepiride) and you're six or more hours late, don't take the delayed medicine — just take the next dose as prescribed.

If the medicine needs to be taken with a meal (for example, metformin, acarbose or miglitol) and you've already eaten — and it's been more than a half-hour since eating — take your next dose with your next meal, when due.

For specific recommendations, check the instructions that came with your prescription, or call your pharmacist or someone on your diabetes care team for advice. They can help you when you're in doubt about what to do.

(Januvia) — increase insulin levels on an as-needed basis. These are relatively expensive medications, and insurance coverage and copay vary based on the plan you have.

These medicines aren't recommended in combination with GLP-1 agonists (such as Victoza, Ozempic, Trulicity, Bydureon BCise and Rybelsus).

Precautions

DPP-4 inhibitors shouldn't be taken if you've had pancreatitis or pancreatic cancer. Likewise, you shouldn't take saxagliptin (Onglyza) if you have had or are at increased risk of heart failure.

These medicines should be used with caution if you have or have had autoimmune joint disease (such as rheumatoid arthritis, lupus-related arthritis or psoriatic arthritis).

DPP-4 inhibitors don't cause low glucose (hypoglycemia) unless they're used in combination with sulfonylurea agents (such as glipizide, glyburide or glimepiride) or insulin.

Possible side effects

DPP-4 inhibitors aren't associated with substantial side effects. The most common side effects are respiratory tract infection, sore throat and diarrhea.

How they're usually given

DPP-4 inhibitors are usually prescribed in a fixed dose, adjusted for the degree of kidney disease, if present.

COMBINATION PILLS

The goal of combination therapy is to maximize the glucose-lowering effects of diabetes medications. By combining medications from different drug classes, the medications may work in two different ways to control your blood glucose. Most combination therapies involve taking two separate drugs. However, the FDA has approved the following combination pills:

- metformin-glipizide
- metformin-glyburide
- metformin-pioglitazone (ACTOplus met)
- metformin-linagliptin (Jentadueto)
- metformin-saxagliptin (Kombiglyze XR)
- metformin-sitagliptin (Janumet, Janumet XR)
- metformin-alogliptin (Kazano)
- metformin-canagliflozin (Invokamet)
- metformin-dapagliflozin (Xigduo XR)
- metformin-empagliflozin (Synjardy)
- metformin-ertugliflozin (Segluromet)
- glimepiride-pioglitazone (Duetact)
- ertugliflozin-sitagliptin (Steglujan)
- pioglitazone-alogliptin (Oseni)
- linagliptin-empagliflozin (Glyxambi)

Although combination pills are convenient because you take fewer pills, there are trade-offs. For example, if you have a side effect, it's harder to tell which medication may be causing it. Or, if you want to change the dose of one, the dose of the other medicine in the pill will also change. In addition, these combination pills can often cost more than the two pills taken separately.

Thiazolidinediones (TZDs)

Thiazolidinediones (thie-uh-zole-uh-deen-DYE-owns), also called TZDs, reduce the need for insulin by making body tissues more sensitive to circulating insulin. As a result, blood glucose levels fall. This class of medications includes the drugs pioglitazone (Actos) and rosiglitazone (Avandia). These are inexpensive medicines. TZDs don't cause hypoglycemia.

Use of pioglitazone is likely associated with a decreased risk of heart attack, stroke and death in those who are at a high risk of such events. Use of TZDs has been shown to reduce liver fat content and reverse fatty liver to some extent.

Precautions

Don't take these medicines if you have a history of heart failure or an increased risk of bone fractures. Pioglitazone also should be avoided if you have a history of bladder cancer since it's been associated with an increased risk of this type of cancer.

If you take pioglitazone, talk to your diabetes care provider about switching to another medication if you:
- Develop swelling of your feet or shortness of breath (at rest or when exerting yourself)
- Experience fractures without a major injury
- Have blood in your urine

Possible side effects

Use of TZDs have been associated with:
- Weight gain, fluid retention, and swelling of feet and face, especially when used in combination with insulin
- Acute heart failure
- Increased risk of fractures
- Anemia

The following signs or symptoms can indicate heart failure. Contact your diabetes care team right away if you experience:
- Shortness of breath
- Sleep problems, such as waking up short of breath
- Weakness or tiredness
- Rapid weight gain (from fluid retention)
- Swelling (edema) in your legs, ankles or feet

How they're usually given

TZDs are typically given as a fixed dose once a day.

Sulfonylureas

Sulfonylureas (sul-fuh-nul-yoo-REE-uhs) have been used for decades to regulate blood glucose. These drugs work by stimulating beta cells in your pancreas to release more insulin.

Glimepiride (Amaryl), glipizide (Glucotrol) and glyburide (DiaBeta, Glynase) are the most commonly used sulfonylureas. Glipizide is available in two forms: a short-acting version and an extended-release (XL) version. Sulfonylureas are inexpensive medicines.

Precautions

Glyburide, although frequently used in the past, is much less used now since safer sulfonylureas are available. Glyburide should be avoided if you have cardiovascular disease.

Possible side effects

Hypoglycemia can be a very serious side effect of sulfonylureas. Hypoglycemia is more likely to happen if you:
- Started taking a sulfonylurea within the last few weeks
- Have impaired liver or kidney function
- Start a new medicine that interacts with sulfonylureas

- Skip a meal or exercise more than usual
- Drink alcohol while on sulfonylureas

Sulfonylurea medicines are more likely to cause hypoglycemia if combined with DPP-4 inhibitors (Tradjenta, Januvia, Onglyza, Nesina) or GLP-1 agonists (such as Victoza, Ozempic, Trulicity, Bydureon BCise andRybelsus).

If you develop hypoglycemia (or even symptoms strongly suggestive of low glucose) while on these medicines, reduce or skip the very next dose of the sulfonylurea medicine and let your diabetes care team know.

Taking a sulfonylurea may be associated with moderate weight gain (2 to 4 pounds).

How they're usually given

Sulfonylureas are typically started at a very low dose and increased very slowly. Your diabetes care provider will likely recommend that you monitor your blood glucose at home.

The dose may need to be reduced if your blood glucose levels start going below 90 milligrams per deciliter (mg/dL). Do not take an extra pill for any reason.

It's important that you meet with your diabetes care provider at least once a year for a periodic reevaluation of your medication use and adjustment of your doses, if needed. Make sure your pharmacist knows what your current regimen is, as well.

INSULIN THERAPY

Insulin is a hormone your body uses to move blood sugar (glucose) from your bloodstream into your cells. When you're not eating, your body maintains a low but constant base supply of insulin. After you eat, your blood glucose level spikes as your digestive system absorbs the food you just ate. In response, your pancreas produces (secretes) additional insulin to escort the extra glucose into your cells. Once your blood sugar returns to a normal level, your pancreas reduces the amount of insulin it produces as well.

Diabetes disrupts this dynamic interplay between blood glucose and insulin and causes havoc with the rest of the body.

Type 1 diabetes is an autoimmune condition that reduces the ability of the pancreas to produce insulin, leaving little to no insulin available and no way for glucose to leave the bloodstream. So, insulin therapy is a must for people with type 1 diabetes. You might hear this type of insulin therapy referred to as replacement insulin.

In type 2 diabetes, the pancreas may still produce some insulin, but it's not enough to meet the body's needs. There is also resistance at the tissue level to the effect of insulin, so that often more insulin is needed to overcome that resistance. There are a few ways to treat this kind of insulin deficiency. A balanced diet, regular exercise and a healthy body weight, as well as certain medicines, can reduce the body's overall need for insulin. Other medicines can trigger the release of insulin from the pancreas, increasing its supply in the bloodstream. Over a period of time, however, people living with type 2 diabetes may not respond as well to these medicines and may need supplemental insulin therapy.

Many types of insulin are available, including rapid-acting, short-acting and long-acting insulin, and intermediate options. They vary by:
- How long they take to begin lowering blood glucose (onset)
- When they reach their maximum effect (peak)
- How long the overall effect lasts (duration)

These aspects of insulin also can be affected by other factors. For example, exercise of the injected area can speed up onset and maximum effect, as can local massage or heating the injection area. A higher dose of insulin takes effect quicker and lasts longer than a lower dose. In addition, fat and scar tissue at the site of repeated insulin injections (lipohypertrophy) can make the onset, the maximum effect and the duration erratic.

Intermediate-acting and long-acting insulins are typically given once or twice a day to help your body maintain the necessary constant level of insulin (basal insulin). Rapid-acting and short-acting insulins are usually given before a meal (bolus insulin) to assist with glucose uptake into tissue cells.

Insulin can't be taken by mouth to lower blood sugar because stomach enzymes interfere with insulin's action. Insulin is

Pre-mixed insulins	
Humulin 70/30; Novolin 70/30; Novolin/ReliOn 70/30	30% short-acting insulin and 70% intermediate-acting neutral protamine hagedorn (NPH) insulin
NovoLog Mix 70/30	30% rapid-acting insulin aspart and 70% intermediate-acting NPH insulin
Humalog Mix 75/25	25% rapid-acting insulin lispro and 75% intermediate-acting NPH insulin
Humalog Mix 50/50	50% rapid-acting insulin lispro and 50% intermediate-acting NPH insulin

Pre-mixed insulin combines rapid-acting or short-acting insulin with intermediate-acting insulin. This is convenient if you need two types of insulin but have trouble drawing up insulin out of two bottles, or you have poor eyesight or have arthritis or other problems with your hands. Because you're getting two types of insulin, the onset, peak and duration of each type will differ but overlap. Follow the directions of your diabetes care team. Typically if the pre-mixed product has short-acting insulin, you'll inject it 30 minutes before a meal; if the product has rapid-acting insulin, you'll inject it no more than 15 minutes before your meal.

usually injected in the fat under the skin using a syringe, insulin pen or insulin pump.

Which insulin is best for you depends on a number of factors, including the type of diabetes you have, how much your blood sugar changes throughout the day and your lifestyle.

Depending on your needs, your diabetes care provider may prescribe a mixture of insulin types to use throughout the day and night. For an overview of insulin medicines, see page 302 in the appendix at the back of this book.

Insulin regimens

There are many ways insulin can be used in a diabetes treatment plan, either as a supplemental therapy or as a complete replacement therapy.

Supplemental insulin plan

When noninsulin medications aren't enough to effectively manage type 2 diabetes, the next step your diabetes care provider will likely recommend is a long-acting or intermediate-acting insulin to supplement natural insulin secretion.

The supplemental insulin dose is added to the other diabetes medicines.

Supplemental insulin is usually taken once or twice a day on a schedule and not necessarily before a meal. As long as the dose of long-acting insulin is appropriate, the dose usually remains the same whether you're eating or not.

INSULIN AND TYPE 2 DIABETES

Insulin is an effective medication for treating type 2 diabetes. You may take insulin alone, or you may use it in combination with a noninsulin medicine. Your diabetes care provider may recommend insulin injections if your pancreas isn't making enough insulin or your body isn't responding to other medications. Your provider may turn to insulin first if one or more of the following is true:

- Your blood glucose level is markedly high — more than 300 milligrams per deciliter (mg/dL) — especially if your ketones levels are high.
- You have a markedly high blood glucose level and are dehydrated.
- You have gestational diabetes that can't be managed with diet alone.
- You have a high blood glucose level and you're sick, especially if you're hospitalized.
- You have high blood glucose and noninsulin medicines are unable to bring glucose to a reasonable range.

Supplemental insulin plus some meal insulin

Over time, type 2 diabetes can wear out the pancreas so that it secretes less and less insulin and the combination of noninsulin medicines plus some supplemental insulin is no longer sufficient to keep blood glucose within the goal range. Often, an injection of short-acting insulin given before meals is added to the regimen at this point. Noninsulin medicines are often scaled back when additional insulin is added to the regimen.

Alternatively, a pre-mixed insulin injection may be used; it provides both a short-acting mealtime insulin and a long-acting insulin in the same dose. Pre-mixed insulin needs to be taken before a meal (once or twice a day) — 30 minutes before a meal if containing short-acting insulin or 15 minutes before a meal if containing rapid-acting insulin.

Replacement insulin plan

In people with type 1 diabetes, insulin production ceases completely early on in the disease process, making replacement insulin necessary. In some people with type 2 diabetes, insulin production also stops, usually later in the course of disease.

To give your body the insulin it needs, you use a long-acting insulin once or twice a day to provide basal needs through day and night.

In addition, an injection of a short-acting insulin is given before each meal to meet the sudden increase in need for insulin after eating.

Sometimes pre-mixed insulin containing both short-acting insulin and long-acting insulin may be taken before the morning and evening meal.

Usually, short-acting or rapid-acting insulin injections aren't given other than at mealtimes. They would not be given at bedtime, for example.

In people with type 2 diabetes, a noninsulin medicine may be continued along with the insulin injections.

To minimize injections, people who need replacement insulin often use a small portable insulin pump that can be programmed to deliver insulin through a small catheter inserted in the abdomen. An insulin pump provides constant or variable basal insulin as well as a manual or calculated bolus of insulin for meals through buttons on the pump that are pressed by the user (see page 166).

Insulin dosage options

There are several ways of dosing insulin so that your body gets the right amount at the right time.

- ***Single or split dose of intermediate-acting or long-acting insulin only.*** You inject a dose of intermediate-acting or long-acting insulin once each day. Sometimes the insulin is split into two doses.
- ***Mixed and pre-mixed dose.*** You inject rapid-acting or short-acting insulin and

intermediate-acting insulin — mixed in one syringe, or available as a mixture in a vial or a pen. This can be taken once a day or twice a day before eating.

- **Intensive therapy.** This regimen involves multiple daily injections of insulin. Alternatively, many people use an insulin pump to reduce the number of injections (see next page).

Injection methods

When you first learn that you need to take insulin, you may feel nervous about injecting yourself with the medication. That's understandable. Going through the process with a certified diabetes care and education specialist (CDCES) or your diabetes care provider and doing it a few times will help you feel more comfortable.

Insulin needs to be delivered underneath the skin (subcutaneously) into the fat tissue. From there it's absorbed into your bloodstream. There are several ways to inject insulin. Your method of choice depends on a number of factors, including your insulin needs, what type of insulin you take and your personal preferences. Your diabetes care team can help you determine which method is best for you.

Syringe

This method is usually the least expensive. Syringes are marked in units and come in several sizes to accommodate different doses of insulin. Sizes range from small-volume (30-unit) syringes marked in half-unit increments to large-volume (100-unit) syringes marked

in two-unit increments. Don't use syringes that aren't specific to insulin medication and be sure to use syringes appropriate to the dose or concentration. For example, only use U-500 syringes when drawing up U-500 insulin, a more concentrated form of insulin, from a vial. Two compatible insulin types can be mixed in the same syringe and injected at the same time, allowing for one injection instead of two.

Insulin pen

An insulin pen requires fewer steps to inject insulin. Some insulin pens can deliver doses in half-unit increments. Smaller doses of insulin are more likely to be accurate, which makes an insulin pen preferable for people with type 1 diabetes who need very small doses. Some insulin pens can keep track of prior doses, which is helpful in avoiding extra doses and making insulin dose adjustments.

Disposable delivery patch

This wearable once-daily device (V-Go) does away with multiple daily injections by delivering insulin through a patch on your skin. V-Go provides a constant supply of basal insulin as well as insulin on demand at mealtimes when you click on a button. You change the patch once a day.

Injection port

An injection port (i-Port Advance) can also help reduce the number of daily injections. This is an injection site that inserts under your skin like an insulin pump infusion site, but is used to inject all of your daily injections for syringe or insulin pen use. You can keep it on for up to three days.

Insulin pump

An insulin pump eliminates the need for multiple injections throughout the day. It is essentially a syringe of rapid-acting insulin driven by a motor. It injects a small amount of insulin throughout the day (basal insulin) and can also provide additional insulin for meals (bolus insulin). Read about insulin pumps on page 166.

Alternative methods of delivery

People with arthritis, visual disabilities and disabilities of the hand may find one insulin delivery method more acceptable than the others. Discuss device options with your diabetes care team to determine which method is best for you.

For people who have trouble with needles, an insulin jet injector may be an option. This device uses high-pressure air to send a fine spray of insulin under your skin. There may be some discomfort and possible bruising. Keep in mind that this device may not be as accurate as other methods because some of the insulin can be lost during injection. Jet injectors are more expensive than pen injectors and are currently available only in certain countries. Talk to your diabetes care team to find out more.

Selecting an injection site

Insulin may be injected into any area of your body where a layer of fatty tissue is present and where large blood vessels, nerves, muscles and bones aren't close to the surface.

One of the best locations to inject insulin is the abdomen because this location allows for quick and consistent absorption. However, avoid the 2-inch radius around your belly button (navel), which doesn't absorb as well.

If appropriate, your diabetes care team may recommend alternative areas for injection, such as your upper arms, thighs or buttocks. See the illustration on page 146 for recommended injection sites.

Be sure to rotate between injection sites to avoid or reduce indentations in your skin, thickened skin or hard lumps from the injections.

If you take daily showers or baths, it's not necessary to clean the skin with an alcohol wipe before an injection. If you've cleaned the site with alcohol, be sure to let it dry before giving the injection.

Using a syringe

Using a syringe to inject yourself with insulin may make you feel a little anxious, but you won't have to do it alone the first time. You'll learn how to use a syringe with the help of your diabetes care provider or a CDCES. There are several steps to injecting yourself with insulin.

INSULIN INJECTION SITES

Generally, the abdomen is the best injection site. Within the abdominal area, change locations for each injection to avoid irritating or scarring the tissue. The thighs and upper arms as well as the buttocks (shaded areas) also are potential injection sites.

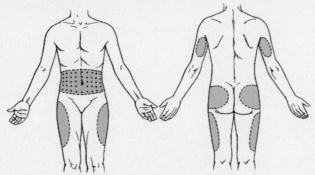

Once you select a region, try to use that same area for specific daily injections. Changing from the abdomen to the thigh, arm or buttocks from one day to the next isn't recommended. This means, for example, that you inject every morning dose of meal insulin in the same area. Avoid giving the morning dose of meal insulin one day on the abdomen, the next day on the thigh and the next day on the arm. Consistency is best. Nonetheless, it's important to rotate injection sites within the area (see dots in abdominal area, for example).

Drawing insulin into the syringe

With time and practice, the process of drawing insulin into a syringe becomes routine and may no longer seem so daunting. Here's how to do it (for illustrated instructions, see page 304):
- Gather your supplies: bottle of insulin, syringe, alcohol wipe, and a covered, puncture-resistant container for needle discard.
- Check the label on the insulin bottle for the type, concentration and expiration date. Use the same type of insulin every time, unless your diabetes care provider tells you otherwise. Changing insulin types may affect glucose management.
- Check the insulin bottle for any changes in the insulin. Make sure no clumping, frosting, precipitation, or change in clarity or color has occurred, which may mean that the insulin has lost potency.
- Wash your hands with soap and water.
- Clear insulin doesn't need to be mixed. However, cloudy insulin should be

mixed by gently rolling the bottle between your hands. (Don't shake the bottle — that may decrease the insulin's potency.) Then, check to make sure there are no particles at the bottom of the bottle.

- Wipe off the top of the insulin bottle with an alcohol wipe.
- Remove the needle cap from the sterile syringe.
- Pull the plunger to draw in an amount of air equal to the amount of insulin that you need.
- Insert the needle through the rubber stopper and push the plunger so that air goes into the bottle. This equalizes air pressure in the bottle, making it easier to withdraw the insulin.
- While keeping the needle in the bottle, turn the bottle upside down.
- Pull the plunger on the syringe and withdraw insulin, not air, slightly past the number of units needed. Air isn't dangerous, but it reduces the amount of insulin in the syringe.
- If there are air bubbles, remove them. Push the insulin back into the bottle (without taking the needle out of the bottle) and draw it again.
- Recheck the syringe for air. If air is present, repeat the previous step.
- Double-check the amount of insulin in the syringe.
- Pull the needle out of the bottle.

Injecting the insulin

Once you have the right amount of insulin in the syringe and you've removed the needle from the bottle, it's time to inject the insulin. To do so:

- Hold the syringe like a pencil. Quickly insert the entire length of the needle into a pinched fold of your skin at a 90-degree angle (with small, 4-millimeter needles skin does not need to be pinched).
- If the skin was pinched, release the pinch. Inject the insulin by gently pushing the syringe's plunger all the way down at a steady, moderate rate.
- Pause for ten seconds, then withdraw the needle from your skin at the same angle it went in.
- Don't recap the needle. Discard it in a covered, puncture-resistant container.

Needle disposal and safety

For safe use and disposal of needles:
- Use a new needle for each injection.
- If you're using a pen and you can't dial the dose you need, check to see if there's enough insulin in the reservoir.
- Don't leave a needle on the pen between uses.
- When throwing away a disposable insulin pen, remove the needle first. Throw away the pen with regular trash.
- Don't throw needles or lancets directly into the trash. Use a puncture-resistant sharps disposal container to collect the needles and lancets. Check with your local waste disposal company about the rules for disposing of medical sharps in your community.

Avoiding problems with insulin injections

The following steps can reduce your risk of problems from insulin use.

Stick with the same pharmacy

If possible, buy all of your insulin from the same pharmacy. This will help ensure that you receive the type and concentration of insulin that's prescribed and that you are alerted to changes in your prescription. Check the expiration date on the package, and always keep a spare bottle on hand, if possible.

Store your insulin safely

Store insulin bottles in the refrigerator until they're opened. In general, a bottle it may be kept at room temperature for one month after it's been opened. Check with your diabetes care team about the insulin you're using and its room temperature tolerance. Insulin at room temperature causes less discomfort when injected.

Throw away your insulin after the expiration date or after it's been kept at room temperature for the recommended period of time for your specific insulins.

For safe storage of insulin pens:
- Store unopened insulin pens in the refrigerator until you use them. They can stay in the refrigerator until the expiration date noted on the pen.
- After you open an insulin pen, don't put it back in the refrigerator. Keep it at room temperature until your next injection.
- Many insulin pens expire around 28 days after they're opened. Consult manufacturer guidelines for your specific insulin, as some expire before or after 28 days to a month.

- Never leave an insulin pen in a hot car or other place where it could get overheated.

Avoid temperature extremes

Never freeze insulin or expose it to extremely hot temperatures or direct sunlight.

Look for changes in appearance

Check your insulin before using it. Throw away insulin that is discolored or contains solid particles.

Speak up

To avoid possible drug interactions or drug side effects, make sure your pharmacist, dentist and other health professionals who may not be familiar with your medical history know that you take insulin.

Avoid injection site discomfort

To reduce discomfort and pain from injections, you can take the following steps:
- If you use alcohol to wipe the injection site, allow the site to dry before injecting insulin.
- Make sure the insulin is at room temperature.
- Relax your muscles in the area of the injection.
- Penetrate your skin quickly with the needle.

WHEN TO MONITOR YOUR BLOOD GLUCOSE

If you use...	Test this many times daily...	At these specific times*...
Long-acting insulin once or twice a day	2	• Morning • Bedtime • If bedtime is missed, at about 2 to 3 a.m.
Intermediate-acting insulin every morning	2	• Morning • Before the evening meal
Intermediate-acting insulin every evening or at bedtime	1	• Morning • Before the evening meal
Short-acting or rapid-acting insulin before a meal	2	• Before a meal • Before the next meal
Premixed (short-acting or rapid-acting insulin plus intermediate-acting insulin) once a day before breakfast	3	• Morning • Before the noon meal • Before the evening meal
Premixed (short-acting or rapid-acting insulin plus intermediate-acting insulin) twice a day before breakfast and before the evening meal	4	• Morning • Before the noon meal • Before the evening meal • Bedtime
Multiple dose insulin injection plan (short-acting or rapid-acting insulin plus once-daily or twice-daily long-acting insulin)	4	• Morning • Before the noon meal • Before the evening meal • Bedtime

*Always test your blood glucose in a fasting state (4 or more hours after the last meal or snack).

- Don't change the direction of the needle.
- Don't reuse the needle. These needles are so fine that they begin to dull after a single injection. A dull needle can contribute to discomfort.

Wear diabetes identification

Wear an identification necklace or bracelet that identifies you as an insulin user. In addition, carry an identification card that includes the name and phone number of your diabetes care provider or other member of your diabetes care team. Also, list all of the medications you're taking, including the kind of insulin. In case your blood glucose drops too low, this will help people know how to respond.

Check all medications

Before taking any medication other than your insulin, including over-the-counter products, read the warning label. If the label says you shouldn't take the drug if you have diabetes, check with your diabetes care provider or pharmacist before taking it.

Avoid scar tissue buildup

Some people develop scar tissue — soft or hard lumps, thickened skin, or indentations — in areas where they inject insulin (insulin lipodystrophy). This happens from repeated injections in the same place. Don't use areas of lipodystrophy for insulin injection because the insulin won't absorb reliably. Avoiding these areas as injection sites may clear away these problems over 3 to 6 months. You can prevent the development of insulin lipodystrophy by not injecting insulin in the same spot more than once within 2 to 3 weeks.

Adjusting insulin to find the right dose

Using insulin medications to mimic the way your body naturally balances glucose and insulin can be a challenge. If your blood glucose levels aren't staying within your target range, you may need to adjust your insulin doses.

Finding the right dose of insulin to keep your blood glucose stable depends on the type of insulin you use. In most cases, your diabetes care team will teach you how to safely adjust your insulin to get within your target blood glucose range.

Following are details on how to safely and effectively adjust insulin when necessary. But be sure to ask your diabetes care team for help if you have any questions or concerns.

Adjusting the dose of long-acting insulin

If you're using long-acting insulin along with short-acting or rapid-acting insulin at each meal, adjust the dose of long-acting insulin first.

The purpose of long-acting insulin is to prevent your blood sugar from going up when you're not eating. Long-acting insulin should not cause your blood sugar to fall. If the dose is right, it should hold your blood glucose steady anytime you fast or don't eat. Keep in mind that this type of insulin is meant to be your foundational insulin, not to cover meals or any food that you eat. Long-acting insulin should be taken daily whether you're eating or not.

To determine whether you're using an appropriate dose of long-acting insulin, check your glucose as outlined below. Repeat your testing at least three times to assess for a true pattern. Be sure to do so with an empty stomach, and don't eat, drink or use rapid-acting insulin during your assessment time. Choose one of the following methods to check the effectiveness of your dose:

- Check glucose late at night (four or more hours after the last meal or last snack) and then again the next morning.
- Or check glucose at midnight and then again at least six hours later.
- Or use continuous glucose monitoring to assess your glucose level while fasting overnight. For your safety, note that this may not be as accurate as using traditional finger stick readings.

Compare your bedtime reading to your morning reading. Ideally, you shouldn't see your blood glucose levels go up or down more than 40 mg/dL from your bedtime reading. If needed, you can adjust your basal insulin dose up or down to ensure that the glucose concentration remains steady between the two readings. Adjust your current dose no more than 10% for safety. If you do make an adjustment, wait 3 to 4 days to see the effect of that change before making further adjustments.

Adjusting the dose of intermediate-acting insulin

A dose of intermediate-acting insulin can be adjusted by assessing a four-hour fasting glucose level, measured about 8 to 12 hours after the insulin injection. For example, if you take this insulin twice daily and want to determine if your morning insulin dose is correct, measure your glucose before the evening meal. For the evening (or bedtime) insulin dose, measure glucose in the morning before breakfast. Remember blood sugar values are like mirrors and reflect back on your previous dose of insulin.

If your glucose level is within your target range, no change is needed. If it falls out of your target range (too high or too low) at the corresponding glucose check, you will need to make a 10% adjustment.

Again, make your adjusment based on pre-meal glucose values taken over three days. Don't adjust your insulin dose based on a single blood glucose level, unless it is below 70 mg/dL for unknown reasons or you've been directed to adjust it by your diabetes care team.

After adjusting the dose of intermediate insulin, wait a minimum of three days to determine whether the new dose is right before making any further changes — unless your glucose level is repeatedly low, in which case you should adjust the very next dose.

If taking this insulin only once daily in the morning, use both your pre-breakfast and pre-evening meal glucose levels to assess your dose. Both should show the same three-day pattern to warrant a dose adjustment. Contact your diabetes care team if you have any questions about adjusting your dose.

If your blood glucose reaches hypoglycemic levels, reduce your next dose and maintain that lowered dose to prevent the low from happening again.

Adjusting the dose of short-acting or rapid-acting insulin for meals

The main purpose of short-acting or rapid-acting insulin (also called mealtime insulin) is to bring blood sugar back to where it was before eating. It can also be used to correct a high blood sugar level, but for this section the focus is on the mealtime function of these insulins.

The appropriateness of the mealtime insulin dose can be best determined after you know that your dose of long-acting insulin is keeping your blood sugar steady when you're not eating.

Typically, rapid-acting insulin is taken before eating, and the dose depends on a set amount of carbohydrates to be eaten. If you skip a meal or eat a meal without carbohydrates, such as a plain salad with grilled chicken, you usually won't need your meal dose (bolus dose) of insulin. In fact, taking insulin in this situation could potentially cause low blood sugar 1 to 5 hours later.

Remember that your mealtime insulin dose is "married to your meal," and that your meal should include some carbohydrates to prevent hypoglycemia. Mealtime insulin works best when you use set doses for each meal along with eating a consistent amount of carbohydrates for each of those meals.

For example, if you take 5 units of insulin at breakfast every day, those 5 units won't work as well if your breakfast carbohydrate intake varies widely between meals, such as a slice of toast with eggs on one day and four pancakes with maple syrup the next.

To find out if your insulin dose for breakfast is right, eat the same breakfast for a few days in a row. Check your blood sugar in the morning before breakfast and 4 to 5 hours later (before the noon meal) with no snacks in between. Take a fixed dose of meal insulin before eating breakfast. If the breakfast insulin dose is appropriate, your blood glucose before the noon meal will be within your glucose target range.

Repeat this testing three days in a row and see if you observe any trends in your pre-noon meal blood glucose levels. If your observations show a pattern of glucose values that aren't within your target range, make the necessary insulin adjustment and then reassess in 3 to 4 days.

Once you find the correct dose for those specific breakfast items, try and see if the same dose works for other breakfast foods with roughly the same carb count. Then do the same assessments for noon and evening meals. Remember that general consistency in carbohydrate intake is important and that higher fat or protein intake may impact your test results.

The assessment for the insulin to carbohydrate ratios is a bit different, so review the next section if you use a ratio for your mealtime dosing.

Be careful when taking mealtime insulin while nauseous. In this case, for safety's sake, wait to take your dose until you know you won't vomit. And when eating at a restaurant, wait to take your dose until you've confirmed that the server has brought you the meal you requested.

Adjusting an insulin to carbohydrate ratio of rapid-acting or short-acting insulin

The insulin to carbohydrate (I:C) ratio is another way of dosing rapid-acting or short-acting insulin before a meal or snack.

This ratio regimen is ideal if you are searching for more flexibility in carbohydrate intake at mealtimes. This method should not be used with split-mixed insulins or long-acting insulins.

As with set doses of mealtime insulin, the dose is taken before eating, but the number of units is entirely dependent on the amount of counted carbs you plan to eat. Work with

---

SAFETY CONSIDERATIONS FOR ALL INSULIN DOSE ADJUSTMENTS

When adjusting your insulin dose, keep these factors in mind:
- Don't adjust a dose up or down more than 10% of your current dose. For example, if you take a 20-unit dose of long-acting insulin once daily, you would adjust this dose up or down only 2 units at a time based on your need.
- Don't adjust a dose based on just one day of blood glucose values. Monitor your values for three days to assess for a true pattern requiring adjustment.
- But don't wait to assess hypoglycemic levels. If your blood glucose level is below 70 mg/dL (hypoglycemia) for unknown reasons, plan to reduce the corresponding insulin dose the very next time you take it. Continue this lowered dose and follow up with your diabetes care team.
- If you take more than one dose of insulin a day and need help deciding which dose to adjust, don't guess. Reach out to your diabetes care team for help.
- Only use four-hour fasting blood glucose levels to assess insulin doses. Don't eat or drink anything with calories four hours before you check your blood sugar. This will ensure that you're safely adjusting your insulin based on clear blood sugar levels — not levels that are affected by food or drink digesting in your stomach.

your diabetes care team to obtain a ratio or ratios that will work for your various mealtimes throughout the day. You'll need to be trained in carb counting prior to safe and effective ratio use.

To adjust your I:C ratio, follow these steps:
- Choose a time when your blood sugar is in target range and you haven't eaten for four hours.
- Choose a low-fat meal to eat for the test, and count the carbohydrates within it.
- Use your I:C ratio to determine the dose and administer it before eating.
- Check your blood sugar at two and then four hours after eating. At two hours after eating, your blood sugar shouldn't be higher than 40 to 80 mg/dL above where your pre-meal blood sugar level was. At four hours after eating, your blood sugar should return to within your goal range.
- Repeat this testing at least three days in a row for each mealtime.

When assessing the appropriateness of your I:C ratio, consider the following factors:
- If you see that your blood sugar rises above 80 mg/dL but returns to goal range by four hours, you may simply need to take your insulin dose earlier compared with when you eat your meal. Remember, rapid-acting insulin takes roughly 15 minutes to start working in your system and short-acting insulin takes up to 30 minutes.
- If you see that your blood sugar level at four hours after eating has dipped below your target range, you likely need

to decrease the ratio. As long as your blood sugar isn't dipping below 70 mg/dL, test the ratio twice more at those mealtimes to find a pattern before adjusting the ratio. If your blood sugar goes below 70 mg/dL, decrease the ratio right away.
- If your blood sugar at four hours after eating has risen above your target range, you likely need to strengthen the ratio. Test the ratio twice more at that mealtime to find a pattern and only increase the ratio by 10%.

An important safety note: When adjusting an I:C ratio, remember that the smaller the number of grams in the ratio, the more insulin you will dose. For example, 1 unit of insulin to 15 grams of carbohydrate (1:15) is not as strong of a ratio as a 1 unit of insulin to 5 grams of carbohydrate (1:5) ratio. You get more insulin per meal using a 1:5 ratio than you would using a 1:15 ratio. Be very careful when adjusting these ratios. Work closely with your diabetes care team to receive guidance that will keep you safe.

Adjusting a correction dose of rapid-acting or short-acting insulin

If your regimen of long-acting insulin keeps your blood glucose steady when you're not eating and your regimen of rapid-acting insulin brings glucose back to where it was before eating, your glucose numbers will likely stay within your goal range.

For various reasons, however, your blood sugar may be high (or low) before eating.

In this situation, you can temporarily adjust the rapid-acting insulin dose you take before your meal so that your glucose level before the next meal is in your goal range. This is often done using a correction scale (see the sample correction scale on this page). The correction dose of short-acting or rapid-acting insulin is added to or subtracted from the meal dose before eating.

You can think of this correction scale as a temporary bandage to help you correct your pre-meal blood sugar in the moment. If you need to use your correction scale frequently at a particular mealtime or at all meals, you likely need to adjust your set mealtime doses.

Using the correction scale frequently is often the first sign that your doses of insulin or carbohydrate amounts need to be reassessed. Ultimately, your insulin and self-care regimen should help you prevent high and low blood sugars, as well as react to them.

Your diabetes care team will help you tailor your scale to your insulin needs and your blood sugar goal range.

Adjusting a correction dose of inhaled insulin

Inhaled insulin is meant to be used at mealtime or as a corrective measure only. The dosing cartridges come prefilled with doses of 4 units, 8 units or 12 units. You can take this insulin before the meal or after based on the directions of your diabetes care team.

Dose adjustment is not possible without new cartridges and prescriptions since they come in set amounts. Talk with your CDCES before you use more than one cartridge at a single mealtime. Know how to use inhaled insulin safely not only for mealtime insulin but also for correction doses as needed.

Noninsulin and insulin combination treatment

Combining insulin with a noninsulin medicine can help both drugs work more effectively, and often with fewer side effects and a simpler treatment plan. The combination can also lower your daily insulin requirements and may limit weight gain associated with insulin therapy alone. However, a simultaneous use of pioglitazone and insulin can cause significant weight gain.

Sample Correction Scale

Glucose levels	Bkfst	Lunch	Supper
0 to 69	-2	-2	-2
70 to 89	-1	-1	-1
90 to 99	-0	-0	-0
100 to 140	0	0	0
141 to 200	+1	+1	+1
201 to 260	+2	+2	+2
261 or higher	+3	+3	+3

Glucose goals

Talk with your diabetes care team about what your target glucose levels should be. These are individualized based on how you might benefit from blood sugar management and the risks associated with your treatment plan. Here are a few examples:

• A 40-year-old with diabetes diagnosed within the last five years, no complications from diabetes and no other illness will likely target fasting and pre-meal glucose goals between 80 and 130 mg/dL. This should bring glycated hemoglobin (A1C) below 7%.

• An 80-year-old with diabetes diagnosed about 50 years back and now with chronic kidney failure and coronary artery disease will want to avoid hypoglycemia episodes as much as possible and target fasting and pre-meal glucose goals between 100 and 160 mg/dL. This should bring A1C below 8% or even 8.5%.

• A 20-year-old with type 1 diabetes and no complications who is planning a pregnancy will likely aim for fasting and pre-meal glucose goals below 120 mg/dL, and a A1C of less than 6.5%, so long as it can be safely achieved.

Drawbacks of intensive insulin therapy

Intensive insulin therapy has two possible drawbacks: low blood sugar (hypoglycemia) and weight gain.

When your blood sugar is already close to standard, hypoglycemia can occur even with minor changes in your routine, such as an unexpected increase in activity. You can counter this risk by being aware of changes in your routine that increase your risk of hypoglycemia.

It's also important to recognize the signs and symptoms of low blood sugar and respond quickly when you begin to experience them (see page 125).

When you use insulin to manage your blood sugar, more glucose gets into your cells so less is excreted in your urine. This is a good thing as it keeps you healthy. Glucose that's not used by your cells for fuel accumulates as fat. Weight gain can occur when you use insulin. The key is to maintain a balance between calorie intake and circulating insulin.

If you have type 2 diabetes and are taking insulin, talk with your diabetes care provider to see if less intensive insulin therapy or a therapy plan without insulin would be appropriate for you. With a less intensive plan, you'll likely need to measure your blood glucose level less often, and need fewer injections of insulin.

Healthy eating and exercising remain key components of diabetes management. Addition of certain medicines can be helpful in other ways — aiding with weight loss, preventing progression of kidney disease to kidney failure, and preventing acute heart failure, heart attacks, strokes and premature death.

LONG-TERM BENEFITS

Most of the discomfort of diabetes, at least initially, results not from symptoms but from the management of diabetes — the cost of treatment, monitoring supplies, blood tests and clinic visits; and medicine side effects. Then there's the sheer work involved: poking your fingers, counting carbs, thinking about dosing adjustments, and countless other physically and mentally taxing requirements.

Over the years, though, your hard work will pay off. Though not every complication can be prevented, managing your diabetes now can help significantly reduce, by up to 60%, the risk of serious complications later. Several landmark clinical trials in people with type 1 and type 2 diabetes, including the Diabetes Control and Complications Trial (DCCT), the United Kingdom Prospective Diabetes Study (UKPDS) and the Steno-2 study have shown the protective effects of keeping blood sugar levels within the standard range. Keep in mind that people without diabetes also develop kidney failure, blindness, heart attacks strokes and amputations.

Your diabetes care team will help you monitor your health by performing certain tests periodically, including an eye exam, to determine if there's any evidence of developing complications. If so, problems can be treated in a timely-manner and progression of these complications can be reversed or slowed.

CHAPTER 7

Using technology
to manage diabetes

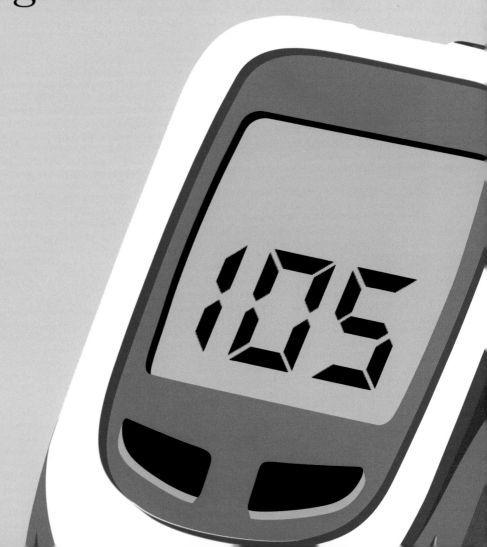

A VISIT WITH ANNA KASPER, R.N., CDCES

"As diabetes technologies continue to expand and advance, it can feel a bit intimidating to decide whether or not these tools can be a good fit for you. Diabetes technologies encompass a wide array of devices and seeking nonbiased information is important to ensure that what you choose adds positively to your life."

As with everything in diabetes self-care, technology use is a highly individual choice. The options available are ever-expanding and becoming more sophisticated. There are phone apps, increasingly dynamic glucose meters, smart pens, insulin pumps, continuous glucose monitors (CGMs), combination systems and DIY systems. In today's technology environment, you can be creative in meeting your needs and you can use various tools without committing to any others, should you wish.

For many people, starting with a phone app or a smart insulin pen can be a great introduction into diabetes technology use. CGM technology is also a great starting point because this tool can afford you a 24-hour window into your blood glucose levels and trends.

I've traveled around the world with my various diabetes technology tools and they have helped me live the life I wish to create. I have summited a volcano, enjoyed lazy beach days, slept under the stars and gardened to my heart's desire. These diabetes tools, coupled with professional education, can allow you to live the life you wish and to do so with increased ease.

A certified diabetes care and education specialist (CDCES) can help you review diabetes technology in a balanced manner. Though today's devices are wonderful, they're not a cure. You'll still need to manage them on a daily basis. There will be frustrations, of course. You could be attached to the "latest and greatest" devices, but if something is amiss, you need to be willing and able to troubleshoot the situation to get back on track with your diabetes self-care.

But that's where your diabetes care team can truly help you to succeed. They can provide education and support so that you can more easily troubleshoot problems and potential barriers. They can also assist you in deciding if this is the right time in your life to take on something new and help you assess the support networks you have available to you. This consideration is especially important when working with children and their parents or guardians.

Diabetes technology can provide increased flexibility, spontaneity, and safety to many people living with diabetes. Work together with your diabetes care team to make sure you move into the future as positively and seamlessly as you can while living with diabetes.

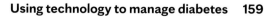

Tools to manage diabetes have come a long way since the first blood glucose meter was introduced in 1970. For people who monitor blood sugar (glucose) regularly and need multiple daily injections of insulin, technology can make life a little easier.

Today's devices are convenient to use, less invasive and help simplify treatment regimens, which can lead to fewer disease complications and an improved quality of life. Within the wide array of choices available are glucose sensors that continuously monitor blood sugar levels, insulin pump devices that more seamlessly deliver insulin when needed, and systems that can integrate both blood sugar monitoring and insulin delivery.

While these advancements have been helpful to many people living with diabetes, there are a few factors to consider before diving in. Most devices require a certain amount of time and money, and there's often a learning curve as you incorporate technological tools into your diabetes management plan.

Every person living with diabetes is different in how they experience and manage the disease, so there's no one-size-fits-all solution. But this chapter can help you sort through your options and find the tools that best fit your needs.

IS DIABETES TECHNOLOGY FOR ME?

Diabetes treatment is complex and can be challenging for people with diabetes, as well as their care teams. Whether some-one is newly diagnosed or has been using insulin therapy for years, it's a balancing act to keep blood glucose in the target range 24 hours a day, seven days a week.

Insulin is a powerful and life-sustaining hormone. Errors with insulin dosing — including missed or delayed doses or accidental overdosing — can happen, sometimes with serious consequences. In addition, blood sugar levels and insulin needs can fluctuate significantly with various activities, such as during exercise versus sleep, or in times of illness and stress. Knowing how to adjust your medications to match your needs isn't always intuitive.

Today's devices are geared to help with these day-to-day changes and considerations. Together with your diabetes care team, you can determine whether combining one or more of these technologies might benefit your management plan.

For example, living with diabetes typically requires a blood glucose meter to measure and display the amount of sugar in your blood. You're probably familiar with the basic models that require a fingerstick and drop of blood to determine your blood sugar levels at that moment. (See Chapter 5 for a full guide regarding this important diabetes self-care tool.) There also are more-advanced models that monitor blood sugar continuously through the day via a sensor placed under your skin.

Glucose sensors may be used alongside insulin administration tools such as traditional vials with syringes, insulin pens, smart insulin pen devices that help calculate and track doses, or insulin pumps.

Some insulin pumps and sensor systems can work together to allow for automatic delivery of extra insulin, as well as a temporary change in insulin delivery ranging from a full suspension of insulin to an increase in insulin delivery. All of these functions are based on blood sugar fluctuations and the algorithm used in the combined system.

When deciding whether technology may benefit you, consider your current routine, needs and abilities. Think about:

- *Hypoglycemia episodes.* Do you have frequent hypoglycemia? Do you ever have unrecognized low blood sugars? If it's a challenge to keep blood sugar levels within your target range, you may benefit from continuous monitoring technology with customizable safeguards and real-time data features.
- *Lifestyle.* Are you looking for greater flexibility in dosing that doesn't interfere with your lifestyle? Technology that provides customizable and dynamic insulin dosing may be a good option. Smart insulin pens and phone apps can allow for this increased flexibility in your management plan. Sensors may allow you more peace of mind as you are busy living your life.
- *Costs.* Diabetes management devices aren't always covered by insurance, which may make cost a consideration. There are a range of price options on the market today, including free phone apps, so ask your diabetes care team to help you find the right fit.

- *Individual needs.* Are there special considerations in your diabetes health picture — such as episodes of high blood sugar in the early morning hours (dawn effect) — that require an insulin adjustment? A pump and sensor system that can automatically adjust insulin delivery during this time is a possible solution. Even a standalone insulin pump (without a sensor system) can allow you to further refine your dosing to meet your sleep and daytime needs. Do you have vision problems or dexterity issues? A technology tool or two may assist you further in living well with diabetes.
- *Technological savvy.* Are you comfortable troubleshooting problems and being resourceful in navigating the daily use of various diabetes management tools? Are you willing to learn how to use new technology and adjust to it? Learning to use a device does take some time and patience especially if you're accustomed to low amounts of technology use or haven't had a lot of exposure to technology. Depending on your circumstances, simpler tools without all the bells and whistles may be all you need to achieve your goals. Sometimes less truly can be more depending on your needs and abilities.

The importance of a diabetes care team

A key part of your success in adopting diabetes technology is having a supportive diabetes care team (see page 7 for more on who makes up a diabetes care team). Having an objective care team that's well versed on the range of diabetes devices available and that can provide a thorough education — including helping you understand the pros and cons of each device — is crucial.

A supportive diabetes care team considers your preferences, lifestyle and circumstances when helping you choose devices. This team can support you in living comfortably year-round with technology as well as make sure you're able to continue doing the activities you enjoy while using the devices. Without this ongoing support, it can be difficult to get the full benefit of the technology available.

You also play a pivotal role in your own diabetes management. Currently, no devices on the market take complete control of diabetes management. That means you can't just press a few buttons and forget about your blood sugar and insulin levels. But if you're willing to learn how to use these devices and take part in ongoing education with your diabetes care team, these tools can be extremely helpful in keeping your blood sugar levels where you need them to be while giving you a little more freedom and flexibility.

WHAT ABOUT TECHNOLOGY FOR KIDS?

Many families have found diabetes technology to be very helpful. The considerations for children using insulin therapy are a lot like those for adults. Children who require insulin need access to a diabetes care team skilled in providing support and tools that fit the unique needs of younger people. For example, team members can offer parents tips on how to best help young children cope with sensor or infusion site insertions, and they can help teens learn how to manage their devices throughout the school day and while playing sports, or while transitioning toward independence.

Other things to think about when considering diabetes technology for children:

- *Dosing flexibility.* Look for a device that's able to address glucose fluctuations that come with the hormonal and developmental changes common in childhood.
- *Lifestyle disruptions.* Alarms, alerts, calibration requests and other features available on some devices can be disruptive to schooling, child care and playtime. Some children may appreciate devices that aren't worn on the body, while others may prefer more-discreet devices continuously worn on the skin. Student athletes may have a sense as to which system interferes the least with their sports. Some teens may feel empowered by constant data availability, while others may prefer less.
- *Caregiver education.* Babysitters, grandparents and others who look after your child need to be well versed on what to do when problems arise, such as a malfunction in a device or specific alarms.
- *Existing delivery system.* Is your child taking multiple daily injections successfully and are blood glucose targets regularly being met? There may not be a need to switch if your child isn't ready to change routines or isn't expressing interest after learning about technology options.

For more on kids and insulin pumps, see page 170.

TECHNOLOGY TYPES

Technological tools dedicated to diabetes management typically fall into two categories: devices that help you monitor your blood sugar and devices that deliver insulin. There's also the ability to combine these various tools into systems that communicate and function together.

Continuous glucose monitor

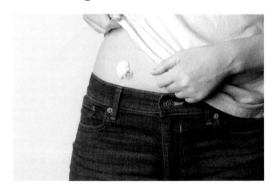

Continuous glucose monitors (CGMs) — sometimes called sensors for short — provide a 24-hour window into blood sugar levels. Typically placed on your abdomen, lower back or back of the arm, the system features a sensor inserted into fat tissue under your skin and a transmitter that relays blood sugar values every few minutes. A receiver device displays the current and recent glucose readings, and an arrow that predicts whether glucose levels will likely go up or down. The sensor sites under the skin typically need to be changed every 7 to 14 days. Some models feature sensors that can be worn up to several months.

The CGM parts that are worn on your body are waterproof when placed correctly. No needle is left under the skin with any of the CGM systems. Only a small wire, or implantable sensor capsule, is placed into fat tissue to read your blood sugar level. You don't remove it until it expires. These sensors continue to become smaller and easier to insert.

Many CGMs use real-time readings. This means they continuously report blood sugar levels on a receiver, insulin pump, smartphone or smartwatch, and alert you to the possibility of your blood sugar dipping too low (hypoglycemia) or rising too high (hyperglycemia).

CGMs often provide customizable alerts that offer peace of mind when blood sugar levels fluctuate. With many products, the associated software offers the option of sharing real-time glucose values and alarms with someone else, such as a parent or partner.

With these systems there are often additional software options that allow your diabetes care team members to have a look at your data as well. This can be very helpful when they work with you to adjust your medication regimen.

Other CGMs take a more bare-bones approach, such as providing data only on demand and leaving out customizable alarms. With these systems, you check your blood sugar by waving a receiver over the sensor. These more-basic devices are typically recommended as backup for adults who are self-monitoring their blood sugar levels and require frequent glucose testing. They serve as a great way to lessen the need for traditional fingersticks and are most often recommended for adults who don't have a history of low blood glucose or who have a lower risk of experiencing hypoglycemia.

Is a CGM right for me?

Given the amount of data they automatically collect, CGMs can be a powerful tool to help you understand how your blood sugar responds to your lifestyle. They can give you a broad view of your own personal trends over time.

The built-in alerts can also be helpful for children and adults who aren't always aware of when their blood sugar levels drop too low (hypoglycemia unawareness). When used correctly, CGMs have been shown to help people reach their blood sugar targets, lower A1C levels and reduce episodes of hypoglycemia.

And of course, most CGMs reduce the number of traditional fingersticks you need to perform in a day. Some CGMs still require fingerstick checks with a traditional blood sugar meter to calibrate the monitor. Your device's user guide can tell you if you need to calibrate it and, if so, how often you need to perform these checks. Review with your diabetes care team or product representative what "calibration" means if you have questions after your initial training.

Keep in mind that, regardless of the CGM system you use, you'll always need to keep your meter with you for back up in case of CGM system failure or errors. Blood glucose values from finger sites continue to be the most accurate capture of your blood glucose in the moment. This is because it's measuring true blood glucose, not the glucose circulating in your interstitial space, such as what the CGM sensor reads.

There are many ways to ensure that you're comfortably able to exercise, travel and be intimate while using CGM therapy. Talk with your diabetes care and education specialist about safety during travel, and with X-rays, CT scans and MRIs. Also, work with your diabetes care team to discuss what CGM options may work best for your needs.

Factors to keep in mind when considering a CGM include:
- **Reliability.** CGMs are gaining in accuracy, but it's still important to manually double-check your blood sugar levels when in doubt of a CGM reading, dehydrated, experiencing rapidly falling or rising levels, or when taking medications known to interfere with CGM system accuracy.
- **Emotional health.** You might want to consider whether you're comfortable having technology attached to your body 24 hours a day, 7 days a week. Note that you can take technology breaks safely with the support of your team. Also, be sure to speak with your team regarding healthy ways to cope with continuous glucose data. Remember these devices are tools meant to

build positively onto your regimen, not contribute additional anxieties or stressors. If continuous data flow is causing you anxiety or too much stress, reach out to your diabetes care team for support.

- **Skin sensitivity.** Some people experience skin sensitivity with the adhesive that's worn on the body. If this is an issue for you, talk with your diabetes care team about it. There are many skin preparations that you can try to lessen skin sensitivity. There are also many products available to assist with greater adhesion or easier removal of the sensor adhesive patches.
- **Troubleshooting.** Even if a CGM model doesn't require fingersticks for calibration, it's essential to keep a meter kit handy, just in case the CGM system stops displaying readings or fails.
- **Medication interference.** Certain medications, such as acetaminophen (Tylenol, others), albuterol (Proair HFA, Ventolin HFA, others), and lisinopril (Prinivil, Zestril, Qbrelis), may interfere with the accuracy of some CGM systems, particularly with older models. Readings on newer sensor systems don't seem to be affected by standard doses of acetaminophen (up to 1,000 milligrams a day for an adult).

Your diabetes care team can help. If you need to take medications that may affect the accuracy of the readings, your team may recommend double-checking your results with a standard blood sugar meter. Pregnancy, dialysis or a critical illness also can affect CGM system readings. CGM systems may not be Food and Drug Administration (FDA) approved for these circumstances, so check with your team about CGM use in these situations.

Smart insulin pen

Smart insulin pens work like standard insulin pens in that they're a convenient, portable way to deliver rapid-acting insulin when you need it, such as at mealtime. The devices are about the size of a large ink pen and feature a needle, a cartridge that holds the insulin, a dosage dial and a button that administers the insulin. Each injection requires a new needle.

In addition, a smart insulin pen typically offers several advanced features. One of its primary advantages is that it can connect wirelessly to a smartphone app to record information such as insulin dose and time, active insulin tracking and glucose data. It can also help with dose reminders, mealtime dosing calculations and assessments to share with your diabetes care team.

Recent innovations in smart pen technology include add-on devices that can be

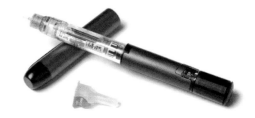

A smart pen (shown with disposable needle) calculates and delivers insulin doses.

retrofitted to a standard insulin pen to track real-time dosing behavior, including dose amount, time and insulin type. If desired, the information can also be sent to diabetes care providers via a smartphone app.

Is a smart insulin pen right for me?

Are you looking for some of the mealtime assistance of an insulin pump, but don't know if you want to wear one yet? A smart insulin pen may help you achieve your goals. It allows for similar dosing calculation assistance that an insulin pump can give you, but is not attached to your body.

Using a smart pen is also a great way to build up your knowledge base and comfort prior to adding other types of diabetes technology into your regimen.

Other advantages of a smart pen include more-finetuned dosings for those times when you need extra insulin (bolus), customizable reminders, and a digital record of your insulin doses and glucose data. This information can be helpful to you and your care team in making treatment decisions and goals.

Current smart pens communicate with a corresponding app. As a result, you'll need access to a smartphone or tablet that's able to exchange data wirelessly with the pen (using Bluetooth, for example). Having both components is vital to getting the maximum benefits. But in case of a lost phone, the pen can still be used as a standard insulin delivery device.

Insulin pump

Does your treatment plan include multiple daily injections of different types of insulin? Do you have difficulty fine-tuning your regimen so that your blood sugar levels are within your target goals? Insulin pump therapy may be a dynamic way to help you better meet your 24-hour insulin needs.

An insulin pump is a computerized device that's about the size of 1 to 2 decks of cards. You program it to deliver specific amounts of insulin continously and also when you eat, eliminating the need for daily shots. Some pumps are worn on your belt or in your pocket, while others stick to your skin.

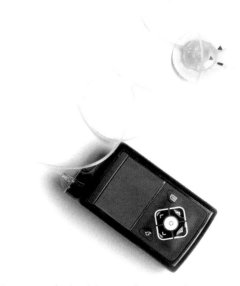

An extended tubing-style pump has a custom-length tube that connects the reservoir of insulin to a customizable infusion set that's inserted under the skin.

How it works

Based on settings that you and your diabetes care team program into the device, an insulin pump delivers a continuous (basal) infusion of insulin. A pump also allows you to deliver a customized dose of insulin (bolus) before meals to cover food intake, as well as to correct dosing when blood sugar levels are high.

In all insulin pumps there is a calculator function designed to reduce bolus amounts when blood sugar levels are low or if you have insulin still active in your body (insulin on board) from a previous bolus.

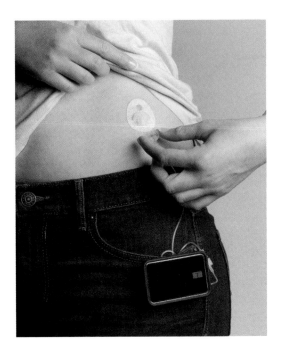

The infusion set (attached to the skin) can be easily disconnected from the tubing for activities such as showering or swimming.

Insulin pumps can provide different customized delivery rates of both basal and bolus insulin, depending on your specific needs. For example, your needs for insulin may be different during the daytime than during nighttime or in the morning hours.

Basal insulin is meant to hold your blood glucose levels steady during times of fasting or sleeping; it's not meant to supply increased insulin needs when you eat. Sometimes, though, your need for basal insulin may increase when you're sick. Or it may decrease when you're exercising. In situations such as these, you can temporarily adjust the basal insulin rate on your insulin pump.

Boluses, on the other hand, are meant to supply additional insulin to cover your food intake and to correct glucose levels when needed. Certain pump features allow you to extend the timing of your bolus delivery. A meal with high fat or protein content, for example, may slow down your digestion, warranting a slowed insulin delivery of the corresponding bolus.

Another feature lets you split your single bolus into a dual-wave style bolus. This allows part of your bolus to be delivered right away and the other part to be delivered over a customized time frame.

It's important to know how to make an insulin pump fit your lifestyle. Work with your certified diabetes care and education specialist (CDCES) to learn how to use these customization tools safely and effectively.

How you use it

There are a couple of pump styles that are commonly used. An extended tubing-style pump is worn in a pocket or on a belt and uses a soft, flexible tube to transport insulin to an infusion set attached to your skin. The infusion set contains a small, thin catheter (cannula) that goes under your skin. A patch-style pump doesn't require tubing. It's worn as a patch right on your skin. It also contains a cannula that is inserted under your skin.

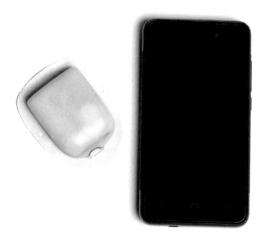

A tubeless-style pump doesn't have the extended tubing that runs between the pump and the infusion set. Instead, this system allows you to wear a small patch-style pump (left) on your skin that is changed out every 2 to 3 days. This pump has a built-in reservoir for insulin. The infusion set is inserted using a remote control-style device, which is also how you would make changes to pump settings or deliver boluses.

Both pump styles deliver insulin to your body at a spot called an infusion site. Sites that have fat tissue under the skin — on your abdomen, back of your arms, outer thighs, upper buttocks and lower back — are good infusion site options.

You can use any fat tissue site that's free of scar tissue, tattoos, body hair, boney prominences or moles. You'll also want to avoid the space near your bellybutton by 2 to 3 inches. Don't place the infusion set near your CGM sensor site, if you're using a CGM.

Every second or third day you'll need to change the infusion set, tubing, insulin and reservoir. Don't reuse these components. To change the setup, you pull out the infusion set and insert a new one at a different site. It's recommended that you rotate the infusion site every time.

The insulin used in all of these pumps is either rapid-acting insulin or short-acting insulin. Work with your diabetes care team to ensure safety regarding the choice of insulin in your pump. Don't place long-acting, intermediate-acting or pre-mixed insulins into your pump. Many pumps also feature capabilities to store and share data to help guide treatment decisions and goals.

If you decide to use an insulin pump, you'll typically receive thorough training in all aspects of pump use. During this training you'll learn how to determine your insulin requirements, how to program your pump to safely administer the insulin, and how to insert the infusion set and care for the infusion site.

Is an insulin pump right for me?

Insulin pumps can help if you're using multiple types of insulin and are having trouble maintaining blood sugar levels with injection therapy, even when you've been making refined dosing adjustments. If you don't need both bolus and basal insulin replacement, insulin pumps usually aren't warranted.

Pumps can help refine continuous basal insulin delivery, as well as corrective and mealtime bolus dosages. Pumps can provide more convenient as well as flexible dosing when compared with traditional injection regimens. Also, there may be less variation in the amount of insulin absorbed with pumps than with needles and syringes, and pens.

Because a pump releases a constant flow of insulin into the body, it's especially popular with people who have an unpredictable schedule. The greater flexibility pumps provide is considered one of their most significant advantages, with research showing that they can improve quality of life among both adults and children compared with insulin injections. Separate studies have linked pump usage to lower rates of diabetes complications and heart complications, as well.

While insulin pumps work well for many people, there are a few factors to consider before committing to one. Some points to think about:

- **Time investment.** Insulin pumps are not a cure and still require a lot of user input and care. When using a pump, you may still need to monitor glucose levels several times a day and program the pump for when you eat, are physically active or get sick. You'll need to change the infusion setup every 2 to 3 days, as previously outlined, and charge or change the pump's batteries intermittently, depending on the model.
- **Emotional health.** Some people find it difficult to wear a pump all day, every day. Work with your diabetes care team to assess your needs as well as review your options for living well with this technology.
- **Cost.** Pumps and their continuing supply requirements can be costly and may not be covered entirely by your insurance. Work closely with your insurance company and diabetes care team to assess these costs and your options. There may be company assistance programs or nonprofit organizations that can help with the costs as well.
- **Complications.** Pump infusion failures can occur and may be due to detachment, tubing becoming kinked, leaking around the infusion set, prolonged infusion site use, site infection, physical pump damage or battery problems. Such disruptions increase the risk of ketone buildup and diabetic ketoacidosis (see page 124) and should be addressed immediately.
- **Discontinuation.** Though discontinuing the use of a pump is less likely with today's advanced technology options, those users who do discontinue cite reasons such as cost, the discomfort of wearing a pump, and problems with blood sugar management. Some of these reasons may be rooted in lack of educational resources and support.

Self-advocacy with pump use is important to success. If you're in a location with limited diabetes self-management resources, seek out virtual support from technology company educators and reliable online resources.

Insulin pumps for children

Insulin pump therapy is a potential option for all children and adolescents with type 1 diabetes to help them reach optimal target blood glucose readings while reducing the risk of diabetes complications. In some cases, pumps may be the preferred choice, including in children under the age of 7, as a pump may provide the refined dosing that's often required in small children.

Children who experience the following may be good candidates for insulin pumps:
- Regular episodes of severe low blood sugar (hypoglycemia)
- Hard-to-manage blood sugar levels or patterns
- Difficulty adhering to current injection regimen
- Need for additional flexibility in diabetes self-management

Clinical trials comparing outcomes with pump technology and multiple daily injections in young people have shown modest improvements in blood glucose measurements in pump users. There's also evidence that pumps may help reduce the risk of severe hypoglycemia compared with injections, and the risk of diabetic ketoacidosis as well as diabetes complications such as eye damage (retinopathy) and nerve damage (peripheral neuropathy).

Stopping pump therapy isn't uncommon in adolescents. Many times, this can be traced back to problems wearing the pump. For example, pumps can serve as a constant reminder of having diabetes. Pumps can also get in the way of daily activities, such as sports, and make young users feel self-conscious about wearing them.

Having a supportive diabetes care team can help ease some of these concerns and assist you and your child in navigating some of your child's perceived hurdles. Remember flexibility is key. Your child may decide to take pump breaks throughout life. Or he or she may start insulin pump therapy and continue with it into the foreseeable future.

You can help your child get the most out of using a pump by addressing some common areas of concern:
- **Tube versus tubeless.** Children, particularly young athletes, may find that tubeless pumps interfere the least with their activities and sports. Other children may prefer the discreetness of a tubeless design.
- **Notifications.** Tactfully involve school staff so that they know about your child's pump settings and what the alarms indicate. If you and your child use a shared app that sends you notifications when your child's blood sugar is high or low, have a clear system of communication in place to alleviate concern and help you avoid hovering.

DIY TECHNOLOGY

Do-it-yourself artificial pancreas systems (also referred to as "looping") have been gaining popularity worldwide. Users of looping systems take FDA-approved insulin pumps and CGMs and use these to build their own "closed-loop" systems. Free software is available for download through various open-source sites and provides an algorithm that predicts glucose trends and automatically infuses insulin. Devices such as smartphones and experimental apps allow for some control of insulin infusions.

Looping systems are gaining in popularity among some users. But it's important to keep in mind that these systems aren't FDA-approved or regulated. Other potential drawbacks include investment of time to learn how to set them up, additional financial burden for parts not covered by insurance, potential voiding of pump and CGM warranties, and lack of research to assess systems' safety and effectiveness. Most who are part of the looping community are highly tech savvy and have access to additional resources should their technologies fail.

For example, your child could text you a code word or emoji to show that he or she has noticed the alarm and taken corrective measures.

- *Dietary expectations.* Help your child understand the importance of following a regular meal plan with consistent carb intake throughout the day. You may need to remind your child that having an insulin pump doesn't mean permission to eat without mindfulness.

Automated insulin delivery system

Automated insulin delivery systems take diabetes technology to the next level by combining the data from a CGM with smart software (algorithms) to automatically deliver appropriate amounts of insulin via an insulin pump. Common names for this type of system include a hybrid closed-loop system or an artificial pancreas.

These systems function thanks to a few key interactions.

- An insulin pump is connected to a CGM.
- The CGM tracks real-time blood sugar measurements.
- The measurements are fed into a software system that features sophisticated algorithms.
- Using data such as CGM readings, target glucose values, the amount of insulin on board, foundational pump settings and various activity modes, some algorithms direct the pump to

adjust insulin delivery to avoid high or low blood sugar levels. Some systems can only shut off insulin delivery when low glucose is predicted. Others work by increasing or decreasing basal insulin delivery to keep glucose levels stable. Additional corrective boluses can be delivered in a current algorithm as well.

- Activity modes for exercise or sleep also are available in some hybrid-closed loop systems to help you navigate your daily schedule.
- Additionally, software actions can sometimes be viewed on multiple devices, such as a computer or cell-phone, in addition to the pump screen.

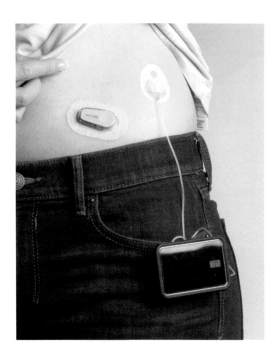

An automated insulin delivery system integrates a continuous glucose monitor (patch on left) with an insulin pump (right).

Is automated insulin delivery right for me?

People who already use a CGM and an insulin pump may be good candidates for an integrated system, particularly if they have frequent low blood sugar despite intensive therapy. Many of the benefits of CGMs and insulin pumps apply to this technology, with the addition of having automatic algorithm-based dosing adjustments to help get blood glucose close to goal range.

It's important to realize that these systems aren't fully automated. They rely heavily on smooth functioning and input of the CGM and insulin pump, as well as input from you, the user. You still need to stay tuned to your overall regimen and in particular, those occasions where you need extra insulin.

For example, you'll still need to program extra insulin before a meal or when your glucose is high. You may also need to periodically confirm blood sugar levels — in some cases, through a fingerstick — so that the system can automatically adjust insulin delivery throughout the day.

These hybrid-closed loop algorithms can assist your blood glucose management in unexpected situations, such as during sudden stress or injury. They can also help with more gradual hormonal shifts such as during menses.

If you already keep your glucose within a tight range without the use of automated insulin delivery, you might find that you generally outperform an automated system. Automated systems can reduce the mental load of diabetes management and reduce the risk of hypoglycemia, but they may not be the best at achieving the tight glucose levels you desire.

Alternatively, you may choose to run the algorithm only during certain times, such as overnight for safety or during exercise. These algorithms aren't necessarily one-size-fits-all.

Currently these algorithms aren't approved for use during pregnancy. This is related to the systems not being capable of reaching the glucose ranges desired during pregnancy.

Speak with your diabetes care team about your current management, preferences, and whether or not you would benefit from this technology.

USING TECHNOLOGY WISELY

Diabetes technology can be really helpful for a lot of people living with diabetes. But it can also be confusing, and it can be difficult to discern which options would work best in your current situation.

Be sure to talk about your goals and concerns with your diabetes care team. A certified diabetes care and education specialist is an objective and well-positioned professional that can help you consider your choices, find the best fit for you, help you with training and follow-up questions, as well as keep you up to date on the latest changes or advances that may benefit you.

FUTURE OF DIABETES TECHNOLOGY

Diabetes technology is rapidly expanding. Here are some anticipated developments:

- *Refined algorithms.* These will build on previous versions, becoming more robust and responsive to the wearer's needs. They'll likely offer more functions, including newer algorithms to help with hyperglycemia and mealtime and carbohydrate management. They may also offer advanced responses and algorithm tools for activities or stress responses.
- *Noninvasive CGMs.* These are being developed to be more comfortable and convenient. Some of these devices will use transmitters and needleless skin-mounted patches outfitted with a sensor. The instruments will be designed to measure glucose molecules just below the skin and transmit readings frequently to a smartphone app.
- *Multihormone automated systems.* These systems aim to dynamically deliver insulin when you have elevations in blood sugar and glucagon when you're experiencing a drop in blood sugar. The dual hormone systems will be designed to further improve glycemic control and improve quality of life.
- *Convertible insulin pumps.* These will be able to switch from an extended tubing-style pump to a patch-style pump that can be worn on your skin.
- *Longer-use infusion sets.* These aim to lengthen the wear time of typical infusion sets beyond the limit of a few days. The hope is to safely extend wear time and minimize the need to change them frequently.

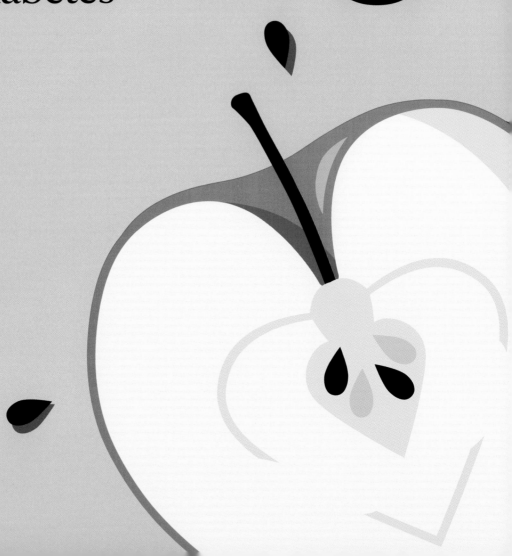

If your child has diabetes

A VISIT WITH ANA L. CREO, M.D.

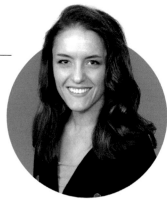

"While many people think of diabetes as an adult disease, children can develop diabetes, too! Fortunately, with the rise of technology, diabetes diagnosed in childhood is becoming easier and easier to manage."

Diabetes is one of the most common chronic diseases in children and adolescents in the U.S. About 215,000 people below the age of 20 live with diabetes. People living with diabetes mellitus fall into two broad groups: those who have a deficiency of insulin (type 1) and those with a diminished effectiveness of insulin (type 2).

Type 1 diabetes is a condition where the body can't make the insulin that's needed to carry glucose into cells. It accounts for the majority of diabetes seen during childhood in the United States. For every 1,000 children between ages 0 and 19, two live with type 1 diabetes. Each year, about 20,000 young people are diagnosed with type 1 diabetes.

Type 2 diabetes begins when the body develops a resistance to insulin and no longer uses insulin properly. As the need for insulin rises, the pancreas gradually loses its ability to produce sufficient amounts of insulin to regulate blood sugar (glucose).

Type 2 diabetes, previously known as adult-onset diabetes, is becoming more common in children and adolescents. The epidemic of childhood obesity and the low level of physical activity among young people are major contributors to the increase in type 2 diabetes during childhood and adolescence.

This chapter discusses a number of issues related to childhood diabetes, including diagnosis and treatment, how to create a diabetes care plan, and how to help your child thrive while living with diabetes.Since type 1 diabetes is characterized by insulin deficiency, all kids living with this condition must take insulin delivered by injection or a pump. Treatment for type 1 diabetes is a lifelong commitment of monitoring blood sugar, taking insulin, maintaining a healthy weight, eating healthy foods and getting regular exercise.

For children living with type 2 diabetes, eating a healthy diet, exercising regularly and maintaining a healthy weight are crucial for managing the condition. Medications also may be considered, including insulin therapy.

Keeping blood sugar levels within the target range developed for your child can help prevent dangerous blood sugar highs and lows. Blood sugar management can also help prevent long-term complications and promote healthy growth and development during childhood.

If your son or daughter was recently diagnosed with diabetes, chances are you're feeling the need to find out everything you can about the condition. It can be overwhelming, especially in the beginning. Suddenly, it seems, you and your child must learn how to manage a chronic illness that involves giving regular injections, keeping tabs on food intake and closely monitoring blood sugar levels.

It's important to learn as much as you can about diabetes and its management. Know that as you gain knowledge and experience, you'll also gain confidence that your child can still thrive while living with diabetes. It takes time to understand what it means for your child to have diabetes and to develop the best treatment plan for your child. Your starting point will depend on whether your child is living with type 1 or type 2 diabetes.

TYPE 1 DIABETES

More than 20,000 children are diagnosed with type 1 diabetes each year in the United States. While the incidence of type 1 diabetes is increasing in all age groups, more and more new cases are affecting younger children between the ages of 1 and 4.

As noted in Chapter 1, in type 1 diabetes the pancreas produces little if any insulin. Without this hormone available to move blood sugar (glucose) into the body's muscles and tissues, too much glucose stays in the bloodstream. This can cause serious organ damage and even death.

Type 1 diabetes is not caused by eating too much sugar, candy or high-calorie foods.

Signs and symptoms

Signs and symptoms of type 1 diabetes usually develop quickly — over a period of weeks — in children and teenagers. The first indication in babies and young children may be a yeast infection that causes a severe diaper rash. If your child already is using the toilet, you may notice a reversal in toilet training and new bed-wetting. Fatigue or irritability is common and should raise your suspicion when it occurs along with other common warning signs:
• Frequent urination
• Intense thirst
• Constant hunger
• Unexplained weight loss

Testing

If your child's health care provider suspects type 1 diabetes, there are several tests that can help with a diagnosis:

Random blood sugar test

This is the primary screening test for type 1 diabetes. Random means any time of day, without fasting. Your child's provider will probably obtain this blood test at your initial visit to check for a high level of glucose. A result of 200 milligrams per deciliter (mg/dL) or greater will confirm the diagnosis in a child who has signs and symptoms of diabetes.

Glycated hemoglobin (A1C) test

This test indicates your child's average blood sugar level for the past three months. It works by measuring what percentage of hemoglobin, the oxygen-carrying protein in red blood cells, is coated with sugar. The higher your child's blood sugar levels, the more hemoglobin he or she will have with sugar attached. An A1C level of 6.5% or higher on two separate tests indicates diabetes and may be helpful when symptoms are mild.

Fasting blood sugar test

In some circumstances, a health care provider may recommend a blood glucose test done after a period of fasting (fasting blood glucose test). Before having blood drawn for this test, your child will be instructed not to eat or drink for at least eight hours — typically, overnight. After a fast, a blood glucose level under 100 mg/dL is considered to be within the standard range. A glucose level from 100 to 125 mg/dL is considered prediabetes, which indicates a high risk of developing diabetes. A glucose level of 126 mg/dL or higher indicate that a diagnosis of diabetes is likely. If symptoms are mild or absent, a second test may be requested to confirm these results.

Antibody test

If diabetes seems likely, your child's provider may order another blood test, one that checks for antibodies that are commonly found in people with type 1 diabetes.

This test may help distinguish between type 1 diabetes and type 2 diabetes, which is important because treatment strategies differ by type. However, not having these antibodies doesn't rule out the possibility of having type 1 diabetes.

ALWAYS KEEP EMERGENCY INFO NEAR YOUR CHILD

When your child has diabetes, he or she needs to have his or her emergency information quickly available at all times, regardless of age. This might be an identification (ID) tag about diabetes in the form of a necklace, dog tag or bracelet (for the wrist or ankle). Let your child choose one that appeals to him or her. Even shoe tags for toddlers are available. You can search online for a variety of styles and prices, and many pharmacies carry them.

If your child has a smartphone, a helpful option might be to set up a medical ID button on your child's phone. On many smartphones, you can find this by tapping Settings, then Health and Medical ID. You set it up so that the necessary information can be viewed even when the phone is locked.

Ketones test

If a child's symptoms are severe or include signs and symptoms such as a fruity-smelling breath, drowsiness or lethargy, the health care provider may want to do a urine or blood test to check for the presence of ketones.

Ketones are toxic acids that the body produces when insulin is very low and the body isn't getting enough glucose, so it resorts to breaking down stored fat. Excess ketones can cause a life-threatening condition called diabetic ketoacidosis (kee-toe-as-ih-DOE-sis), or DKA.

With prompt treatment, this condition can be reversed. Children with DKA initially need treatment in a hospital. However, some children with mild DKA may be quickly and effectively treated with insulin therapy without the need for hospitalization.

If your child is diagnosed with type 1 diabetes, it's best to have an evaluation by an experienced diabetes care team, including a pediatric endocrinologist — a doctor who specializes in treating children who have diabetes.

TREATMENT

Treatment for type 1 diabetes is lifelong and includes blood sugar monitoring, insulin therapy, healthy eating and regular exercise — even for kids. As your child grows and changes, so will his or her diabetes treatment plan. And your child will learn to do more on his or her own.

If managing your child's diabetes seems overwhelming, remember to take it one day at a time. Some days you'll manage your child's blood sugar perfectly, and on other days, it may seem as if nothing works well. Don't forget that you're not alone.

You'll work closely with your child's diabetes care team to keep your child's blood sugar level as close to the desired target range as possible (see page 7 for potential members of your child's care team). This effort often requires a delicate balancing act among meals, activity, monitoring blood sugar and taking insulin. But advances in technology have made it easier to achieve target blood sugar ranges. Your child's care team will choose a blood glucose target range according to your child's medical needs and individual situation.

Blood sugar monitoring

Frequent testing is the only way to make sure that your child's blood sugar level remains within his or her target range — which may change as your child grows and changes. See Chapter 5 for more detailed information on blood sugar monitoring.

You'll need to check and record your child's blood sugar at least four times a day. Many families find it helpful to use a continuous glucose monitor (CGM). This device measures your child's blood sugar every few minutes using a temporary or implanted sensor inserted under the skin. Chapter 7 has more information on CGMs.

Insulin therapy

All people living with type 1 diabetes, adults and children alike, depend on insulin therapy to live. Your child may take insulin with a syringe, an insulin pen or an insulin pump (see *Insulin therapy* on page 140.

Many types of insulin are available (see the table in the appendix on pages 302 and 303). Insulin types are often categorized based on how quickly they start having an effect on the body.

The initial insulin dosage for your child is based on weight, age, activity level and whether puberty has started. With the help of your diabetes care team, you and your child will learn how to make adjustments to insulin doses to manage expected changes in insulin needs as your child grows. In children and teens, there are a few insulin regimens that are most often used.

Multiple daily injections

This regimen consists of a rapid-acting or short-acting insulin taken before meals and snacks as well as a long-acting insulin taken once a day to provide a baseline amount throughout the day.

Split-mixed program

This is a mixture of rapid-acting or short-acting insulin and intermediate-acting insulin in one injection, usually given twice each day.

Insulin pump

An insulin pump is a small device worn outside the body that's programmed to deliver specific amounts of insulin continuously throughout the day and also when your child eats.

Studies show that insulin pumps are as safe and effective as injections are, even for many infants and toddlers. In fact, insulin pumps may be more effective in younger children when injections can't be fine-tuned enough to achieve target goals. Ask your child's diabetes care team how well the pump has worked for other children the same age as your son or daughter. Some devices combine the functions of blood sugar monitoring and insulin delivery. See Chapter 7 for more on diabetes technology. You'll find specific information on the use of insulin pumps in children on page 170.

TYPE 2 DIABETES

Type 2 diabetes used to be considered an adult disease. It was even referred to as adult-onset diabetes. Not anymore. Today, a significant number of children are diagnosed with type 2 diabetes. Why? Obesity plays a major role.

Over the past three decades, the rate of childhood obesity has more than doubled for children and teenagers. Those extra pounds carry an increased risk of type 2 diabetes. Today, most children and teenagers diagnosed with type 2 diabetes are overweight. Other factors that may contribute include the following.

PUBERTY AND DIABETES

Just when you think you have a pretty good handle on helping your child manage blood glucose, along comes puberty. Suddenly you're dealing with unpredictable moods and unpredictable blood glucose readings.

Some teenagers may start neglecting diabetes care as part of an overall drive for independence. This can play a role in unexplained high and low blood glucose readings during puberty. In addition, growth hormone and sex hormone surges typically cause increased insulin resistance. Your teenager will probably need more insulin during puberty, along with more-frequent blood glucose tests to make sure that a mood swing isn't caused by hypoglycemia.

If your teenage daughter has higher blood glucose levels around the time of her period, talk to her health care provider. The provider may adjust her treatment regimen to compensate for the influence of the menstrual cycle. Other options that might help stabilize blood sugar levels during periods include continuous dosing birth control pills or an intrauterine device (IUD).

Your teen's self-sufficiency may tempt you to turn diabetes care entirely over to your teen. But don't tune out. While it's important for your child to assume more responsibility for diabetes management, parental guidance and support remains crucial to managing diabetes throughout the teen years. By the end of high school, most teens should be fully prepared to take over their diabetes care so that they're ready to handle it at college or wherever life takes them.

- *Family history.* Risk increases if a parent, sibling or blood relative has type 2 diabetes. But it's difficult to tell if this is learned behavior, genetics or both.
- *Race and ethnicity.* African Americans, Latinos, Native Americans, Asian Americans and Pacific Islanders are at higher risk for unclear reasons.
- *Signs of insulin resistance.* This includes high blood pressure, polycystic ovarian syndrome or irregular levels of blood fats (lipids).

Signs and symptoms

Unlike type 1 diabetes, in which symptoms typically develop quickly, the signs and symptoms of type 2 diabetes often appear gradually. These may include:
- Frequent urination
- Fatigue
- Intense thirst
- Blurred vision
- Constant hunger
- Frequent infections

- Unexplained weight loss
- Slow-healing sores

Some children living with type 2 diabetes have patches of dark, velvety skin in the folds and creases of their bodies, usually in the armpits and neck. This condition, called acanthosis nigricans, is a sign of insulin resistance and increases the probability that your child has type 2 diabetes. Still, many children living with type 2 diabetes don't have any symptoms.

To diagnose the disease before it does serious damage, experts recommend testing all children and adolescents who are at high risk, even if they're symptom-free. One key risk factor is having a body mass index (BMI) greater than the 85th percentile for your child's age and sex. BMI is a measurement based on a formula that takes into account weight and height to determine if your child has an unhealthy percentage of body fat.

Screening

If your child is overweight and has any two of the risk factors previously noted — family history, high-risk race or ethnicity, or signs of insulin resistance — ask your health care provider about scheduling a diabetes screening.

Health care providers usually use a fasting blood glucose test and an A1C test to diagnose type 2 diabetes in children. Your child will need to avoid food and liquid for at least eight hours before having blood drawn. If your child has a blood glucose level of 126 mg/dL or higher on two separate tests, your child has diabetes. An A1C test result higher than 6.5% also is an indication of diabetes. See page 176 for more on these tests.

Prediabetes

If a fasting blood glucose test indicates a level from 100 to 125 mg/dL, your child may have prediabetes. Many people with prediabetes eventually develop type 2 diabetes.

Studies show that adults with prediabetes who make improvements to their lifestyle, including eating healthier foods and exercising more, may prevent type 2 diabetes from developing. Children and teens with prediabetes can reduce their risk by making these same changes.

Ask your child's health care provider for guidance. In addition, ask how often your child should be screened for diabetes. Whether your child has prediabetes or diabetes, developing healthy eating habits, increasing physical activity and getting regular exercise are vital to prevention and disease management.

Treatment

Treatment for type 2 diabetes is lifelong and includes:

Healthy eating

Because kids are still growing, the focus is on slowing down weight gain instead of losing weight. Your child's dietitian will likely suggest that your child — and the rest of the family — consume fewer animal products and sweets. See page 188 for more on healthy eating.

Regular physical activity

Physical activity lowers blood sugar. Encourage your child to get regular aerobic activity for at least an hour a day. Better yet, exercise with your child. Activity time doesn't have to be all at once — you can break it down into smaller chunks of time. For more on physical activity, see Chapter 4.

Blood sugar monitoring

Your provider will let you know how often you need to check and record your child's blood sugar. Children who take insulin usually need to test more frequently, possibly three times a day or more. See more on monitoring in Chapter 5.

Medications

Many children also need medications to help manage type 2 diabetes. The decision about which treatment is best depends on the child, the level of blood glucose and whether the child has other health problems.

There are three medications that have been approved by the Food and Drug Administration for treating type 2 diabetes in children — metformin, liraglutide (Victoza) and insulin. Metformin is a pill and liraglutide and insulin are taken by injection.

Metformin reduces the amount of sugar a child's liver releases into the bloodstream between meals and helps the body's cells use insulin more effectively. Liraglutide helps the body release more insulin from the pancreas after meals, when blood sugar levels are higher. Both drugs may have digestive system side effects, such as nausea or diarrhea.

Sometimes, insulin also may be needed if your child's blood sugar levels are very high. With lifestyle changes and other medications, your child may be able to be weaned off insulin.

There are a number of different insulins, but a long-acting insulin is often used for type 2 diabetes in children. Insulin is typically delivered via a syringe or an insulin pen. An insulin pump programmed to dispense specific amounts of insulin also might be an option for children who need to take insulin more frequently.

Chapter 6 has more information on diabetes medications.

CREATING A DIABETES CARE PLAN

Leaving your child in the care of someone else can be nerve-racking for any parent. If your child is living with diabetes, you might be even more fearful. But both you and your child are likely to feel more secure knowing that people outside the family can be relied on to help manage diabetes with your child. And your child will build self-confidence from handling diabetes care when you're not around. So take a deep breath, and then take action.

Sit down with your diabetes care and education specialist to create a care plan that maps out your child's treatment regimen and how to respond to high or low blood glucose. Then meet with school or child care personnel to go over the plan in detail.

Note the names of adults who will be primarily responsible for helping your child check his or her blood glucose and take medications. This usually involves a talk with the school nurse. Ask the school nurse or an administrator to help you share the plan with all adults who'll be supervising your child during the day, including teachers, office staff, coaches and bus drivers.

Your child's diabetes care team or health care provider may be able to help you train school and child care staff to perform diabetes care tasks if they aren't already able to do so.

Blood glucose monitoring

Regular blood glucose tests are the only way to know with confidence whether your child's treatment program is working. Whether they are living with type 1 or type 2 diabetes, children and teenagers who use insulin may need four or more blood glucose checks each day. Your child's provider can help you determine the best testing schedule.

More and more, using a continuous glucose monitor (CGM) to monitor blood sugar is becoming the standard of care for diabetes in children. CGMs attach to the body using a fine needle just under the skin that checks blood glucose level every few minutes. They're especially helpful for children who have difficulty recognizing signs of low blood sugar (hypoglycemia). Learn more about CGMs on page 163.

Whether you're using fingersticks or a CGM to monitor blood sugar, log the results in a record book each time you run a test. Keep a separate record book at your child's school for tracking results during the day. Young children will need an adult's help to maintain school record books, but children age 8 and older may begin to log results on their own.

The information you record will help you see how food, physical activity, illness and other factors affect your child's blood glucose. You may start to see patterns that will help your doctor develop the best treatment program for your child.

Young children in particular may have a hard time recognizing the signs and symptoms of low blood glucose (hypoglycemia), explained on page 25. Teach your child — and any caregivers — that if there's any doubt, check the blood glucose levels.

Regardless of your child's age, getting used to frequent glucose checks can be challenging for him or her — and for you. Focus on reassuring (rather than scolding) your child when he or she resists testing

BLOOD SUGAR VS. BLOOD GLUCOSE

You'll likely hear the term *blood sugar* more often than the term *blood glucose.* The terms mean the same thing.

If you decide to use the term *blood sugar,* make sure that your child understands what it means (explained in Chapter 1). Eating other types of carbohydrates — not just sugary foods — can make blood sugar (glucose) rise. Even some adults who've lived with diabetes for many years still think they can't eat any sugar. But they don't realize they're eating too much of other foods that can make their blood glucose rise. The key is moderation. For the full story on healthy eating, see Chapter 2, including *The real scoop on sugar,* page 49.

because it's uncomfortable. Consider simple rewards, such as stickers (not food) for every test accomplished; your child can put them in your record book. Allow even your young child to make some decisions, such as choosing the spot for the glucose check.

As children gain independence, they are sometimes tempted to cut corners or forge numbers to bypass glucose checks. Be wary if you begin to see too many of the same glucose numbers. Usually these are repeating even numbers, such as 180 or 150 several times in a row, or a pattern of even then odd glucose values.

Many children also start to pick up on their parents' emotional reactions to numbers that are outside of the normal range. As a parent, try not to get upset when your child or teen tells you of a blood sugar that's out of range. If you show a lot of disappointment or anxiety,

your child may be tempted to report a "better" but inaccurate number in the future to avoid such a reaction. Instead, be matter-of-fact and encourage your child to continue managing his or her diabetes in a positive way.

If you need help, don't hesitate to ask your child's diabetes care team about how to approach this task, including how to deal with the emotional challenges you may face.

Involving your child

Encourage your child's active participation in meetings and discussions about diabetes care. Eventually, your child will need to take on total responsibility for managing diabetes. You can start working toward that goal from the beginning by asking your child to help with care tasks in age-appropriate ways.

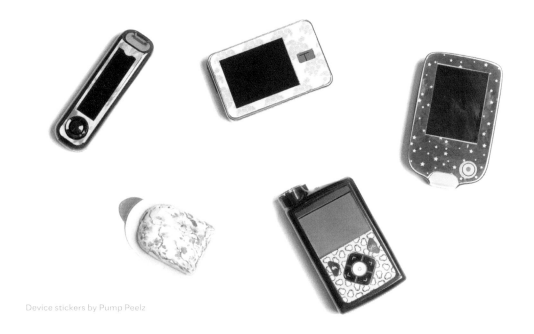

Device stickers by Pump Peelz

Glucose meters, sensors and insulin pumps can be customized with different stickers.

The extent to which your child is ready to participate depends on his or age, abilities and willingness. Here's a general idea of what you can aim for, but ask your child's primary care provider for guidance because children develop at different rates.

Ages 2 and 3

Even as a toddler, your child can help with certain decisions. Your child may be able to pick out a test strip for a blood glucose test, choose between two places for an insulin injection or wipe off the injection site with a swab. If you use an insulin pump, your child could choose the infusion site and stickers that can be applied to the pump.

Ages 4 through 7

Your child may be able to help keep blood glucose records and may enjoy helping plan healthy meals and games that encourage physical activity for the family. At this age, children can also learn to identify CGM alarms and talk an adult through changing a CGM site or infusion site.

Ages 8 through 11

With your supervision and support or that of another trusted adult, your child may be able to perform a fingerstick blood glucose test by age 8 and self-administer insulin by age 10. Children in this age group also can learn to prep a site for a CGM or pump change on their own.

MAKING SMART CHOICES

Your teenager is headed out to a party with friends. Like most parents, you worry about whether alcohol will be served and whether other kids might be doing things like vaping. You want your child to be able to make smart choices when surrounded by risky behaviors.

Have a frank discussion with your teenager about the risks of alcohol and vaping, including risks that relate specifically to diabetes. Both alcohol and vaping increase the risk of hypoglycemia, and the sugar content of many mixed drinks can raise blood glucose. If your teenager experiences high or low blood glucose while partying with friends, they may think your child is drunk and take no action to help. Vaping greatly accelerates diabetes-related complications. It's just not worth the risk to drink or vape. Talk to your child about ways to say no if pressured to make choices that are not in his or her best interest.

Ages 12 through 15

Around the tween and early teen years, your child may be ready to self-monitor blood glucose levels under typical circumstances, using fingerstick checks or a CGM. Most likely, they'll still need help dealing with blood sugar highs (hyperglycemia) and lows (hypoglycemia).

Children who use insulin can probably manage injections or insulin pump infusions with some supervision. They may also be able to do a complete CGM site change and insulin pump setup change with supervision.

Ages 16 through 18

In the later teen years, most children are ready to start managing diabetes care independently and are able to take full responsibility by the end of high school. This includes self-monitoring, completing CGM and pump changes independently and being well prepared to respond to possible complications such as hypoglycemia or hyperglycemia (see page 25).

If you share a CGM app with your child — so that you get notified of your child's blood sugar values — it's usually beneficial to have a clear system in place for managing alarms and notifications. For example, many families set up the expectation that if the parent sees the teen having low blood sugar while out of the house, the teen has 15 minutes to text the parent that the low blood sugar has been treated. This kind of setup improves family communication, helps teens maintain control over their condition and eases parental anxiety.

EMOTIONAL AND SOCIAL ISSUES

Coping with a diagnosis of diabetes is tough for all children and teens. If your child is very young, all the tests and injections may feel like punishment. An older child may be crushed to realize that he or she is different from peers and that diabetes isn't going to go away.

Sadness, anger and withdrawal are all typical reactions. However, feelings of hopelessness that last for weeks call for medical attention.

Encourage your child to talk about feelings. Your preschooler may be able to vent emotions by drawing pictures or role-playing with dolls and stuffed animals. Older children may feel better just having a chance to yell, stomp, kick a pillow or cry. (Parents, too!)

Listen to your child without trying to put a positive spin on diabetes. Let your son or daughter know that you're there to help. Your child may be nervous about telling friends about the diagnosis. Volunteer for practice conversations, and let your child know that whom to tell, when to tell and how much to say is up to him or her — it's a personal decision.

Your child may want to talk with a trusted teacher or school social worker who can help ease the transition to managing diabetes at school. A local support group, online forum or camp (see page 195) for children and teens with diabetes also might make coping easier. Your diabetes care team can provide you with appropriate resources.

When it's more than sadness

Diabetes increases the risk of depression. Every child reacts differently, but keep an eye out for these signs and symptoms in your son or daughter:
- Not caring about the things he or she used to
- Having trouble sleeping
- Staying in bed all of the time
- Eating a lot more or eating less than usual
- Losing or gaining a lot of weight without trying
- Difficulty concentrating
- Feeling anxious a lot
- Crying a lot
- Expressing a desire to inflict self-harm or to die

If you think your child may be depressed, seek help right away. Your doctor or diabetes care and education specialist can refer your child to a mental health professional.

GOOD HABITS FOR STAYING HEALTHY

Healthy eating, increased physical activity and regular monitoring of blood sugar are key steps to managing diabetes. See also Chapters 2, 4 and 5, respectively for more information on these key areas. Many of the principles of diabetes management that apply to adults also apply to children.

Your positive attitude and active participation is a crucial part of helping your child make these permanent lifestyle changes.

ARE TEENAGERS WITH DIABETES AT HIGHER RISK OF EATING DISORDERS?

Yes. Studies show that teens living with type 1 diabetes may be twice as likely as their peers who don't live with diabetes to develop eating disorders. This includes gradually starving themselves (anorexia) and forcing themselves to throw up after eating (bulimia).

It may be that having to pay such close attention to food makes kids with diabetes more likely to obsess about their weight. And insulin can be manipulated to cause weight loss. Eating disorders increase the risk of complications from diabetes. Even in teens without diabetes, eating disorders can be fatal.

Signs that your child may have an eating disorder include:
- Extreme fluctuations in blood glucose that can't be explained
- Frequent problems with high or low blood glucose
- Not complying with insulin needs
- Unexplained weight loss
- Obsession with food or with losing weight
- Avoiding being weighed
- Wearing baggy clothes to hide weight loss
- Avoiding meals with the family
- Binge eating
- Excessive exercising
- Irregular menstrual periods or no menstrual periods

If you think your child may have an eating disorder, call his or her care provider. The provider may arrange for your child to see a mental health professional with special training in eating disorders.

Tips for healthy eating

It's recommended that people living with diabetes follow the same healthy-eating plan recommended for everyone, with moderate portions at regular mealtimes.

That means eating a variety of whole foods, such as fresh fruits and vegetables, whole grains, and lean protein. It also means fewer processed foods, such as burgers, sodas, prepackaged muffins and other convenience foods. See Chapter 3 for more information.

Sometimes people get the impression that all children living with diabetes should follow a low-fat, low-calorie diet. But dietary fat plays an important role in brain development, especially in younger children. Whole-fat dairy is appropriate for toddlers and preschoolers, for example. And children living with type 1 diabetes especially need the right amount of nutrient-rich calories to grow and gain weight.

Whether your child is living with type 1 or type 2 diabetes, focus on foods that contain healthy fats, such as unsaturated fats and omega-3 fatty acids, which can improve blood cholesterol levels. Examples include nuts, avocados, olive oil, and fish such as salmon, cod and tuna. Avoid eating too much food that's high in saturated fat, such as butter and meat. Processed foods tend to be high in saturated fat as well.

Chances are, your entire family would benefit from making the same improvements to fuel up for a healthy, active life.

Launch a family project to find recipes that are healthy and also tempting. Schedule a movie night and set nutritious snacks on the coffee table. Try air-popped popcorn, veggies with hummus dip or fruit with yogurt dip.

Here are some tips for enlisting the whole family in a healthy-eating program:

- Involve your children in helping to prepare meals in age-appropriate ways. They're much more likely to try a new vegetable dish if they helped chop up the ingredients.
- Eat as many family meals together as possible, and keep table conversation to pleasant topics.
- Don't deprive your child or your family of enjoying a dessert, but choose

healthier foods. Modify a favorite recipe with the help of a registered dietitian nutritionist. Try new recipes and always use appropriate portions. A carefully chosen dessert at the end of a balanced meal is fine on occasion, and it can help reduce the likelihood that your child will feel deprived.

- Work with your dietitian to include allowances for foods that your family usually enjoys at celebrations or special occasions.

Eating away from home

Find out if healthy foods are on the menu in your child's school cafeteria. If they're not, pack a lunch that follows the same nutritious standards you're setting for the family dinner table. Then call the school and encourage better options.

Most children and teenagers also need a couple of snacks during the day. Ward off vending machine temptations by slipping tasty, wholesome options into your child's backpack. A few examples of smart snack choices include:

- Mixed nuts
- Whole-grain bread with peanut butter
- Low-fat cheese sticks
- Yogurt
- Fresh fruit

If your child is planning a sleepover at a friend's house, call the other parents and — with your child's input — discuss what food will be served and why you're asking. If they're not planning healthy snacks, tell them you'll send some with your child, and include enough for the other children to enjoy.

NO LIMITS TO ACHIEVEMENT

If you worry that diabetes might limit the dreams your child can reach for, consider Gary Hall Jr.'s story. Gary had four Olympic swimming medals in his pocket and was training for more when, in 1999, he started noticing that he was always thirsty and his vision was blurred. He was soon diagnosed with type 1 diabetes. Gary was shocked. There was no history of diabetes in his family, and he had always worked hard to keep in excellent physical condition.

Gary decided he wasn't going to let diabetes stop him. He found a doctor who believed it was possible for him to continue to train and compete. Under his doctor's supervision, Gary dedicated himself to a rigorous schedule of blood glucose testing and treatment and got back in the pool. At the 2000 Olympic games in Sydney, Australia, Gary won four more medals. And at the 2004 games in Athens, Greece, he took gold in the 50-meter freestyle and became one of the most decorated Olympic athletes in history.

Getting more physically active

Getting active with your child is an essential part of making exercise habits stick, and it will improve your health, too. While regular exercise is important, any physical activity has health benefits. Use these tips to help your kids develop a lifelong appreciation for activities that increase their fitness.

Physical activity has the effect of lowering blood sugar. If your child is on insulin therapy, read up on how to monitor glucose and adjust insulin delivery for sports and physical activity on page 103. This will help your child avoid episodes of low blood sugar (hypoglycemia).

- *Set a good example.* If you want active kids, be active yourself. Talk about physical activity as an opportunity to take care of your body, rather than a punishment or a chore.
- *Limit screen and social media time.* Consider limiting screen time — smartphones, TV, video games and computer time — to two hours a day. Don't put TVs in your children's bedrooms, and keep computers in a family area. Limit the use of smartphones while having family time or during dinner.
- *Choose video games or apps that require movement.* Activity-oriented video games — dance games and video games that use physical movements to control screen action — boost calorie-burning power. In a Mayo Clinic study, kids who traded sedentary screen time for active screen time more than doubled their energy expenditure.
- *Establish a routine.* Set aside time each day for physical activity. Get up early

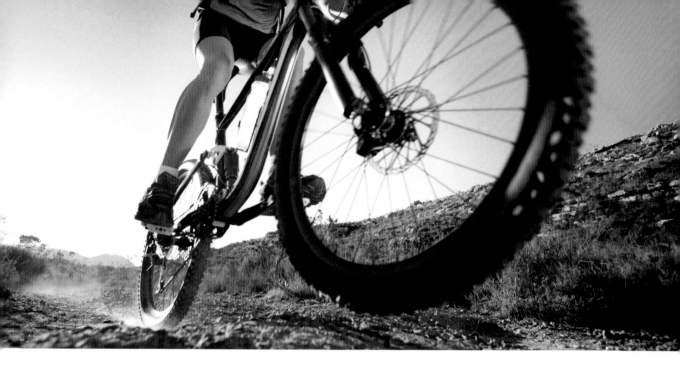

with your children to walk the dog or do jumping jacks together after dinner. Gradually add new activities to the routine as you all become more fit.

- *Encourage your children to walk to school (if feasible).* If school is within walking distance, encourage your older kids to walk there. For younger children, consider talking with parents and others in the neighborhood to see if you can rotate responsibility for walking the neighborhood kids to school.
- *Let your children set the pace.* Organized sports are a great way to stay fit, but they aren't for everyone. What interests your child? If it's reading, walk or bike to the neighborhood library. If it's art, take a nature hike to collect leaves and make a picture. If it's music, dance to your child's favorite music.

Keep it fun

To keep your kids interested in fitness, make it fun for them:

- *Be silly.* Let younger children see how much fun you can have while being active. Run like a gorilla. Walk like a spider. Hop like a bunny.
- *Get in the game.* Play catch, get the whole family involved in a game of tag or have a jump-rope contest.
- *Make chores a friendly challenge.* Who can pull the most weeds out of the garden? Who can collect the most litter in the neighborhood?
- *Try an activity party.* For your child's next birthday, schedule a bowling party, take the kids to a climbing wall or set up relay races in the backyard.
- *Put your kids in charge.* Let each child take a turn choosing the activity of the

day or week. The key is to find things that your children like to do.

- **Get social.** Your children may do better with the encouragement of others. Consider signing them up for a dance club, hiking group or golf league.
- **Join a team.** Sign up for a softball, soccer or volleyball team through your company or through your local parks and recreation department. A team commitment is a great motivator.
- **Join a fitness club.** Sign up for a group exercise class at a nearby fitness club or for virtual exercise sessions. The money you're paying out each month may be an incentive to stick with it.
- **Plan active outings.** Make a date with a friend to hike in a local park, or take a family trip to the zoo.
- **Stay active during errands.** When shopping, park at the back of the lot and walk farther to your destination.

team, you'll learn how your child's blood sugar level changes in response to:

- **Food.** What and how much your child eats will affect your child's blood sugar level. Blood sugar is typically highest 1 to 2 hours after a meal.
- **Physical activity.** Physical activity moves sugar from your child's blood into his or her cells. The more active your child is, the lower his or her blood sugar level. For more details on monitoring blood sugar during exercise, see page 103.
- **Medication.** Any medications your child takes may affect his or her blood sugar level, sometimes requiring changes in your child's diabetes treatment plan.
- **Illness.** During a cold or other illness, your child's body will produce hormones that raise his or her blood sugar level.

Blood sugar monitoring

Depending on your child's treatment plan, you may need to check and record your child's blood sugar several times a day. This requires frequent fingersticks. Regular monitoring is the only way to make sure that your child's blood sugar level remains within his or her target range — which may change as your child grows and changes. Many families opt for a CGM to make the process easier (see page 163 for more on CGMs).

Even if your child eats on a rigid schedule, the amount of sugar in his or her blood can change unpredictably. With help from your child's diabetes treatment

Additional tests

In addition to frequent blood sugar monitoring, your child's diabetes care provider may recommend regular A1C testing to keep tabs on your child's average blood sugar level for the past 2 to 3 months.

Compared with repeated daily blood sugar tests, A1C testing better indicates how well your child's diabetes treatment plan is working. Your child's target A1C goal may vary depending on his or her age and various other factors. An elevated A1C level may signal the need for a change in your child's treatment plan. Many CGMs now provide estimates on

A1C levels, which can be helpful between visits to the doctor.

Other aspects of your child's health that your child's primary care provider or diabetes care provider will want to monitor include:

Thyroid hormone levels

About 10% of children living with type 1 diabetes develop autoimmune thyroid disease, which is the most common autoimmune disorder to occur alongside type 1 diabetes.

Risk of celiac disease

About 5% of children living with type 1 diabetes develop celiac disease, an autoimmune disorder that's characterized by an allergic reaction to gluten, a key component of wheat.

Cholesterol levels

Since diabetes is a risk factor for clogging of the arteries (atherosclerosis), your child's provider will want to make sure that your child's cholesterol levels are healthy.

Potential kidney damage (nephropathy)

Kidney damage related to diabetes can occur in up to 15% to 20% of teenagers. Diabetes care providers often start checking for kidney damage beginning at age 10 and once the child has had diabetes for at least five years.

Eye health

Diabetes can damage the blood vessels of the retina (diabetic retinopathy), potentially causing blindness. Diabetes also increases the risk of other serious vision conditions, such as cataracts and glaucoma.

Growth

Your child's provider will carefully monitor your child's growth, checking it at least twice a year. Blood sugar highs and lows can slow a child's growth and delay development.

Mood disorders

Depression is more common in children, especially adolescents, with type 1 diabetes. As many as 25% of teens with type 1 diabetes have clinically significant depression.

Vaccinations

It's very important that all of your child's vaccines are up to date. This includes yearly flu shots and the pneumococcal polysaccharide vaccine (PPSV23), a vaccine for children and adults with underlying medical conditions that protects against bacterial infections, such as pneumonia and meningitis.

SURVIVING SICK DAYS

Every child has a day here and there when he or she is sick — kids living with diabetes are no exception. How do you care for your child during illness? Follow these tips from the American Diabetes Association.

Continue insulin treatment

Your intuition might tell you to reduce or stop your child's insulin, especially if he or she isn't eating much. Younger or newly diagnosed children could need reduced insulin depending on their blood glucose levels, but other children need just the opposite — extra insulin. Ask your doctor for guidelines for insulin treatment on sick days. Be sure to call the doctor if you're not sure how much insulin to give.

Stay close to the meal plan

You may want to substitute soup and other comfort foods for the usual fare. Just be sure to maintain about the same meal-times and ratio of carbohydrates at each meal and snack as you would on a typical day. If your child has an upset stomach and can't eat, give him or her clear liquids and foods that contain carbohydrates (sports drinks, juices, gelatin, frozen fruit bars).

Give plenty of liquids

Encourage your child to drink water and other noncaffeinated beverages.

Choose medications wisely

Many nonprescription medications contain sugar, alcohol or both. Although there might not be too much sugar in one dose of cough syrup, it can add up if your child takes the medicine every four hours. If you can't find a sugar-free version or if it's too expensive, just account for the medicine's carbohydrates in the meal plan.

Medicines that contain alcohol can lower blood glucose levels. If you give your child a medicine that contains alcohol, have him or her eat something while taking it in order to prevent hypoglycemia. Or look for an option that is alcohol-free.

In addition, certain medications can affect your child's diabetes management. Many decongestants, for example, can raise blood glucose levels. Acetaminophen, the active ingredient in Tylenol, may interfere with older CGMs. Ask your child's care provider what nonprescription medications he or she recommends for common ailments.

Check blood glucose and ketone levels frequently

Diabetic ketoacidosis (DKA) is a danger whenever your child is sick. DKA occurs when a person living with diabetes has too little insulin in his or her system. If left untreated, DKA can lead to coma.

To prevent DKA or catch it early, check your child's blood glucose levels often (every few hours). Also, check your

DIABETES CAMPS

Think your child would savor the chance to hang out with other kids who also are living with diabetes? Look into a diabetes camp provided by the American Diabetes Association. Staff members are trained in diabetes care, and part of their time with campers is focused on sharing tips for good diabetes management. But a lot of time at camp is spent just having fun with friends who'll make your child feel ordinary — in the best possible way. Ask your diabetes care and education specialist to help you locate camps near you.

child's blood or urine for ketones several times a day. If he or she is vomiting or has diarrhea, check ketones even more frequently.

Foods for sick days

When your child isn't feeling well, he or she may not feel like eating much. But it's important for your child to eat in order to keep his or her body from burning fats for fuel (and making ketones) and to keep the body energized so that it can get better fast. Here are a few flu-friendly food ideas for when a bug has your child down. These foods contain between 10 and 15 grams of carbohydrates.

Fluids

- 1 double-stick Popsicle
- 1 cup Gatorade
- 1 cup milk
- 1 cup soup
- ½ cup fruit juice
- ½ cup regular soft drink (not diet)

Foods

- 6 saltine crackers
- 5 vanilla wafers
- 4 Life Savers
- 3 graham crackers
- 1 slice dry toast (not reduced-calorie)
- ½ cup cooked cereal
- ⅓ cup frozen yogurt
- ½ cup regular ice cream
- ½ cup sugar-free pudding
- ½ cup regular (not sugar-free) gelatin dessert
- ½ cup custard
- ½ cup mashed potatoes
- ¼ cup sherbet
- ¼ cup regular pudding

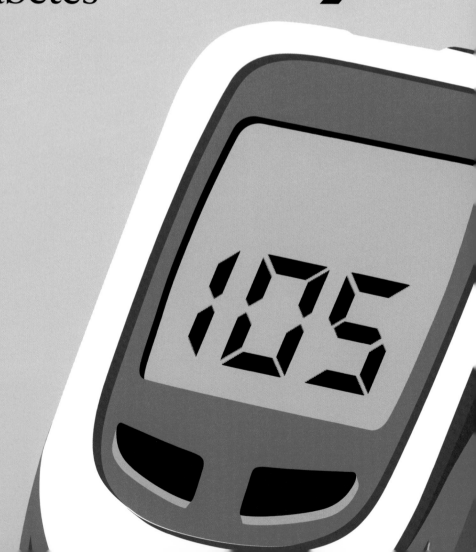

CHAPTER | 9

Living well
with diabetes

A VISIT WITH MARK D. WILLIAMS, M.D.

"When you live with a chronic condition such as diabetes, you can expect to have both negative and positive thoughts about your experience. It's good to acknowledge both kinds of thoughts. But you get to choose which ones you want to highlight."

It's common for people who've recently been diagnosed with diabetes to be coping with a mixture of emotions, such as anger, guilt, sadness, fear, shame or denial. Maybe you are too. Like the weather, these emotions can change from day to day and moment to moment. One minute you're upset about your diagnosis and wondering if life will ever be the same again. The next moment you feel a hint of hope and better days to come.

Personal factors, including your age, gender, stage of life, social support system and cultural background, can affect how you respond and adapt to a diagnosis. If you're a parent whose child has diabetes, you may be facing your own set of emotions and reactions, including worries about your child's immediate and long-term health.

The first thing to know is that whatever you're going through, you're not alone. Countless others have experienced many of the same thoughts and feelings. Diabetes touches so many aspects of life, and so much of the responsibility for managing the condition rests squarely on your shoulders. It's OK to feel daunted by the changes a diagnosis can bring.

During this period of adjustment, you may experience some form of loss — loss of how you see yourself or loss of the freedom to not think about diabetes. It's important to acknowledge and grieve that loss, no matter how great or small.

Allowing yourself to experience all of these thoughts and emotions is an ordinary, even necessary, part of the adjustment process. Whatever you're feeling is what you're feeling and that's OK. But know that you can choose which thoughts and emotions to highlight.

One way to keep your feelings in perspective is to ground yourself in a healthy support system of family and friends. Reach out to those who have been supportive when you've faced challenges in the past. Consider expanding your network to include others who have knowledge of or experience with diabetes.

This is also a good time to seek the professional guidance of a diabetes care team. Understanding your diagnosis and forming a plan of action is one of the best ways to build confidence and move forward. Your diabetes care team also can assist you in finding extra help if the emotional aspects of diabetes become a barrier to self-management.

ADAPTING TO YOUR DIAGNOSIS

Living with diabetes can be a juggling act. Along with daily responsibilities such as monitoring blood sugar or managing medications, you may worry about your diet, long-term health or the impact diabetes has on your family. Sometimes it can feel like diabetes leaves little time for anything else but itself.

But living with diabetes doesn't have to consume your life. There are tips and strategies to help you manage the condition so that it's not overwhelming. In this chapter, you'll find expert suggestions for how to:

- Thrive in your relationships
- Counter diabetes stigma
- Seek positive support
- Nurture your mental health
- Ease the demands of diabetes management
- Avoid diabetes burnout
- Boost your coping skills
- Make the most of the knowledge you gain from your care team, educational programs and peers

Even though diabetes is part of your life, it doesn't have to take center stage. By being proactive, you can overcome challenges, move past obstacles and enjoy your life.

COPING WITH ALL OF THE NUMBERS

Part of adjusting to a diagnosis of diabetes is learning to deal with a lot of data. Depending on your treatment plan, you may check and record your blood sugar as many as four times a day or more. Sometimes, despite making careful choices, the numbers may be too low or too high.

It can be frustrating, stressful and confusing when a number staring back at you doesn't seem to reflect all of the effort you're putting in. You may start to view the numbers as a sign of success or failure, or even a measure of your self-worth.

If you find yourself getting caught up in this way of thinking, remember that the numbers are just numbers. They're not grades or statements of your value but a tool for you to use. Their purpose is to help you and your diabetes care team assess how well your current plan is working and make adjustments as needed.

Show yourself some compassion by remembering that you're doing the best you can and that many people with diabetes have similar struggles. Treating yourself with kindness not only is better for your well-being but also empowers you to better manage your health.

NAVIGATING YOUR RELATIONSHIPS

You don't exist in a vacuum and neither does diabetes. The way that people around you respond to your condition can either help or hinder your progress. Some of the people in your life may be reliable sources of encouragement and support. Others might hold hurtful misconceptions or behave in ways that make it harder for you to prioritize your health. Learning how to respond to negative influences and seek out helpful forms of support can make a big difference in how well you live with diabetes.

Encountering misconceptions and myths

Diabetes is a paradox in that it's both a well-known condition and a commonly misunderstood one. People might have a vague idea that it relates to blood sugar and insulin, but their knowledge often stops there. This lack of understanding often contributes to stigma surrounding diabetes.

Stigma is when someone views you in a negative way because you have a distinguishing characteristic or personal trait that's viewed as a character flaw. Diabetes stigma can take different forms. It can be obvious, such as a family member making a negative remark about your condition or treatment. Or it may be subtle, such as a co-worker's questioning your food choice.

You may encounter misconceptions from family, friends, co-workers and others in your life. You might even harbor some false beliefs about yourself. Where you live, your cultural background and other personal factors also can affect your experience of stigma.

Diabetes stigma can reinforce harmful feelings of shame and self-blame. This can affect your mental health as well as your ability to properly care for yourself. For example, one study showed that people who experienced stigma had greater difficulty managing their blood glucose levels.

The first step may be to challenge false beliefs and misconceptions in your own mind. If you feel that you must be to blame for your condition, challenge the accuracy of that thought. The fact is that diabetes can affect anyone. There are many contributing factors to the disease that you can't control on your own.

On the other hand, if you're feeling like you have no control over your life, reexamine that line of thinking. Things may feel out of control at the moment, but you also have more power to affect your outcome than you might think.

What about dealing with others? How can you respond when someone makes a thoughtless comment about your insulin pump or questions whether it's really OK for you to add sugar to your coffee?

Understandably, your first reaction may be to feel irritated, hurt or angry. You might assume that the person is being intentionally insensitive or willfully ignorant. Rather than act on this assumption, try to keep an open mind. Most of the time, people are well-meaning. They simply don't understand the ins and outs of life with diabetes. You probably didn't either before your diagnosis.

If you feel comfortable speaking up, consider politely countering a false belief with accurate information. If it is someone close to you, point the person in the direction of reliable sources of information about your condition, such as a book or website. Or invite the person to come with you to an appointment with your primary diabetes care provider or another member of your diabetes care team.

If all else fails, you may have to accept that some people just aren't capable of changing their mindset. It's OK to protect yourself from negative or critical people, but don't let one person cause you to cast blame on yourself or doubt your ability to cope. Ultimately, this is about you being able to thrive and live well with diabetes.

Seeking positive support from loved ones

Like you, your loved ones may have a range of reactions to life with diabetes. Some family members may rally around you, shoring up your confidence with encouragement and support. Others may dwell on fears about your health, second-guessing your decisions or nagging you about your self-care. Others still may question the seriousness of your condition, failing to understand the responsibilities and pressures it brings.

Unwanted input or dismissive attitudes can be painful and lead to feelings of

---

DIABETES MYTHS

These are some misconceptions about diabetes that contribute to stigma:
- People with diabetes are to blame for their condition.
- Only someone who is overweight can develop diabetes.
- Type 1 diabetes is the "bad" kind because it's the most severe.
- Type 2 diabetes is the "good" kind and isn't that serious.
- Living with diabetes requires a person to eat a special diet.
- People with diabetes shouldn't ever eat sugary foods or drinks.
- People who need insulin have failed to take proper care of themselves.
- There are certain jobs and activities that a person with diabetes can't do.
- Diabetes can be contagious.

The truth is that diabetes is a complex condition with a variety of causes, and each person's experience with it is unique. There's no good or bad kind of diabetes, just as there isn't a one-size-fits-all way to manage it.

anger and resentment. A lack of positive support can also affect your confidence in your ability to cope, making it harder to reach your health goals. Conversely, research has shown that positive support from family and friends can:

- Help you come to terms with and accept your diagnosis
- Improve your commitment to your treatment plan
- Boost your confidence in your ability to cope
- Encourage a more positive attitude
- Increase your happiness and well-being

If those closest to you aren't offering the kind of support you want and need, begin by recognizing that they aren't inside your body. They don't have the same level of understanding about your condition

WORDS MATTER

Words have power. They can reinforce negative stereotypes or promote a more positive perspective. The people in your life can help push back against diabetes stigma by making conscious choices about the language they use. The same holds true if you're a parent of a child with diabetes. Experts recommend using neutral or compassionate language that avoids labeling or shaming.

Instead of	Say
He's a diabetic. He suffers from diabetes.	He has diabetes.
She has to control her diabetes.	She manages her condition.
He doesn't have good control of his blood sugar.	He's doing his best to manage his blood sugar.
She has the bad kind of diabetes.	She has type 1 diabetes.
You're lucky your diabetes isn't that bad.	I know having diabetes can be hard work. I'm here to help or just listen if you need it.
Your blood sugar is out of control. You need to do better.	I know how demanding it is to manage blood sugar levels. Is there anything I can do to support you?

that you do. Some of them may be eager to offer positive support but need some coaching on what you find helpful — and not so helpful.

Here are some ways you can ask your family and friends for support.

Encourage them to understand diabetes

One of the best steps your loved ones can take is to learn about diabetes as it relates to you. Invite loved ones to tag along to diabetes education programs and diabetes appointments. Make sure they know the warning signs of high blood sugar (hyperglycemia) and low blood sugar (hypoglycemia) and how to respond in a crisis. Also help them understand how important a consistent diet and regular exercise are to managing your diabetes.

Invite them to partner with you

You're more likely to make healthy lifestyle changes if your loved ones are willing to make some of them with you. Plan meals as a family or try out a new healthy recipe. Go on regular walks together or sign up for a fitness class.

Remind them that they don't have to be the food police

If you are a young person living with diabetes or are newly diagnosed, you may find that you benefit from friendly reminders as you navigate food choices. But if you have a firm grasp of what it takes to manage your condition, com-ments or advice on food may feel like criticism, even if your loved ones are well-intentioned. To head off this type of "food policing," let your family know how it makes you feel. Then suggest positive ways your family can support you.

Ask for patience

Managing diabetes is hard work. It takes time and effort to process what can be an overwhelming amount of information and recommendations.

Those closest to you can support you by being patient with the extra time you may need to read labels, count carbohydrates, monitor blood glucose, administer medications and perform other duties of self-care.

Request that they ask rather than assume

What your loved ones think will be supportive may actually be hurtful or stifling. Encourage them to discuss with you how they can be helpful rather than assume they know what you need.

Ask them to help you reduce stress

Stress is part of life, but too much stress can cause your blood glucose levels to increase. Family members can help you relax by looking for ways to assist you in routine chores when you're feeling overwhelmed. They can also join you in stress-busting activities, such as taking a walk or doing yoga.

Remind them to take care of themselves

Everyone has limitations. Your loved ones can't be helpful if they're exhausted or overly stressed. Encourage them to share how they feel and take time for themselves. If they put everyone else's needs before their own, they risk depleting their emotional and physical reserves. For more about caregiver self-care, turn to page 206.

Managing romantic relationships

Just as your family relationships can impact your life, so can your romantic ones. Whether you're just venturing onto the dating scene or entering a long-term relationship, it can be hard knowing how to approach the subject of diabetes. When to open up and how much to share is a personal decision that is yours to make. Here are some suggestions to consider.

Dating

Navigating the dating world can be as daunting as it is exciting. Adding diabetes to the mix often brings another layer of complication.

It can help to come to a date prepared, especially if you use insulin. If you're eating out, look at the restaurant's online menu before you arrive so that you can preview your options and plan out your meal. Bring along some candy or glucose tablets or gel in case you need to quickly stabilize your blood sugar.

If you use an insulin pump, have a backup plan in case the pump stops working. For example, bring a syringe and extra insulin supplies with you.

You may also worry about when to reveal that you have diabetes. Some people prefer to bring it up on the first date. That way, they don't feel a need to avoid or conceal diabetes-related tasks. Other people prefer to wait until a few dates have passed, opening up about their condition once a relationship begins to develop.

Regardless of when you raise the issue, pay attention to how the other person responds. Is your dating partner curious and open to learning about your situation? Does he or she cling to misconceptions about diabetes or seem dismissive? These reactions and attitudes can help you determine whether someone might be a good — or not so good — fit.

Long-term relationships

If you are entering or are involved in a committed relationship, keep the lines of communication open. Encourage honest conversations about diabetes and the way it affects your lives. Be willing to express your needs while also answering your partner's questions and discussing his or her concerns.

You might also consider involving your partner in your diabetes regimen so that you can face problems that arise together. Research shows that when couples manage diabetes as a team, they often strengthen their relationship. Sharing the load with your significant other can also improve your well-being and your ability to cope with the ups and downs of your condition.

Nurturing your relationship with yourself

Perhaps no relationship has the potential to impact your health more than the one you have with yourself. When you treat yourself the way you'd treat a good friend — with care, kindness and compassion — you put yourself in a much better position to handle life's challenges.

In some cases, though, people with diabetes turn against themselves and become their own worst critic. They may question their ability to monitor their blood sugar or eat a balanced diet. They may feel guilty about not managing diabetes "perfectly" or about the effect of their condition on their loved ones.

These negative feelings can ebb and flow, depending on what else is going on in life. Times of stress can affect how you view yourself and your coping skills, as can major life transitions, such as setting off for college, getting pregnant, experiencing the loss of a loved one or losing a job.

Studies show that when people with diabetes hold negative attitudes about themselves, they're less capable of following their treatment plan. They're also more likely to struggle with lower self-esteem and depression. In contrast, developing an attitude of self-compassion can lead to improved mental health and

the ability to manage diabetes more successfully. Practicing self-compassion may even help improve A1C levels and other health outcomes.

What is meant by self-compassion?

One way to nurture a compassionate relationship with yourself is to notice the conversation going on in your head. If you observe that you're speaking negatively to and about yourself, try to back up and broaden your perspective. You may be dealing with some negatives in your life, but what positives also are present? Which do you want to highlight in your mind?

Instead of saying, "I didn't exercise today. I'm such a failure!" remind yourself, "I've gone on four walks this week. That's pretty great." Instead of, "I messed up my carb count again. Why can't I get this right?" say, "Lots of people with diabetes struggle with this, and I'm pretty accurate most of the time." Instead of, "My condition is such a burden for my family," say, "All families have their struggles, and I enjoy a lot of good times with mine."

Practicing this type of self-compassion doesn't mean you ignore or gloss over the real challenges you may be facing. You can acknowledge the obstacles while also choosing to highlight the positive over the negative.

Learning to treat yourself with greater kindness and compassion takes time, practice and patience. Eventually, your self-talk will automatically contain less self-criticism and more self-acceptance, benefiting your health and well-being.

TENDING TO YOUR MENTAL HEALTH

You're late for work and racing out the door when the questions start. Did I eat too much breakfast or not enough? Did I take too much insulin or too little? Have I remembered to pack all my supplies? When will I find time to fit in a workout?

Life with diabetes can be demanding. There are periods when you're up for the challenge and other times when you may feel overwhelmed or discouraged. You might even feel at times that diabetes has sucked the enjoyment out of life. It's important to recognize the signs of trouble so you know when to reach out for support.

Diabetes distress and burnout

Many people feel stress about the challenges of dealing with diabetes and other chronic conditions. Sometimes, these feelings can be overwhelming. Some people develop what experts call "diabetes distress" or "diabetes burnout." Although these terms are often used interchangeably, they refer to two different but related experiences.

Diabetes distress

If you notice you're often worried, frustrated, angry or stressed out because of diabetes, you may be experiencing diabetes distress. Diabetes distress is linked to not feeling in control or on top of your condition. It can develop when the demands of diabetes seem to overwhelm your energy, resources, time or knowledge.

As one person describes it, diabetes distress "is like constantly fighting with my body in a battle that I'm not winning no matter what I do." Even as you continue to do your best to care for yourself, negative feelings about the never-ending pressures of your condition drag you down and affect your sense of well-being.

Diabetes burnout

If you feel worn out by the demands of self-care and want to be "done" with diabetes, you may be experiencing burnout. As one person put it, "I'm just really exhausted, and I don't want to do anything with it. ... I don't care if my blood sugar is high, I don't care if I don't have enough insulin." Diabetes burnout can take different forms at different times in your life. For example, you might stop caring about your diet or even purposely sabotage it. You may check your blood sugar less regularly or stop checking it altogether. Or you could become lax about taking insulin or other medications.

Some people describe diabetes burnout as coming in waves. Sometimes they feel perfectly capable of carrying on, while at other times they want to quit and may even step back from engaging in self-treatment.

Burnout and distress aren't a sign of failure but a common response to life with diabetes. They can feed into one another and affect your motivation, making it hard to manage your condition. This can lead to setbacks, which can lead to more burnout or distress.

By being proactive, you can overcome this cycle of burnout and distress. Try these suggestions to regain your equilibrium.

Get professional support

If you've been struggling with feelings of distress for several weeks or are starting to pull back from your self-care routine, it may be time to seek help from your diabetes care team.

Be honest about the struggles you're experiencing and the burdens that diabetes places on you. Your team can

---

CAREGIVER BURNOUT

Burnout doesn't happen solely to people with diabetes. It can also occur among those caring for a loved one with diabetes. Caregiver burnout is the feeling of being overloaded, drained and unable to continue offering diabetes-related support. It can develop when caregivers become so focused on their loved one that they don't make an effort to care for themselves. People who experience caregiver burnout can be vulnerable to changes in their own physical and mental health. That's why it's important for caregivers to take breaks, engage in enjoyable activities, and share their worries and frustrations with others. Here are some additional suggestions for caregivers to prevent or overcome caregiver burnout:

- *Accept help.* Caregivers can reach out to their own network of friends and family members for emotional support and practical help, such as running an errand, picking up groceries or cooking a meal.
- *Set realistic goals.* Break large tasks into smaller steps that can be done one at a time. Prioritize, make lists and establish a daily routine.
- *Get connected.* Take advantage of caregiving resources online or in the community, such as in-person and online support groups for parents, partners or spouses of those living with diabetes.
- *Don't forget the basics.* Establish a good sleep routine, find time to be physically active on most days of the week, eat a healthy diet and drink plenty of water.
- *Seek professional support.* If burnout is impacting the ability of a caregiver to support a loved one or affecting the caregiver's health and well-being, he or she may benefit from talking to a doctor or mental health provider.

help you develop strategies to ease those burdens and work through barriers. They may also recommend a therapist who can help you cultivate a more positive attitude and greater confidence in your ability to handle life's hurdles.

Share what you're going through

Don't isolate yourself when you're having a bad day or bottle up your worries, anger or sadness. Talking to family, friends or other people with diabetes can relieve your distress and help you see the bigger picture. It can be as simple as telling them you need to vent a little after a stressful day or that you need a bit of extra support at the moment. Most people will be happy to lend a listening ear.

Share the load

During challenging times, some people living with diabetes find it helpful to involve their loved ones in their daily care. At your request, family members can remind you to take your medications, help you monitor your blood glucose levels, count your carbohydrates at meals or change your insulin pump. This type of hands-on support can give you a break while bringing you closer to your loved ones.

You might also consider asking extended family members for assistance with meal prep or the costs of diabetes medications or devices. Even just discussing how to handle costs with someone you trust can help sometimes.

Simplify what you can

With the guidance of your diabetes care team, you may be able to change your medication regimen or introduce new technologies into your care routine. Devices such as a continuous glucose monitor and an insulin pump can make it easier to maintain your blood sugar. For more on devices, see Chapter 7. For tips on food management, see Chapter 2.

Make changes one at a time

If you need to make changes to your eating habits and physical activity, for example, choose the one that will be easiest for you to achieve and tackle it first. Then move on to the next one when you're ready.

Be kind to yourself

No one gets it right 100% of the time. If you have a bad day, or stretch of bad days, forgive yourself and move forward.

Depression and anxiety

Everyone gets blue or stressed sometimes. These emotional ups and downs are a part of life. Temporary bouts of sadness or worry may arise from diabetes-related circumstances, such as a recent diagnosis, the development of diabetes-related complications or conditions, a change in your insurance coverage, or disappointing A1C test results. With help from your care team and support system, you can often find ways to deal with disappointments or difficult situations and restore a sense of well-being.

But for some people, these struggles develop into depression or anxiety. They experience persistent sadness and worry, and a loss of interest in things they once enjoyed doing. These symptoms impact quality of life and daily functioning.

Diabetes is linked to an increased risk of depression and anxiety, both of which can affect your enjoyment of life and ability to cope with your condition. Although the reasons for this increased risk aren't clear, the demands of coping with diabetes management likely play a role.

Symptoms of depression

When you have depression, symptoms usually are severe enough to cause noticeable problems in daily activities, such as work, school, social activities or relationships with others. Depression signs and symptoms are ongoing, lasting two or more weeks, and may include:
- Loss of interest in things you usually enjoy
- Feeling sad, irritable or empty
- Sleep problems
- Lack of energy
- Feeling helpless, trapped, hopeless or worthless
- Changes in weight or appetite
- Feeling restless and fidgety or, conversely, feeling like you're moving in slow motion
- Difficulty concentrating
- Thoughts of death or suicide

Symptoms of anxiety

Anxiety is a part of life, but it can become more than a simple reaction to a difficult day. When symptoms of anxiety like those below are happening most of the time over two or more weeks — especially if the anxiety is impacting your functioning — it could mean a need to get some help. Symptoms may include:
- Persistent nervousness, worry or feeling on edge
- Worry about a variety of concerns
- Fear that something terrible may happen
- Inability to set aside or let go of a worry
- Difficulty relaxing
- Trouble sleeping
- Increased irritability
- Restlessness and difficulty sitting still

Keep in mind that depression and anxiety are not the same as diabetes distress or diabetes burnout, though they may share some similarities. For example, someone with diabetes distress may be anxious, but the anxiousness is focused on coping with the diabetes. In contrast, a person with anxiety will be anxious about many things beyond diabetes.

Similarly, a person experiencing diabetes burnout may notice certain symptoms in common with depression, but depression tends to be longer lasting and related to more than diabetes.

If you think you might be experiencing depression, anxiety or both, talk to someone on your diabetes care team. Ask about reliable and effective psychiatric and psychological services in your area.

DIABETES-RELATED FEARS

For some people, living with diabetes brings up intense fears related to their condition. While people who are more vulnerable to anxiety are more likely to develop diabetes-related fears, anyone can experience these fears. Family members also may struggle with similar fears and worries for a loved one living with diabetes.

People with diabetes or their loved ones may develop a fear of:

- *Hypoglycemia.* For some people, the fear of developing low blood sugar is so intense that they purposely maintain high blood sugar levels. But high blood glucose has its own set of problems. Intense worry about hypoglycemia can negatively impact a person's quality of life and cause long-term health complications.
- *Hyperglycemia.* On the other hand, fear of serious health complications from high blood sugar can cause some people to purposely maintain low blood sugar levels. This can cause serious problems, including seizures or unconsciousness, that require emergency care.
- *Needles and pricks.* No one enjoys the needles and pricks that go along with glucose monitoring. But some people with diabetes harbor an intense fear of one or both of these aspects of their self-care. That can pose a significant barrier to managing their diabetes.
- *Discrimination.* People with diabetes who harbor an intense fear of being judged or misunderstood by others may avoid social interactions or hide their condition from the people around them. This can limit their social life and sense of belonging. It also prevents friends, co-workers and others from recognizing a crisis, such as hypoglycemia and hyperglycemia.

Diabetes-related fears may come and go depending on other stressors that are present at the time. If fear or anxiety about anything is getting in the way of daily life, talk to your diabetes care team about it. Solutions are available to ease these intense fears and make them manageable or even eliminate them.

For example, a phobia of needles is like any other phobia in that the person involved generally knows the fear is out of proportion to what is feared, but feels unable to get past it. Fortunately, simple phobias are among the easiest things to overcome among behavioral health problems. It can take only a few visits with a psychologist to significantly reduce this type of problem.

Your diabetes care team can help you problem-solve and overcome fears and anxieties, and find professional help if you need it.

Medication and a number of other therapies and lifestyle changes can help relieve your symptoms and allow you to enjoy life again.

Some examples of treating diabetes and depression or anxiety together include:

- *Diabetes self-management programs.* Diabetes programs that focus on behavior have been successful in helping people improve their metabolic control, increase fitness levels, and manage weight loss and other cardio-vascular disease risk factors. They can also help improve sense of well-being and quality of life.
- *Psychotherapy.* Similarly, participants in psychotherapy, particularly cognitive behavioral therapy, have reported improvements in depression and anxiety. This improvement can free up a person to direct more energy toward diabetes management.
- *Medications and lifestyle changes.* Medications — for both diabetes and depression — and lifestyle changes, including different types of therapy coupled with regular exercise, can improve both conditions.
- *Collaborative care.* New research shows that both depression and diabetes improve when a nurse case manager supervises treatment and steps up therapy when needed. This type of care may not be available in all health care systems.

Keep your diabetes care provider informed of any treatment you receive for depression or anxiety and how it's working. Often when people start feeling better mentally, they also feel more ready to exercise and make healthy food choices, which can improve blood sugar levels and affect diabetes medication regimens.

KEEPING A HEALTHY RELATIONSHIP WITH FOOD

When you're living with diabetes, food can be a double-edged sword. It provides vital nourishment and enjoyment, but it can also be a source of stress.

Even when you've carefully calculated each bite of food, from the bun on your burger to that squirt of ketchup, your body's response can sometimes be unpredictable. Your blood glucose level may rise unexpectedly. Or it may not rise enough, forcing you to eat or drink beyond fullness to regain balance.

You may also receive unwanted advice from others, putting you and your food choices under an even greater micro-scope. All of this can lead to an intense focus on food.

Some people with diabetes get caught up in needing to be "perfect" with their food choices, avoiding a spike or a dip in their blood sugar at all costs. They may start counting every carb, calorie and mouthful, or avoiding entire food groups to achieve their goals.

Such dietary perfection is impossible, leading in some cases to a swing in the opposite direction. Fed up with a hyper-focus on food, some people stop counting carbohydrates and abandon their dietary plan entirely.

TIPS ON FINDING A MENTAL HEALTH PROVIDER

If you're looking for a mental health provider, congratulate yourself on taking that first step toward finding help. However, it's not always clear where to begin. Here are some suggestions.

- Seek a referral or recommendation from your health care provider or a member of your diabetes care team.
- Check the American Diabetes Association's website. It has a search page for finding mental health providers in your area who specialize in diabetes care.
- Check to see whether your company's employee assistance program or student health center offers mental health services, or ask for a referral.
- Call or connect online with a local or national mental health organization, such as the National Alliance on Mental Illness (NAMI), Veterans Affairs and the Anxiety & Depression Association of America.
- Search the internet for professional associations that have directories of mental health providers, such as the American Medical Association, the American Psychiatric Association, the American Psychological Association, or the Association for Behavioral and Cognitive Therapies.

Before making an appointment, make sure the provider you've chosen is licensed to provide mental health services and covered by your health insurance company. When you find a mental health provider, connect him or her with your diabetes care team so that your care can be coordinated appropriately.

Virtual mental health care

These days, it's possible to meet with a mental health provider virtually rather than in person. This can make scheduling and attending therapy sessions more convenient. There are even computer programs that can provide cognitive behavioral therapy. If this interests you, ask about virtual sessions.

There are also a number of apps designed to help boost mental health. Some focus on tracking factors that influence mental health, such as sleep or exercise. Other apps can help you learn techniques such as mindfulness or meditation.

Keep in mind that apps aren't a substitute for professional therapy, especially if you're experiencing burnout, distress, depression or anxiety. But they can support you in maintaining healthy coping skills and a positive outlook. One Mind PsyberGuide is an organization that reviews apps based on criteria that mental health experts have developed.

Other people develop disordered eating habits that can significantly impact the body's ability to get appropriate nutrition. This can include severely restricting calories or skipping meals, eating excessive amounts of food, or purging after eating. Girls and young women with type 1 diabetes are often the most likely to develop disordered eating. But the problem can develop in anyone, at any age and with any form of diabetes. Turn to page 188 to learn about warning signs of disordered eating.

Living well with diabetes means having a healthy relationship with food and your body. To sustain a balanced diet and reduce stress around food, consider these tips.

Plan ahead

Some people find it helpful to create a daily or weekly meal plan that includes the foods they intend to eat and approximately when they'll be eating. Meal plans can take some of the guesswork out of counting carbs and managing medications or insulin. But avoid making your meal plan too rigid. Life doesn't always go to plan, and flexibility is also important.

Simplify where possible

To reduce the amount of thought that goes into your food choices, look for shortcuts. Buy individual-sized snack packs to reduce the need to count and calculate. If a favorite food doesn't come in pre-portioned packages, consider measuring it out yourself into smaller bags or containers that you can grab on the go.

Take advantage of technology

Apps and websites that calculate carbs in foods can do some of the work for you. Look for options that are trustworthy and easy to use.

Cut yourself some slack

Everyone deserves the chance to indulge now and then — without guilt. Make room in your diet for foods you enjoy, such as dessert with friends or a bit of chocolate at the end of a long day. To compensate, you can adjust your insulin dose, other food choices or physical activity.

If you eat something you regret or slip in your carb counting, don't beat yourself up. Remember, you're human. Practice self-compassion and move forward. Every meal is a new meal and every day is a new day.

Seek support

A registered dietitian nutritionist or certified diabetes care and education specialist (CDCES) can offer practical suggestions and provide you with skills to make food choices more manageable.

If you think you may be developing disordered eating behaviors, reach out to your primary care provider, someone on your diabetes care team or a mental health provider. Early treatment can help you regain healthy habits and prevent long-term health problems.

CULTIVATING COPING SKILLS

Diabetes has a way of throwing curveballs, whether it's an unexpected blood glucose level, a change in your condition or an adjustment to your treatment. Some people are able to roll with the punches with relative ease. Others struggle to restore a sense of well-being and get back to life as usual.

The ability to withstand and bounce back from setbacks and challenges is known as resilience. When you have resilience, you harness inner strength that helps you rebound from adversity. Resilience doesn't make problems go away, but it can help you cope with them more successfully and find enjoyment in life.

Resilience can also benefit your health. Studies in people with diabetes suggest that high resilience levels are related to lower A1C levels, indicating better blood glucose management.

In contrast, people who lack resilience might dwell on problems, become overwhelmed and struggle to keep up with their treatment plan. This can impact both their physical and mental health.

The good news is that anyone can learn to become more resilient and boost their coping skills. Try these strategies.

Nurture optimism

A positive attitude can boost your resilience and improve your ability to cope with the demands of diabetes. Like resilience, optimism can be cultivated. Start by noticing what's going well in your day-to-day life. Celebrate the triumphs. This could be a new job promotion or a great A1C result. Acknowledge the small victories, such as a trip to the gym or a blood sugar reading within your goal rand. Appreciate joyful moments, such as a child's graduation or a beautiful sunset. You may even want to keep a gratitude journal to record these moments.

Another way to nurture optimism is to search for the silver lining, especially when it comes to diabetes. Perhaps you've met a wonderful new friend through a diabetes class or discovered a newfound love of walking. Maybe you've learned that you're braver and stronger than you ever thought possible. There is usually something to be grateful for if you pay attention and take the time to look.

You can also practice projecting more positivity onto the future. Instead of imagining that the worst will happen, picture how things might go well for you. Try to proceed in life with that positive expectation, trusting you'll be able to adapt as needed. This positive mindset can often lead to positive outcomes.

Promote a sense of purpose

When you can identify and incorporate a personal sense of meaning into your daily life, even in small ways, you're better able to handle everyday stress and times of challenge or upheaval.

Your purpose doesn't need to be lofty — just take small steps to discover what makes you feel more energized and connected. What are your strengths? What experiences or interactions bring you fulfillment and meaning? Perhaps it's your role as a parent. Or maybe you find fulfillment in your career or in your spirituality or creativity.

Deepen that sense of purpose by building on it. If you love being a parent, make time to enjoy your children. Maybe arrange your schedule so that you can have breakfast together before everyone's day begins, or set aside time in the evening to read together. If you find joy in using your creative side, volunteer for a new project at work or explore a hobby, such as painting or photography.

Be proactive

Research shows that when people with lifelong health conditions proactively engage in decisions about their health care, they're better able to cope with their condition and engage in their treatment plan.

One of the best ways to take charge is to set realistic, achievable goals with the guidance of your diabetes care team. Identifying and working toward those goals can be empowering and build your self-confidence. For suggestions on how to establish realistic goals, turn to page 217.

Expect and accept change

Life isn't static and neither is diabetes. Your condition may change over time, causing your treatment plan to change along with it. Strive to accept what you can't control and aim to take charge of what you can. Have faith in your ability to deal with and adapt to whatever situations you encounter.

Strengthen your support system

Having a robust social network helps you build resilience and improves your ability to cope with diabetes and other difficulties. To strengthen your support system, make time for the people in your life that are important to you.

As your schedule allows — and without creating additional stress — accept invitations from friends and attend family gatherings. Make a point to check in with those close to you. Be willing to give as well as receive. One of the keys to maintaining supportive relationships is to accept support but also offer kindness and attention in return.

If you'd like to expand your social network, try making a list of people you can reach out to in person or online. Don't limit yourself to the most obvious options. A neighbor or co-worker may be a great walking partner or have a loved one with diabetes. Connect with new people by participating in local or virtual activities or classes through a recreation center, gym, place of worship or community education program.

Practice mindfulness

At its simplest, mindfulness involves staying focused on the present moment. It requires you to focus your awareness on what you're experiencing in an open, interested and nonjudgmental way. The goal of mindfulness is to create a space between what you experience through your senses and your judgment about that situation or feeling.

For example, instead of reacting immediately to a disappointing blood sugar reading, you might step back and simply observe the thoughts and feelings that the number evokes. This moment of nonjudgmental awareness gives you the space to react more thoughtfully and calmly.

Some studies indicate that practicing mindfulness may reduce stress in people with diabetes and improve diabetes distress, depression and blood glucose management.

It can be hard to slow down and notice things in a busy world. Aim to carve out some time each day to experience your environment with all of your senses — touch, sound, sight, smell and taste. For example, when you eat a favorite food, take the time to smell, taste and truly enjoy it.

Another good time to practice mindfulness is when you have negative thoughts or emotions. Try to still yourself. Focus on your breath as it moves in and out of your body. Observe your thoughts and feelings as if they're passing clouds. Allow them to come and go without labeling them as good or bad or grabbing onto them. Practicing this kind of mindfulness for even just a minute can help.

Mindfulness can be a powerful way to reconnect with and nurture yourself. Try practicing mindfulness every day for about six months. Over time, you might find that it becomes more effortless and natural.

THRIVING WITH DIABETES TECHNOLOGY

Devices such as continous glucose monitors (CGMs) and insulin pumps have many benefits. But even people who love the convenience, information and control these technologies provide sometimes struggle with the drawbacks.

Alarm fatigue

Do you find yourself obsessively checking your CGM, trusting it over your own body's cues? Do you jump to attention at every alert and alarm? Or are the frequent alarms straining your patience? Some people become overly focused or dependent on their diabetes devices. Others find the alarms more draining or irritating than helpful. Parents and partners of those living with diabetes also may develop these reactions to diabetes technology.

Such acute awareness can be exhausting, resulting eventually in alarm fatigue. When alarm fatigue creeps in, you may delay your response to the beeps and blips or ignore them altogether.

MINDFULNESS EXERCISES

Focused exercises are a good way to practice mindfulness. Set aside some time when you can be in a quiet place without distractions or interruptions.

You might choose to practice this type of exercise early in the morning before you begin your daily routine or at night before going to bed.

- **Body scan meditation.** Lie on your back with your legs extended and arms at your sides, palms facing up. Focus your attention slowly and deliberately on each part of your body, in order, from toe to head or head to toe. Be aware of any sensations, emotions or thoughts associated with each part of your body.
- **Sitting meditation.** Sit comfortably with your back straight, feet flat on the floor and hands in your lap. Breathing through your nose, focus on your breath moving in and out of your body. If physical sensations or thoughts interrupt your meditation, note the experience and then return your focus to your breath.
- **Walking meditation.** Find a quiet place 10 to 20 feet in length and begin to walk slowly. Focus on the experience of walking, being aware of the sensations of standing and the subtle movements that keep your balance. When you reach the end of your path, turn and continue walking, maintaining awareness of your sensations.

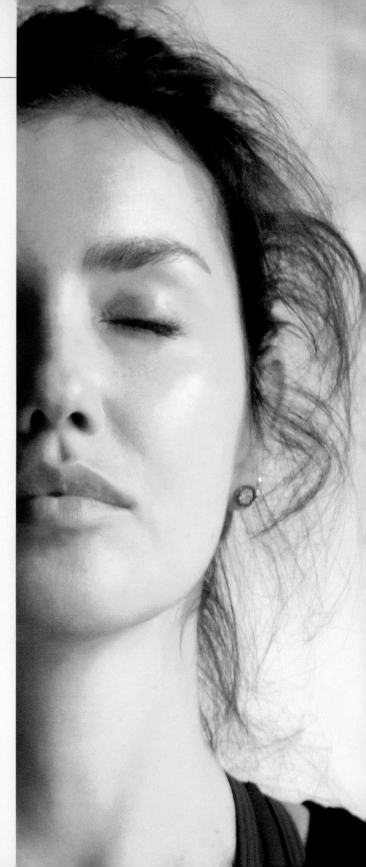

Attachment considerations

It can be hard living with a device stuck to your body at all hours of the day and night. CGMs and insulin pumps can get in the way when you're dressing and undressing or during certain physical activities. They may cause skin irritation or draw unwanted attention. The result can be that you begin to resent having to wear these devices.

If any of this sounds familiar, reach out to your diabetes care team for support. They can help you cope with common issues and troubleshoot problems. If you continue to feel overwhelmed by your diabetes devices, it may be time to consider a "technology vacation." This involves removing your CGM, insulin pump or both for a few hours, days or longer and instead manually monitoring your blood sugar or administering insulin injections.

Before taking this sort of break, talk to your diabetes care team. The team can help you safely prepare and plan for the change in your self-care routine.

EMPOWERING YOURSELF WITH KNOWLEDGE

A key to living well with diabetes is arming yourself with knowledge. When you deepen your understanding of your condition and learn new strategies for managing it, you boost both your skill level and your confidence. This can also be a strong antidote to diabetes distress. By learning more ways to handle a specific problem or need, you'll increase your sense of control and feel more capable of facing changes and challenges. Diabetes knowledge can come from a variety of places, both in health care settings and in the larger community.

Your diabetes care team

Your team may include a variety of providers, such as a primary diabetes care provider, an endocrinologist and other specialists, a registered dietitian nutritionist, a certified diabetes care and education specialist (CDCES), a mental health provider, and a social worker. (Turn to page 7 for more information about the people who make up a diabetes care team.) Each team member brings knowledge and expertise that can help you navigate your self-treatment plan and overcome any hurdles you encounter along the way. The team can help support you in several ways.

Setting realistic goals

Your care team can partner with you to set SMART goals that fit within your lifestyle and reflect your priorities. SMART goals are:

- *Specific.* A good goal includes specific details. For example, a goal to exercise more is not specific, but a goal to walk 30 minutes after work every day is specific. You're declaring what you will do, how long you will do it and when you will do it.
- *Measurable.* If you can measure a goal, then you can objectively determine how successful you are at meeting it. A goal

of eating better is not easily measured, but a goal of eating an extra serving of vegetables each day can be measured.

- *Attainable.* An attainable goal is one that you have enough time and resources to achieve. For example, if your work schedule doesn't allow spending an hour at the gym every day, then it wouldn't be an attainable goal. Two weekly trips to the gym might be more attainable.
- *Relevant.* It's important to set goals that are relevant and meaningful to you and where you're at in your life right now. Ask yourself what's most important to you, and then work with your team to determine your goals.
- *Time-limited.* Pick your goal and set a deadline accordingly. For example, if you want to lose 10 pounds, circle a reasonable finish line on a calendar and strive for that. Giving yourself a time limit can motivate you to get started and stay on course.

Handling bumps in the road

There may be times when you struggle with a particular aspect of your condition or falter in your goals or diabetes regimen. For example, your ability to deal with diabetes may shrink when you're facing a crisis in another area of life or transitioning from one phase of life to another.

Don't be afraid to lean on your diabetes care team during these tough times. Members of the team can help you reassess where you are, adjust your goals and find solutions to problems so that you can continue to adapt and thrive.

Health education programs

Whether you're newly diagnosed or need a refresher, health education programs can give you a leg up on diabetes.

Some of these programs focus on self-management skills. They may take place in health care settings or be available online. They cover topics such as eating a healthy diet, being physically active, monitoring blood sugar and coping with stress. The skills they teach can help you lower your A1C levels and risk of diabetes-related complications, reduce your medical costs, and increase your overall quality of life.

Other health education opportunities may be offered by local organizations such as your community center, place of worship or workplace.

Diabetes networks

Talking to other people with diabetes can be invaluable. These peers can share coping techniques, provide emotional guidance and offer an understanding ear. Studies show that this kind of support can also increase your self-confidence and your ability to successfully manage your condition.

Diabetes camp

Summer camps devoted to young people with diabetes allow children and teens to learn self-care strategies, connect with their peers and have fun. Some camps include the whole family, while others are geared toward specific age groups.

Diabetes camps may be offered by the American Diabetes Association, health clinics, hospitals and other organizations. Some camps may be offered virtually. Although less common, camps and retreats for adults with diabetes also may be offered.

Diabetes events

Virtual and in-person conferences and fairs bring people who are living with diabetes together locally and across the country. These events provide education, support and opportunities to expand your diabetes network.

Support groups

An in-person or online support group allows you to hear from others who have dealt with issues similar to the ones that you're experiencing. Support group members can offer advice, cheer on your triumphs and relate to your struggles. They may even provide information on topics such as experienced babysitters or places to eat that have helpful staff.

Ask your diabetes care team for support group recommendations. The team may be able to help you find a group that meets your cultural and religious needs. If one support group isn't the right fit, try another until you find a good match. Support groups for partners or spouses of people living with diabetes exist, too.

Advocacy groups

Organizations such as the American Diabetes Association, the JDRF and the International Diabetes Federation have local or national chapters that bring people together virtually or in person. They also provide information, advice and support for people living with diabetes and their families.

Diabetes books

Books such as this one, geared toward people living with diabetes, can be another invaluable resource. Look for publications from reputable sources, such as those written by health care providers or produced by reliable organizations such as the American Diabetes Association.

CHAPTER 10

Staying healthy

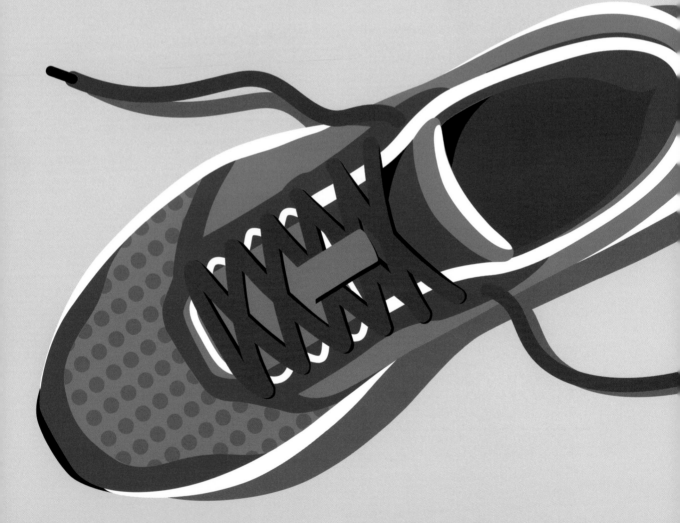

A VISIT WITH VINAYA SIMHA, M.D.

"Staying healthy and reducing your risks of chronic disease is like riding a bicycle. You are the one that provides the energy to better health by operating the pedals of self-management."

Staying healthy while living with diabetes involves implementing effective self-management behaviors to prevent or slow the progression of complications. The pedaling of your diabetes management bicycle includes nutrition, exercise, medications, self-monitoring, problem-solving, risk reduction and psychosocial adjustment.

The bicycle's frame is important in supporting your self-management efforts. It includes family, friends, work and the health care system.

Members of your diabetes care team are experts in helping you set realistic goals, and they act as the guiding front wheel. The framework of the bike that connects you to your health care team often leads to collaboration and productive interactions. Your diabetes care team provides guidance and direction, but they don't provide the energy. It's up to you to pedal the bike.

This chapter emphasizes the importance of regular checkups and preventive care. Creating an action plan is a good way to start. Make certain the plan is realistic and can be part of your life. Periodically, reassess that action plan and ask yourself, "Am I still meeting the goals that I set?" If not, problem-solve with family, friends and your diabetes care team to help redirect your diabetes self-management efforts.

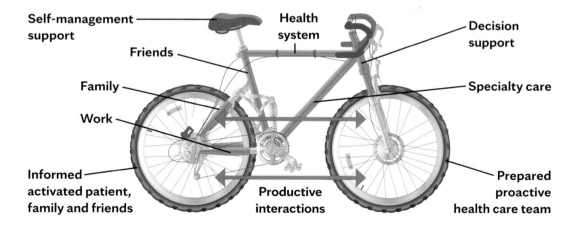

Self-management support · Health system · Decision support · Friends · Family · Specialty care · Work · Informed activated patient, family and friends · Productive interactions · Prepared proactive health care team

Within weeks to months after your diagnosis, managing your diabetes will likely become routine. You'll gradually develop a pattern for testing your blood sugar (glucose), taking your medications, exercising and eating.

But you may often wonder, "How am I doing?" You'd like to know if your efforts at managing your blood glucose are paying off. You can find out the answer by keeping in regular contact with your diabetes care team and making sure you receive appropriate tests during your checkups. These tests can give you a big picture of your blood glucose patterns and spot potential problems or complications that may arise. Regular checkups also provide an opportunity to hear suggestions from your diabetes care team on how to meet your goals.

How often you should see your diabetes care provider or other members of your diabetes care team depends on what's happening with your health. If you're having trouble keeping your blood glucose levels down or if you're changing medication, you may need to contact a member of your diabetes care team weekly. You may even need to check in more often.

In general, though, if you're feeling good and keeping your blood glucose within the range that you and your diabetes care team have agreed upon, you probably won't need to see your diabetes care provider more than four times a year. If you reach and are able to maintain your blood glucose goals, the visits may be less frequent.

YEARLY CHECKUPS

Even as you manage your diabetes self-care, it's important that you also see your diabetes care team at least once a year. During a yearly checkup, your team can check for potential complications and you can discuss how your treatment plan is working.

You'll probably see your primary diabetes care provider, but you may also meet with a certified diabetes care and education specialist and other members of your diabetes care team as needed. See *Meet your diabetes care team* on page 7.

What to expect

Your diabetes care provider will likely begin your exam by asking you questions about your blood glucose readings and overall health:

- How have you been feeling?
- Have you been experiencing any new symptoms or problems?
- Have you been able to keep your blood glucose within your target range?

It's very helpful to bring your daily log of blood glucose readings with you to your appointment so that your provider can review it. Or maybe you share your glucose meter results electronically with your diabetes care team. Be sure to discuss any episodes of high or low blood glucose and how often they occur. Your diabetes care team can help you determine what may have caused these episodes and how to prevent them from happening in the future.

Other issues you may want to cover with your diabetes care team include:
- Temporary adjustments you made to your treatment program, including changes in medication, to accommodate for high or low blood glucose readings
- Problems you may be having in following your treatment program
- Emotional or social difficulties you may be experiencing
- Changes in your use of tobacco or alcohol

During your checkup, a member of your care team may also check your blood pressure, weight and feet and collect blood and urine samples.

Blood pressure check

High blood pressure (hypertension) can damage your blood vessels, and you're at increased risk of blood vessel disease if you're living with diabetes. Diabetes and high blood pressure are often associated, and when present together they significantly increase your risk of complications. Managing high blood pressure can help prevent complications.

Weight check

If you have diabetes and you're overweight or obese, losing weight can help you manage your blood glucose. Gaining more weight will make it harder to manage your glucose. If you take a diabetes medication, weight loss may reduce your need for medication.

Foot check

Each time you visit your health care provider, it's important to have a brief examination of your feet to check for healthy nerve sensation and any open sores or abrasions that may have gone unnoticed. At least once a year make sure you have a thorough foot exam.

During a thorough foot exam, here's what your provider is looking for:
- Breaks or scrapes in the skin, which could lead to an infection
- Pulses in your foot, which indicate if you have good blood circulation in the foot, and a sense of touch, which indicates if sensory nerves in the foot are working properly
- Typical range of motion, to make sure there is no muscle or bone damage
- Bony deformations or evidence of increased pressure, such as calluses, which may indicate that you need different shoes

If a problem is identified, examine your feet regularly to make sure the condition doesn't worsen (see page 233). If you're unable to examine your feet yourself, recruit the help of a family member or a close friend.

Blood and urine tests

Simple blood and urine tests can detect early signs of diabetes complications, such as kidney disease. The earlier you discover and treat emerging problems, the better your chances of stopping, or at least slowing, the damage.

IMPORTANT TESTS

The following four tests are especially important to people living with diabetes. Three of them examine your blood, and one checks your urine.

A1C test

An A1C test, also known as a hemoglobin A1C or glycated hemoglobin test, is a tool for assessing your blood glucose levels over time. This blood test is different from a fasting blood glucose test or a daily fingerstick, both of which only measure your blood glucose at any given moment. An A1C test indicates your average blood glucose level over the past 2 to 3 months.

How it works

Some of the glucose in your bloodstream attaches to hemoglobin, a protein found in red blood cells. This is known as glycated hemoglobin (A1C).

To check your A1C level, blood is usually drawn from a vein in your arm, and the sample is sent to a laboratory for analysis. Although some home test kits are available, it's important that this test be done correctly. Test results indicate what percentage of your hemoglobin is sugar-coated (glycated).

Usual ranges for A1C results may vary between laboratories, but most commonly:
- A level of 4% to 5.6% is typical for people who do not have diabetes.

- A level of 5.7% to 6.4% generally indicates prediabetes. Or if you've been previously diagnosed with diabetes, it indicates that you're keeping your blood glucose in a healthy range.
- Less than 7% is an ideal goal for most people living with diabetes.
- More than 8% is a concern and may indicate a need for a change in your treatment plan.

Talk with your diabetes care provider to find out your specific goal. Although an A1C level under 7% is a common target, your provider may recommend a level as close to 6% as possible if you are pregnant or need a stricter goal for other reasons.

Less than 8% is appropriate for people at risk of low blood sugar (hypoglycemia) and older adults. Less than 8% is also appropriate for people who have other illnesses and in whom the risk of hypoglycemia may outweigh the benefit of a lower goal.

If you've had testing done elsewhere and you're seeing a new diabetes care provider, it's important that he or she take this possible variation into account when interpreting your test results.

How often should you have it done?

If your therapy has recently changed or you're not meeting your blood glucose goals, your diabetes care team will likely recommend an A1C test every three months. If you're meeting treatment goals, an A1C test is recommended at least twice a year.

How does it help?

An A1C test can help in many ways. Say, for instance, you're having difficulty meeting your blood glucose goals and your diabetes care provider is deciding whether to prescribe medication or allow more time for diet and exercise to work. Your provider may have you increase the amount of time you exercise for two or three months and then have you come in for another A1C test. If the test shows an improved reading, then increased exercise may be all that you need to manage your blood glucose, and your provider may not prescribe medication.

In addition, the test is a way to alert you and your diabetes care provider to potential problems. If you've had optimal A1C readings for several months or years and suddenly you have an unusual reading, this may be a sign that your treatment plan needs a change, including more-frequent blood glucose testing. Results of the A1C test also indicate your risk of complications from diabetes — generally, the higher your test result is, the greater your risk.

Lipid panel

A lipid panel measures the fats (lipids) in your blood, including cholesterol and triglycerides. Blood is drawn from a vein in your arm and sent to a lab. To get an accurate reading, it's best to fast for 9 to 12 hours before blood is drawn. The measurements can indicate your risk of having a heart attack or other heart disease. The panel typically includes:

- *Total cholesterol.* Cholesterol is a waxy substance that serves many essential functions in the body. However, too much cholesterol can increase the risk of heart disease, though this risk depends on the type and number of small particles carrying cholesterol in the blood.
- *Low-density lipoprotein (LDL) cholesterol.* Cholesterol in the LDL particles is often referred to as "bad" cholesterol as it promotes accumulation of fatty deposits (plaques) in the arteries. These plaques reduce blood supply to the heart and other vital organs.
- *High-density lipoprotein (HDL) cholesterol.* Cholesterol in the HDL particles is considered "good" cholesterol since it helps protect against heart disease by helping clear excess cholesterol from your body. This keeps the arteries open and the blood circulating more freely.
- *Triglycerides.* This measurement represents fat being transported across different organs including intestines, liver, muscle and fatty tissue. Some amount of these blood fats is needed for good health to help the body store fat that's later used for energy. But high levels of triglycerides increase the risk of heart and blood vessel disease.

How often should you have it done?

People who don't have diabetes need a lipid panel at least every five years — more often if their blood-fat levels are above the healthy range or they have a family history of elevated blood fats.

If you have diabetes, it's important to have a lipid panel at least once a year, but more often if you're not achieving your lipid goals.

If your lipid values are at low-risk levels — LDL less than 100 milligrams per deciliter (mg/dL), HDL higher than 50 mg/dL, triglycerides under 150 mg/dL — a lipid panel every two years may be enough. However, if you have cardiovascular disease, your diabetes care provider may recommend a goal of less than 70 mg/dL for LDL cholesterol with the use of a cholesterol-lowering drug called a statin. Talk with your provider about your target lipid goal.

How does it help?

A rising level of blood fats can alert your diabetes care provider to an increased risk of blood vessel damage. That's because diabetes can accelerate the development of clogged and hardened arteries (atherosclerosis), which increases your risk of a heart attack, stroke, and poor circulation in your feet and legs.

Knowing your blood-fat levels also helps your diabetes care provider determine whether you might benefit from medication to help lower your cholesterol or triglyceride levels. Diet and exercise are the first defenses against unhealthy blood-fat levels, just as they are in managing diabetes.Your provider may prescribe lipid-lowering medication if these steps aren't effective or if your LDL or triglyceride levels are above your target goals.

Serum creatinine test

A serum creatinine (kree-AT-ih-nin) test measures the level of creatinine in the blood. The test is used to assess how well the kidneys are functioning.

Creatinine is a waste byproduct of creatine, a protein that supplies energy for muscle activity. The kidneys filter creatinine from the blood so that it can be eliminated in the urine.

If the creatinine level in your blood is above the standard range, it's a sign that your kidneys have been damaged and aren't able to function properly (renal insufficiency). The higher the creatinine level, the more advanced the kidney disease.

Typical values of serum creatinine vary, depending on your sex, muscle mass and other factors, so ask your diabetes care team what's normal for you. Different labs may have slightly different standard ranges.

At Mayo Clinic, standard ranges are:
- 0.9 to 1.4 mg/dL for men
- 0.7 to 1.2 mg/dL for women

How often should you have it done?

A serum creatinine test is recommended once a year. If you have known kidney damage or you're taking medications that could have a harmful effect on your kidneys, your diabetes care team may recommend that you have this test done more often.

How does it help?

Knowing the health of your kidneys is important because kidney function influences many decisions regarding your medical care, including which medications are safe for you to take and how best to manage your blood pressure.

Urine test for protein

A urine test that detects tiny amounts of protein (albumin), called a urine microalbumin test, also is used to assess kidney health.

When the kidneys are functioning as expected, they filter out wastes in the blood. These wastes are removed through urination. Protein and other helpful substances remain in the bloodstream. When the kidneys become damaged, the reverse occurs — waste products remain in the blood and protein leaks into the urine.

The preferred method to screen for protein leakage is called a spot collection, a method that uses about the same amount of urine provided during routine urine testing (urinalysis). This easy collection, done at a medical visit, generally provides accurate information. An alternative collection method for this test is to save all of the urine produced over a 24-hour period in a jug provided by the health care provider. The urine jug is returned to the provider's office, where it's sent to a laboratory and analyzed.

In the initial stages of kidney damage, typically only tiny amounts of protein escape. More-advanced stages can occur after you've been living with diabetes for many years.

URINE TESTING AT HOME

Different types of home urine test kits are available, but they vary in quality — and some types aren't reliable. Depending on the kit, you can test for:
- Ketones
- Glucose and ketones
- Microscopic amounts of protein (microalbuminuria)

Ketone kits, also available in strip form, detect some ketones, but not all of them. Ketone test strips reveal results through color changes.

Some health care providers recommend checks for microalbuminuria in which you mail a urine sample to a lab. A doctor must interpret the results. Ask your diabetes care team for more information.

Typically, here's what the urine test results will mean, measured as milligrams (mg) of protein leakage over 24 hours:

- Less than 30 mg is standard
- 30 to 299 mg (microalbuminuria) indicates early-stage kidney disease
- 300 mg or more (macroalbuminuria) indicates advanced kidney disease

Protein in the urine can occur for reasons other than diabetes, so if your test results are higher than expected, you may be tested again to confirm that you have kidney disease.

How often should you have it done?

A urine protein test is recommended once a year, starting five years after the diagnosis of type 1 diabetes or when type 2 diabetes is diagnosed. The test is also recommended during pregnancy for women with diabetes.

How does it help?

A urine test for protein can alert you and your diabetes care team to kidney damage. By keeping your blood glucose level within a standard or near-standard range, you can help prevent the progression of kidney disease.

Managing high blood pressure is also important in preventing further kidney damage. Blood pressure medications called angiotensin-converting enzyme (ACE) inhibitors often are prescribed to people with kidney damage because these drugs help protect kidney function.

Other classes of blood pressure drugs can also be beneficial, and you may need more than one type.

Eating a low-protein diet may improve protein leakage by reducing the workload on your kidneys. Your diabetes care team can give you advice on a low-protein diet if you need one.

CARING FOR YOUR EYES

Diabetes is the leading cause of new cases of blindness in people ages 20 to 74. The American Diabetes Association (ADA) recommends an initial comprehensive eye exam by an eye specialist (ophthalmologist or optometrist) shortly after diagnosis if you have type 2 diabetes and within five years after onset if you have type 1 diabetes. After that, have an eye exam by a specialist yearly — or more often if you have eye damage (retinopathy) that's getting worse.

If your diabetes is hard to manage, you have high blood pressure or kidney disease, or you're pregnant, you may need to see an eye specialist more than once a year. If your eyes appear healthy after an exam and your blood sugar is in your target range, your eye specialist may recommend an eye exam every 2 to 3 years.

Don't wait for vision problems to develop before you see an eye specialist. Typically, by the time symptoms emerge, some permanent damage has already occurred. Choose an eye specialist who has expertise and experience in diabetic

EXAMS, TESTS AND QUICK CHECKS

If you have diabetes, you'll need regular exams and tests to watch for current or potential health problems. Test results may indicate a need to change your treatment plan.

Which test	How often
Blood pressure check	At every visit with your diabetes care team
Weight check	At every visit with your diabetes care team
Foot exam	Brief check at every visit with your diabetes care team; thorough exam at least once a year
Eye exam	At least once a year, but more often if you have eye problems, difficulty meeting glucose targets, high blood pressure or kidney disease or if you're pregnant
A1C test	At least two times a year if you're meeting treatment goals and blood glucose is stable; about every three months if you're not meeting glucose goals or your treatment changed
Lipid panel (cholesterol and triglyceride levels)	At least once a year, but more often if needed to achieve your goals; every two years if lipid values are at low-risk levels (LDL less than 100 mg/dL, HDL higher than 40 mg/dL for men and higher than 50 mg/dL for women, triglycerides under 150 mg/dL)
Serum creatinine test	Once a year, but more often if you have kidney disease or are taking medications that could have a harmful effect on your kidneys
Urine test for protein (urine microalbumin test)	Once a year, starting five years after the diagnosis of type 1 diabetes, or starting when type 2 diabetes is diagnosed (also recommended during pregnancy for women with diabetes)

In addition to monitoring your blood glucose, you also need to pay attention to your blood pressure and blood cholesterol.

Monitor your blood pressure

People living with diabetes are about twice as likely to develop high blood pressure than are individuals who don't have diabetes. Living with both diabetes and high blood pressure is serious. Similar to diabetes, high blood pressure can damage your blood vessels. When you have both of these conditions and they're hard to manage, you increase your risk of a heart attack, stroke or other life-threatening complications.

Blood pressure is a measure of the force of circulating blood against the walls of the arteries. The higher the blood pressure, the harder the heart has to work to pump blood to all parts of the body. Blood pressure is measured as two numbers, such as 120/70 millimeters of mercury (mm Hg). The first number (upper number) is the peak pressure at the moment the heart contracts and pumps blood (systolic pressure) to the different blood vessels in the body. The second number (lower number) is the level of pressure when the heart relaxes to allow blood to flow back into the heart (diastolic pressure).

Blood pressure goals and treatment

Adults living with diabetes should strive to keep their blood pressure below 140/90 mm Hg. If you have kidney disease or heart disease, your diabetes care provider may recommend a lower blood pressure (below 130/80 mm Hg). The same healthy habits that can improve your blood glucose — a balanced diet and regular exercise — can help reduce your blood pressure.

If diet and exercise aren't enough to keep your blood pressure in a healthy range, your provider may prescribe blood pressure-lowering medication. The American Diabetes Association recommends drug therapy if systolic pressure is at or above 140 mm Hg or diastolic pressure is at or above 90 mm Hg. If your systolic blood pressure is 130 to 139 mm Hg or your diastolic blood pressure is 80 to 89 mm Hg, your diabetes care provider may encourage you to try lifestyle changes for three months before prescribing medication.

Drugs most often prescribed for people living with diabetes include angio-tensin-converting enzyme (ACE) inhibitors, angiotensin 2 receptor blockers and thiazide diuretics. These medications have a low rate of side effects, and they help protect your kidneys and heart, which are at high risk of damage from both diseases.

Watch your cholesterol
High levels of cholesterol and triglycerides increase your risk of heart attack and stroke. A healthy lifestyle is critically important. Focus on reducing your intake of saturated fats, trans fats and cholesterol and getting regular physical activity. Cholesterol recommendations for people with diabetes are generally as follows:
- Low-density lipoprotein (LDL) cholesterol, also known as the "bad" cholesterol, less than 100 mg/dL of blood
- High-density lipoprotein (HDL) cholesterol, also known as the "good" cholesterol, higher than 40 mg/dL for men and 50 mg/dL for women
- Triglycerides under 150 mg/dL

If you don't achieve your goals, your provider may prescribe a cholesterol-lowering drug called a statin, especially if:
- You're over 40
- You're under 40 and you have other risk factors for cardiovascular disease
- You have cardiovascular disease

Studies, including the Heart Protection Study, suggest that taking statins can lower the risk of heart attack or stroke in people living with diabetes even if they have standard cholesterol levels. Statin therapy isn't recommended for women who are pregnant.

If you have or are at significant risk of cardiovascular complications, research also suggests that taking an aspirin every day can greatly reduce the risk of heart attacks and other cardiovascular complications in people older than age 40 who have type 1 or type 2 diabetes. Ask your diabetes care provider if aspirin therapy would be of benefit to you. A daily aspirin isn't recommended if you have liver disease.

retinopathy. Make sure this person knows that you have diabetes and performs a thorough exam, including dilation of your pupils. Your eye exam may include a number of tests.

Visual acuity test

This test determines your level of vision and need for corrective lenses, and it establishes a baseline measurement for future eye exams.

External eye exam

An external eye exam measures your eye movements, along with the size of your pupils and their ability to respond to light.

Retinal exam

When doing a retinal exam, your eye specialist places medicated eye drops into your eyes to dilate your pupils and check for damage to your retinas and the tiny blood vessels that nourish them. This is an especially important test for people with diabetes because retinal damage is the most common eye complication of diabetes.

Glaucoma test

A glaucoma test (tonometry) measures the pressure inside your eyes. Unusually high pressure is an indicator of glaucoma — a disease that can gradually narrow your field of vision and produce tunnel

vision and blindness. Diabetes increases your risk of developing glaucoma.

Slit-lamp exam

During a slit-lamp exam, your eye specialist evaluates the structures of your eyes, such as the cornea and iris. He or she also looks for cataracts, which cloud your lenses and can make you feel as if you're looking through wax paper or a smudgy window. Diabetes can spur cataracts to develop sooner than they otherwise would.

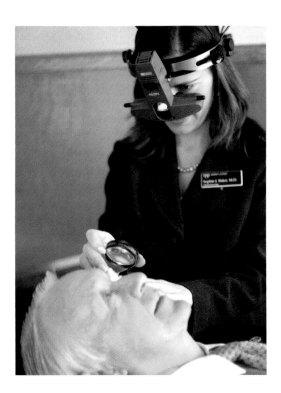

During a retinal exam, you typically lie back while the eye doctor holds your eye open and examines it with a bright light mounted on his or her forehead.

Eye photography

If you have eye damage or suspected damage, your eye specialist may take photos with specially designed cameras. These photos are meant to document the status of your vision and establish a baseline for future exams.

CARING FOR YOUR FEET

Diabetes can cause two potentially dangerous threats to your feet: It can damage the nerves in your feet, and it can reduce blood flow to your feet. When the network of nerves in your feet is damaged, the sensation of pain in your feet is reduced. As a result, you can develop a blister on your foot or cut your foot without realizing it.

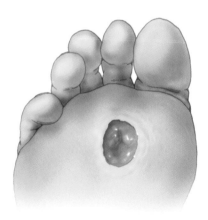

Diabetes can impair blood flow to your feet and cause nerve damage. Without proper attention and care, a small injury can develop into an open sore (ulcer) that can be difficult to treat.

Diabetes can also narrow your arteries, reducing blood flow to your feet. With less blood to nourish tissues in your feet, it's harder for sores to heal. An unnoticed cut or sore hidden beneath your socks and shoes can quickly develop into a larger problem.

Check your feet every day

Use your eyes and hands to examine your feet regularly. If you aren't able to see some parts of your feet, use a mirror or ask a family member or a friend to examine those locations.

Look for these common ailments:
- Blisters, cuts and bruises
- Cracking, peeling and wrinkling
- Redness, red streaks and swelling
- Feet that are a different color than usual

Keep your feet clean and dry

Wash your feet each day with lukewarm water. To avoid burning your feet, test the water temperature with a thermometer. It should be no warmer than 90 F. Or test the water by touching a dampened washcloth to a sensitive area of your body, such as your face, neck or wrist.

Wash your feet with a gentle, massage-like motion, using a soft washcloth or sponge and a mild soap. Dry your skin by blotting or patting. Don't rub because you may accidentally damage your skin. Dry carefully between your toes to help prevent fungal infection.

Moisturize your skin

When diabetes damages your nerves, you may sweat less, leaving your skin dry, especially on your feet. Dry skin can itch and crack, increasing risk of an infection.

Keep the blood flowing

To keep blood flowing to your feet, put your feet up when sitting, then move your ankles and toes frequently. Don't cross your legs for long, and don't wear tight socks.

SEEING A PODIATRIST

Because foot care is especially important to people living with diabetes, your diabetes care team may recommend another team member: A doctor who specializes in foot care (podiatrist). A podiatrist can teach you how to trim your toenails properly. If you have vision problems or significant loss of sensation in your feet, he or she can trim them for you.

A podiatrist can also teach you how to buy properly fitted shoes and prevent problems such as corns and calluses. If problems do occur, a podiatrist can help treat them to prevent more-serious conditions from developing. Even small sores can quickly turn into serious problems without proper treatment. Signs of foot trouble include:

- Ingrown toenails
- Blisters
- Plantar warts on the soles of your feet (flesh-colored bumps with dark specks)
- Athlete's foot
- An open sore or bleeding
- Swelling
- Redness
- Warmth in one area
- Pain (though you may not feel anything if you have nerve damage)
- Discolored skin
- A foul odor
- An ulcer that lasts longer than 1 to 2 weeks
- An ulcer bigger than ¾ inch
- A sore that doesn't quickly begin to heal
- An ulcer so deep you can see the bone underneath

If you, a family member or friend notices any of these signs, call your podiatrist or health care provider promptly.

Wear clean, dry socks

Wear socks made of fibers that pull (wick) sweat away from your skin, such as cotton or special acrylic fibers — but not nylon.

Avoid socks with tight elastic bands that reduce circulation or that are thick or bulky. Bulky socks often fit poorly, and a poor fit can irritate your skin.

It's also a good idea to avoid mended socks with thick seams that can rub and irritate your skin. For people with diabetes, these socks can cause pressure sores.

Trim your toenails carefully

Cut your toenails straight across so that they're even with the end of your toe. File rough edges so that you don't have any sharp areas that could cut the neighboring toe. Be especially careful not to injure the surrounding skin. If you notice redness around the nails, report this to your diabetes care team or your foot doctor (podiatrist).

Use foot products cautiously

Don't use a file or scissors on calluses, corns or bunions. You can injure your feet that way. Also, don't put chemicals on your feet, such as wart removers. See your diabetes care team or podiatrist for problem calluses, corns, bunions or warts.

Wear shoes that protect your feet from injury

To help protect your feet and toes, follow these tips:

Protect against heat and cold

Don't use heating pads on your feet. Use proper footwear to avoid hot pavement in hot weather and to avoid frostbite in cold weather.

Always wear shoes

Wear slippers with soles around the house.

ARE ELECTRIC BLANKETS DANGEROUS FOR PEOPLE WITH DIABETES?

If you have any degree of nerve damage, you may not be able to sense if an electric blanket or a heating pad is too hot — which can lead to inadvertent burns. The same issue applies to water temperature when bathing. If you have diabetes and would like to use an electric blanket, warm up your bed with the blanket before bedtime — then turn the blanket off or remove it from the bed before you climb in.

Check your shoes

Look inside your shoes for tears or rough edges that might injure your feet. Shake out your shoes before you put them on to make sure that nothing is inside, such as a pebble.

Select a comfortable and safe style of shoe

Good shoe design includes the following:
- **Soft leather tops.** Leather adapts to the shape of your foot and lets air circulate. Good air circulation is important because it reduces sweating, a major cause of skin irritation.
- **Closed-toe design.** Shoes with closed toes provide the best protection from cuts and scrapes.
- **Low-heeled shoes.** These shoes are safer, more comfortable and less damaging to your feet.
- **Flexible soles made from crepe or foam rubber.** These soles are the most comfortable for daily wear. They also act as good shock absorbers. The soles of your shoes should provide solid footing and not be slippery.

Have at least two pairs of shoes so that you can switch shoes each day. This gives your shoes time to completely dry out and regain their shape after each use. Don't wear wet shoes because moisture can shrink the material and make your shoes rub against your feet.

CARING FOR YOUR TEETH

High blood sugar can impair your immune system, making it difficult to fight off bacteria and viruses that cause infection. One common site of infection is your gums.

DOES THE SHOE FIT?

When you buy new shoes:
- Make sure the tip of each shoe extends at least a ¼ inch past your longest toe. The shoe tip should be wide and long enough that your toes aren't cramped. Put on both new shoes, and walk around the store to see how they feel.
- If possible, try on shoes in early afternoon. Feet swell as the day goes on. If you buy shoes in the morning, they may feel too tight later on. Getting fitted at the end of the day may give you a fit that's too roomy in the morning.
- If one foot is bigger than the other, buy shoes to fit your larger foot.
- If you have reduced sensation in your feet, take the shoes home and wear them for 30 minutes. Then remove them and examine your feet. Red areas indicate pressure and a poor fit — return the shoes. If no problems occur, increase the time you wear them by a half-hour to one hour each day.

That's because your mouth harbors many bacteria. If these germs settle in your gums and cause an infection, you may end up with gum disease. Untreated gum disease can cause your teeth to loosen and fall out.

In addition, limited research suggests that people with gum infections may be at increased risk of cardiovascular disease. One theory is that bacteria from the mouth gets into the bloodstream and may cause inflammation throughout the body, including the arteries. This may be linked with the development of artery-clogging plaques, possibly increasing the risk of a heart attack or stroke.

To help prevent damage to your gums and teeth, follow these steps.

- See your dentist twice a year for professional cleanings, and make sure your dentist knows that you have diabetes.
- Brush your teeth twice a day, using a soft nylon toothbrush, and brush the upper surface of your tongue.
- Floss daily. It helps remove plaque between your teeth and under your gumline.
- Look for early signs of gum disease, such as bleeding gums, redness and swelling. If you notice any of these signs, see your dentist.

GETTING VACCINATED

Because high blood sugar can weaken your immune system, you may be more prone to complications from the flu

DON'T SMOKE

People living with diabetes who smoke are at least twice as likely as nonsmokers with diabetes to die of cardiovascular disease, such as heart attack or stroke. People with diabetes who smoke are also more likely to develop circulation problems in their feet. Consider these risks:
- Smoking increases your risk of nerve damage and kidney disease.
- Smoking narrows and hardens your arteries. This increases your risk of heart attack and stroke and reduces blood flow to your legs, making it more difficult for wounds to heal.
- Smoking appears to impair your immune system, producing more colds and respiratory infections.

If you have diabetes and smoke, talk to your diabetes care team about methods to help you quit. And don't be discouraged if your first attempts aren't successful. Stopping smoking can take several attempts, but it's vitally important to your health.

(influenza) and pneumonia than are people who don't have diabetes. And if you have heart or kidney disease, you're at an even higher risk of problems.

Annual flu shot

The best way to avoid the flu (influenza) or to reduce its symptoms is to have an annual flu shot (vaccination). In the United States, the best time to be vaccinated is in October or November. This allows your immunity to peak during the height of the flu season, which is generally December through March.

In other parts of the world, the flu season varies: In the Southern Hemisphere, it's primarily from April to September, and in the tropics, you can catch the flu year-round. So take this into account if you're traveling, and get advice from your diabetes care team or a travel medicine specialist.

In the U.S., flu shots are modified annually to protect against those flu strains that are most likely to circulate during the coming winter.

The injectable vaccine contains only noninfectious viruses and can't cause the flu. (Special circumstances need to be considered when taking the intranasal vaccine.) The most common side effect is a little soreness at the spot where the injection is given. Ask your diabetes care team or your primary care provider if there are any other risks in your case.

Pneumonia vaccine

Most diabetes care providers recommend that people living with diabetes receive the pneumonia (pneumococcal) vaccine. For healthy people age 65 or older, generally just one lifetime dose is recommended unless they were younger than 65 when first vaccinated.

However, a one-time booster after five years is often recommended if you have diabetes, renal failure or kidney transplantation. Check with your diabetes care team for advice.

The pneumonia vaccine contains substances that activate your immune system (antigens). These antigens protect you

COVID-19 VACCINE

People with diabetes aren't necessarily more prone to getting coronavirus disease 2019 (COVID-19). But those who do get infected — whether they have type 1 or type 2 diabetes — are at increased risk of more-severe symptoms and quicker progression of COVID-19. If you have diabetes, getting the COVID-19 vaccine is the best thing you can do to reduce your risk of severe disease.

against 85% to 90% of all forms of pneumonia found in the United States. Side effects of the pneumococcal vaccine are generally minor and include mild soreness or swelling at the injection site.

Other vaccinations

Make sure you're up to date on other important vaccinations, such as a tetanus shot and a booster shot every 10 years. Ask your diabetes care provider about getting vaccinated for protection against hepatitis B if you receive hemodialysis. It is also recommended to receive vaccination to prevent shingles if you are over 50.

MANAGING STRESS

When you're under a lot of stress, it becomes more difficult to take good care of yourself. You might not eat well or exercise as you usually would. And you might not take your medication as prescribed.

Stress can also affect your blood sugar directly. Excessive or prolonged stress can increase production of hormones that block the effect of insulin, causing your blood sugar to rise.

The stress response

Stress is your response to an event — not the event itself. Often referred to as the fight-or-flight reaction, the stress response occurs automatically when you feel threatened. The threat can be any situation that is perceived — even falsely — as dangerous, so your perception is a key issue.

When you perceive a threat, your body responds by sending out a flood of hormones, including adrenaline and cortisol, into your bloodstream.

These hormones help focus your concentration, speed your reaction time, and increase your strength and agility. At the same time, your heart rate and blood pressure increase as more blood is pumped through your body, prepping you to do what's required to adapt and survive. This is called your stress response.

Not all stress is bad. Stress can be positive when it results in energy directed toward growth, action and change. This is the type of stress associated with the welcome birth of a child or a job promotion, for example. However, stress can be harmful to your health when you have too much stress, it lasts too long or it's linked with negative experiences.

Individual reactions to stress

Your reaction to a stressful event may be different from someone else's. Some people are more sensitive to stress than others. For most people, different stressors cause different degrees of stress.

Genetic variations may partly explain the differences. The genes that control the stress response keep most people on a fairly even keel, only occasionally priming the body for fight or flight. Overactive or underactive stress responses may stem from slight differences in these genes.

Life experiences may increase your sensitivity to stress as well. Strong stress reactions sometimes can be traced to early environmental factors. People who were exposed to extreme stress as children tend to be particularly vulnerable to stress as adults.

Stop and think about what causes you stress. Then think about whether you can do anything to change the situation. If a hectic day of running from one event to another causes stress, try to reduce your daily commitments. If certain friends or family members cause you stress, limit the time you spend with them. If your job is stressful, look for ways to lighten the load, such as delegating tasks. Also ask your diabetes care team for advice.

Learning to relax

While your stress response may be somewhat linked to genetics, you can still teach yourself to relax. Relaxing means more than getting away from stressors. It means changing your physical and emotional reactions to stress. Here are some techniques that have been shown to help. With regular practice, you can quickly learn how to use these methods whenever and wherever needed.

Relaxed breathing

Ever noticed how you breathe when you're stressed? Stress typically causes rapid, shallow breathing, which sustains other aspects of the stress response, such as a rapid heart rate. If you can get control of your breathing, the spiraling effects of acute stress will decrease.

Practice relaxed breathing (deep breathing or diaphragmatic breathing) at least twice a day and whenever you begin to feel tense:
- *Inhale.* With your mouth closed and your shoulders relaxed, inhale slowly and deeply through your nose to the count of six. Allow the air to fill the muscle between your abdomen and your chest (diaphragm).
- Pause for a second.
- *Exhale.* Slowly release the air through your mouth as you count to six.
- Pause for a second.
- *Repeat.* Complete this breathing cycle several times.

You're breathing deeply when your abdomen — not your chest — moves with each breath. If you're lying down, place a piece of paper on your abdomen. When you breathe in, the paper should rise. When you breathe out, the paper should go down.

Progressive muscle relaxation

A technique called progressive muscle relaxation can help reduce muscle tension. First, find a quiet place where you'll be free from interruption. Position yourself comfortably; lying flat is often easiest.

Following the guide below, tense each muscle group for at least five seconds, and then relax for up to 30 seconds. Note the difference between the tight state and the relaxed state. Relax and repeat before moving to the next muscle group:

- **Upper part of your face.** Lift your eyebrows toward the ceiling, feeling the tension in your forehead and scalp. Relax. Repeat.
- **Central part of your face.** Squint your eyes tightly and wrinkle your nose and mouth, feeling the tension in the center of your face. Relax. Repeat.
- **Lower part of your face.** Gently clench your teeth and pull back the corners of your mouth toward your ears. Show your teeth like a snarling dog. Relax. Repeat.
- **Neck.** Gently touch your chin to your chest. Feel the pull in the back of your neck. Relax. Repeat.
- **Shoulders.** Pull your shoulders toward your ears, tensing your shoulders, head, neck and upper back. Relax. Repeat.
- **Upper arms.** Pull your arms back and press your elbows in toward your body. Try not to tense your lower arms. Feel the tension in your arms and shoulders and into your back. Relax. Repeat.
- **Hands and lower arms.** Make a tight fist and pull up your wrists. Feel the tension in your hands, knuckles and lower arms. Relax. Repeat.
- **Chest, shoulders and upper back.** Pull your shoulders back as if you're trying to make your shoulder blades touch. Relax. Repeat.
- **Stomach.** Pull your stomach in toward your spine, tightening your abdominal muscles. Relax. Repeat.

LISTEN AND VISUALIZE

If you have about 10 minutes and a quiet room, you can take a mental vacation almost anytime. Consider listening to relaxation podcasts or using a relaxation app to help you unwind and rest your mind.

Options include:
- *Spoken word.* These recordings use spoken suggestions to guide your meditation, educate you on stress reduction or take you on an imaginary visual journey to a peaceful place.
- *Soothing music or nature sounds.* Music has the power to affect your thoughts and feelings. Soft, soothing music can help you relax and lower your stress level.

No one recording works for everyone, so try several to find which works best for you. Listen to samples online, or ask your friends or a stress management professional for recommendations.

- *Upper legs.* Squeeze your knees together. Feel the tension in your thighs. Relax. Repeat.
- *Lower legs.* Bend your ankles so that your toes point toward your face. Feel the tension in the front of your lower legs. Relax. Repeat.
- *Feet.* Turn your feet inward and curl your toes up and out. Relax. Repeat.

Perform progressive muscle relaxation at least once or twice each day for maximum benefit. Each session should last about 10 minutes. Your ability to relax will improve with practice. Be patient — eventually you can experience a greater sense of calm.

Meditation

Different types of meditation techniques can calm your mind and reduce your stress level.

Concentration meditation involves focusing your attention on one thing, such as your breathing, an image you visualize or a real image you look at — for example, a candle flame.

Here's a meditation technique that's simple and easy to follow:
- Put on comfortable clothes.
- Choose a quiet space where you won't be interrupted.
- Sit comfortably.
- Close your eyes, relax your muscles, and breathe slowly and naturally.
- For several minutes, slowly repeat a focus phrase (silently or aloud), such as "I am calm" or "I am serene." When

other thoughts intrude, bring your attention back to your focus phrase.
- When you're finished, sit quietly for a minute or two to make the transition back to your regular routine.

The best-known example of meditation is prayer. You can pray using your own words, or you can read prayers written by others.

Meditation may be practiced on its own or as part of another relaxation therapy, such as yoga or tai chi.

Other relaxation techniques

You can choose many other relaxation techniques to help you reduce your level of stress, such as:
- *Tai chi.* Tai chi (TIE-CHEE) involves slow, gentle, dance-like movements. Each movement or posture flows into the next without pausing. Tai chi can reduce stress and improve balance and flexibility. This form of exercise is generally safe for people of all ages and levels of fitness because the low-impact movements put minimal stress on muscles and joints.
- *Yoga.* Yoga typically combines gentle breathing exercises with precise movements through a series of postures. For some people, yoga is a spiritual path. For others, yoga is a way to promote physical flexibility, strength and endurance. In either case, yoga may help you to relax and manage stress. Although yoga is generally safe, some yoga positions can put a strain on your lower back and joints. If you have any

concerns, check with your health care provider before doing yoga.

- **Massage.** Massage is the kneading, stroking and manipulation of your body's soft tissues — your skin, muscles and tendons. It may be used to relieve muscle tension or promote relaxation as people undergo other types of medical treatment. For healthy people, it can be a simple stress reliever. Massage is generally safe as long as a trained massage therapist does the therapy.

Keeping your cool

You can keep your cool and lighten your load by remembering the four A's to managing stress: Avoid, alter, adapt or accept. Here's what you need to know about keeping your cool.

Avoid

A lot of needless stress can simply be avoided:

- Take control of your surroundings. Does rush-hour traffic drive you crazy? Plan to leave earlier for work. Hate waiting in line at the corporate cafeteria? Pack your own lunch.
- Avoid contact with someone who bothers you. If you have a co-worker who causes your jaw to tense, put physical distance between you and this person.
- Learn to say no. You have a lot of responsibilities and demands on your time. Turn down requests that drain your energy and that aren't essential.

Alter

Attempt to change your situation, so things work better in the future:

- Respectfully ask others to change their behavior and be willing to do the same. Small problems often create larger ones when they aren't resolved.
- Communicate your feelings openly. Use "I" statements, as in "I feel frustrated by a heavier workload. Is there something we can do to balance things out?"
- Sometimes inaction creates tension. Vie for the assignment you really want at work. Take a chance. It may feel good, regardless of the outcome.

Adapt

Adapting — changing your standards or expectations — is one of the best ways to deal with stress:

- Adjust your standards. Do you need to vacuum and dust twice a week, or can you accept less often — especially during busy weeks? Redefine cleanliness, success and perfection.
- Focus on positive thoughts. Don't linger on gloomy thoughts. Refuse to replay a stressful situation as negative, and it may cease to be so.
- Use humor. Allow yourself to see a terrible day as comical. Laugh at the lunacy of it all.

Accept

If you have no choice but to accept things as they are, consider the following steps.

SELF-CARE INVENTORY

Are you taking enough time to care for yourself?

Ask yourself	Yes	No	Quick tip
Are you getting enough physical activity and exercise?			Regular physical activity promotes both physical and mental health. Something is better than nothing.
Do you get enough rest and relaxation on a regular basis?			Try to get enough sleep, and consider doing restful activities (such as reading, listening to music or meditating) to help you balance an active day.
Do you challenge yourself mentally?			Keep your mind active with crossword puzzles, word games, writing, a class or anything else that's mentally stimulating.
Are your spiritual needs being addressed?			Depending on how you define spirituality, participate in organized religious activities, experience the beauty of nature, or express yourself in music, meditation or art.
Do you have enough social contact with others?			Consider dining out with friends, having friends over, or joining a musical group or a sports league.
Do you have enough alone time?			Solitary time lets you focus on your inner thoughts and take a break from meeting the demands of others. Read a book, take a walk, write in a journal, meditate, or take some time to look out a window.
Are you using your creative abilities?			Dance, write, paint, cook, play an instrument — do anything that gets your creative juices flowing.
Have you considered service to others?			You might do volunteer work for an agency or a community project, cook or do yardwork for a neighbor, or care for a friend's child.
Is there novelty or adventure in your life?			Experience new things. Consider traveling, hiking, camping, or learning a new skill or hobby. Do something outside of your comfort zone.

- Talk with someone. Phone a friend or schedule a coffee break. You'll feel better after talking it out.
- Forgive. It takes energy to be angry. Forgiving may take practice, but by doing so, you'll free yourself from burning more negative energy.
- Smile. It may improve your mood. Smiles are contagious. Before long, you're likely to see your smile sincerely reflected back at you.

Making time for yourself

Do you take time to focus on yourself and do things that you enjoy? Some people get so used to always working or doing chores around the house that they don't know how to take leisure time. But leisure activities are important. They can reduce your stress and improve your outlook on life. Not taking time for yourself can affect personal relationships and decrease your effectiveness and enthusiasm for your roles at work and home. Taking time for self-care is not selfish. It's a chance to refresh your energy stores so that you can be generous with your attention when it's needed.

Find leisure activities to meet your needs

Leisure activities — what you choose to do during your free time — vary from person to person. What someone else finds interesting and fun may be incredibly boring for you. But if you've been burying your nose in your work, you may not even know what you want to do for leisure. Take the time to find out!

DIABETES AND PREGNANCY

If you're living with diabetes and thinking about becoming pregnant, you may have some concerns about how it will all go and whether diabetes will have an impact on your baby.

It's true that your blood sugar not only affects your health, it also affects your baby's health. But ready for some good news? Women with diabetes who manage their blood sugar before they're pregnant and during their pregnancy have almost the same chance of having a healthy baby as do women who don't have diabetes.

Why it's best to plan your pregnancy

To prevent diabetes-related complications, make sure you're meeting your blood sugar goals before you become pregnant. Ideally, your blood sugar level is in stable condition for 3 to 6 months before you try to get pregnant.

The first 6 to 8 weeks of pregnancy are critical for the formation of a baby's organs. But most women aren't aware of being pregnant until 2 to 4 weeks in.

If during the first 6 to 8 weeks of your baby's development — when heart, lungs, kidneys and brain are being formed — your blood sugar is too high, your baby is at increased risk of health problems. A high level of ketones in your blood (diabetic ketoacidosis) also can cause miscarriage. Later in pregnancy, unmanaged blood sugar can lead to premature birth or stillbirth or other problems.

Fortunately, most of these problems are preventable or treatable.

Planning your pregnancy ahead of time won't guarantee a risk-free pregnancy. But it does allow you to take good care of yourself and do your best to keep your blood sugar levels within your target range. This will substantially reduce your baby's risk of organ damage and set your baby up for optimal health later in life.

To help your baby thrive, your pregnancy care provider (and your diabetes care team) will recommend that you take a multivitamin with folic acid each day, ideally starting three months before you attempt to get pregnant, and a prenatal vitamin throughout your pregnancy.

When you become pregnant

Like most women, you're probably experiencing the ups and downs of being pregnant. One minute you feel excited and energetic, the next tired and anxious. But you may also be concerned about the effects diabetes can have on your body, on labor and delivery, and on the health of your baby.

Having diabetes does present some extra challenges. But the most important aspect of living with diabetes is managing your blood sugar so that you're meeting the target range agreed upon with your health care team. With your team's help, you can keep a close eye on your blood sugar and avoid complications as your pregnancy progresses.

In addition to the people on your diabetes care team, other members of your health care team may include:

- An obstetrician with special training in handling high-risk pregnancies and pregnancies of women with diabetes.
- A pediatrician or neonatologist with expertise in treating babies born to women living with diabetes. A pediatrician specializes in the treatment of children, and a neonatologist is a pediatrician who specializes in the care of sick newborn babies.

If you live in a small town or a rural area and don't have easy access to specialists, ask your pregnancy care provider about his or her experience treating pregnant women with diabetes. Find out if he or she has access to a specialist at a nearby university or metropolitan area. Your provider may consult with the specialist during your pregnancy and have you visit the specialist once during your pregnancy.

Managing your blood sugar

During your pregnancy your chief goal is to keep your blood sugar in your target range. Your diabetes or pregnancy care provider will help you determine what your target blood sugar range is.

If you have type 2 diabetes, you may stop taking oral medications and take insulin to manage your blood sugar while you're pregnant. One reason is that intensive insulin therapy can help you better manage your blood sugar. Another is that the safety of oral diabetes medications for pregnant women and unborn babies is unknown when taken during all nine months of pregnancy.

If you switch to insulin therapy, your diabetes care team will teach you how to take insulin. The team will also tell you how often to check your blood glucose. For many pregnant women, using a continuous glucose monitor (CGM) can be helpful in tracking blood sugar levels. See page 163 for more on CGMs.

What to expect during pregnancy

Here's what can happen as your pregnancy progresses.

1st trimester

During the first 10 to 12 weeks of your pregnancy, you'll probably see your obstetrician fairly frequently. This is the time that your baby's organs are developing, so your blood sugar needs to be as close to standard as possible to prevent birth defects. Frequent or continuous blood glucose monitoring can help you do this.

Because your need for insulin may drop slightly during the first trimester, be alert to signs of low blood glucose (hypoglycemia). If morning sickness makes you miserable, talk with your pregnancy care team about medication to treat nausea.

2nd trimester

The second trimester is when you'll likely receive an ultrasound to check the health of your baby. Your pregnancy care team also will keep track of your weight gain.

If you're at a healthy weight when you start your pregnancy, research suggests a total gain of 25 to 35 pounds is best for you and your baby. If you're too thin, you may need to gain more. If you're overweight, you may need to work with a dietitian to limit your weight gain.

If you take insulin, expect your insulin requirements to rise gradually to about week 20 and then accelerate dramatically. Hormones made by the placenta to help your baby grow block the effect of your insulin, so you'll need significantly more to compensate.

At this stage of your pregnancy, it's also important to see an eye specialist. Damage to the small blood vessels in your eyes can progress during pregnancy.

3rd trimester

During the final three months of your pregnancy, you'll need careful monitoring. Your pregnancy care provider will check for complications that can occur during the late stage of any pregnancy, such as high blood pressure (hypertension), swollen ankles from fluid buildup and kidney problems. Your provider may also recommend that you have your eyes examined again to check for eye damage.

Because women with diabetes are more likely to give birth to babies who weigh more than 9 pounds, you may receive another ultrasound to assess the size and

PREGNANCY AND DIFFERENT TYPES OF DIABETES

It's important to make the distinction between type 1, type 2 and gestational (jes-TAY-shun-ul) diabetes, although all three types require close monitoring and blood sugar management during pregnancy.

Type 1 or type 2 diabetes develops before or after pregnancy. Gestational diabetes refers to diabetes that is diagnosed for the first time during pregnancy. Gestational diabetes is caused by an increased production of the hormones estrogen and progesterone during pregnancy, which make your body less sensitive to the effect of insulin. This type of diabetes also differs in that it generally disappears immediately following delivery. However, gestational diabetes increases your risk of developing type 2 diabetes later in life.

Rarely, some women develop type 1 or type 2 diabetes during pregnancy. In most cases, the condition is initially diagnosed as gestational diabetes. But unlike gestational diabetes, blood glucose levels don't improve after the pregnancy. Blood sugar levels remain high, requiring daily insulin going forward.

health of your baby. At this stage, any potential problem for you or your baby may prompt early delivery.

Labor and delivery

Your health care team will help you determine the best time and safest method to deliver your baby. Delivering your baby at home with a nurse-midwife generally isn't recommended because of the increased potential for problems related to diabetes. As long as your blood sugar stays within target range, and you and your baby don't experience complications, you can expect a typical vaginal delivery.

During labor, your blood sugar will be closely monitored to prevent a large decrease or increase in your glucose levels. Because your body is working so hard and using glucose as energy, you'll likely need less insulin.

If there are complications or your baby is too large for a safe vaginal delivery, your baby may be delivered by C-section through an incision in your lower abdominal and uterine walls. Regardless of the delivery method, the result for most women who've managed their blood sugar during pregnancy is a healthy baby.

Following delivery, your insulin needs will decrease. However, it may take weeks to months before your body changes are complete and you return to your usual medication regimen.

Gestational diabetes

Gestational diabetes only occurs during pregnancy, generally developing in the second or third trimester. Like other forms of diabetes, gestational diabetes causes blood sugar to become too high. If untreated or unmanaged, gestational diabetes can result in health problems for mothers and babies.

During pregnancy, the placenta — the organ that supplies a baby with nutrients through the umbilical cord — produces hormones that prevent insulin from doing its job. These hormones are vital to preserving a pregnancy. Yet they also make cells more resistant to insulin. As the placenta grows larger in the second and third trimesters, it secretes even more of these hormones, further increasing insulin resistance.

Most of the time, the pancreas responds by producing enough extra insulin to overcome this resistance. But pregnant women may need up to three times as much insulin as usual, and sometimes the pancreas simply can't keep up. When this happens, very little glucose gets into cells and too much stays in the blood.

Gestational diabetes usually occurs between week 20 to week 24 of pregnancy, and testing is typically recommended by 24 to 28 weeks of pregnancy. After the baby is born and placental hormones disappear from the bloodstream, blood sugar levels typically return quickly to their usual standards. Most women don't experience any signs or symptoms of gestational diabetes. When they do occur, signs and symptoms may include excessive thirst and increased urination.

Risk factors

Millions of women develop gestational diabetes, but factors that may increase your risk include:
- Gestational diabetes in a previous pregnancy
- Family history of diabetes
- Being overweight before pregnancy
- Having a medical condition associated with diabetes development, such as polycystic ovary syndrome
- Age older than 40
- Certain races and ethnicities, including African Americans, Latinos, Native Americans, Asian Americans and Pacific Islanders (in which type 2 diabetes tends to be more prevalent)
- Unexplained stillbirth
- Previously having delivered a baby that weighed more than 9 pounds

Up to 20% of pregnant women who develop gestational diabetes have no risk factors — one of the reasons why screening all pregnant women for gestational diabetes is generally recommended.

Screening and diagnosis

Screening for gestational diabetes is generally a routine part of prenatal care.

Most women with diabetes (any type) deliver healthy babies. However, untreated blood sugar levels can cause serious problems.

Complications that may affect your baby
Keeping your blood sugar levels within an optimal range can reduce the risk of complications, such as:

- *Macrosomia.* Extra glucose can cross the placenta and end up in your baby's blood. When that happens, your baby's pancreas makes extra insulin to process the extra glucose, and this can cause your baby to grow too large (macrosomia).
- *Shoulder dystocia.* If you have a very large baby, the shoulders may be too big to move through the birth canal, a potentially life-threatening emergency known as shoulder dystocia (dis-TOE-shuh). In most cases, doctors can perform maneuvers to free the baby.
- *Hypoglycemia.* Sometimes, babies of mothers with diabetes develop low blood glucose (hypoglycemia) shortly after birth. That's because they've been receiving large amounts of blood glucose from their mothers, and their own insulin production is high. Hypoglycemia is easily detected and treated.
- *Respiratory distress syndrome.* Babies born prematurely to mothers with diabetes are more likely to develop respiratory distress syndrome, a condition that makes breathing difficult.
- *Jaundice.* Jaundice is a discoloration of the skin and a yellowish discoloration of the whites of the eyes from a buildup of old blood cells that aren't being cleared away fast enough by the baby's liver. This is easily treated but requires careful monitoring.
- *Stillbirth or death.* If the mother's diabetes goes undetected, a baby has an increased risk of stillbirth or death as a newborn.

Complications that may affect you
If you have diabetes, you may be at risk of:

- *Preeclampsia.* A condition called preeclampsia (pre-uh-KLAMP-see-uh) is primarily characterized by a significant increase in blood pressure. Left untreated, it can lead to serious, even deadly complications for mothers and babies.
- *Having to have a C-section.* Having diabetes isn't a reason to schedule a C-section, but your doctor may recommend one if your baby is too large (macrosomia).

To screen for gestational diabetes, most diabetes experts recommend a glucose challenge test.

This test is usually done between 24 and 28 weeks of pregnancy. However, if your pregnancy care provider thinks you're at high risk, he or she may recommend that you test earlier. The glucose challenge test is a modified version of the oral glucose tolerance test, explained on page 24.

Typically, if you receive an irregular result on the challenge test, your health care provider will recommend follow-up glucose tolerance testing, which is done after an overnight fast.

Treatment

Managing your blood sugar is essential to keep your baby healthy and also avoid dangerous complications for you both.

Monitoring your blood sugar is a key part of your treatment program to see whether your blood sugar is staying within your target range. Most women with gestational diabetes are able to manage their blood sugar with diet and exercise, but some may also need insulin or other medications.

Evidence supports that more-intensive treatment in women with gestational diabetes helps decrease the risk of problems during pregnancy and childbirth. This means following a consistent healthy diet, exercising, closely monitoring blood sugar and using insulin when necessary. In addition, some studies indicate that glyburide (DiaBeta, Glynase), an oral drug,

may be safe for women with gestational diabetes after the first trimester. Insulin is still considered to be first line therapy if medications are required for control of diabetes during pregnancy.

After delivery

To make sure that your glucose level has returned to a healthy range after your baby is born, you'll typically have your blood sugar checked often after delivery and again in six weeks. Once you've had gestational diabetes, continue to have your blood glucose tested at least once a year.

The very steps you're taking to control your blood sugar — such as eating a healthy diet and getting regular exercise — may also help prevent you from developing type 2 diabetes in the future.

DIABETES AND MENSTRUATION

Ovaries produce the hormones estrogen and progesterone, which regulate the female reproductive (menstrual) cycle. As the hormone levels fluctuate during the cycle, so can blood sugar.

Most women who have menstruation-related changes in blood sugar notice it in the 7 to 14 days before bleeding begins. Blood sugar generally stabilizes a day or two after the period starts. These changes tend to be more noticeable in women with premenstrual syndrome (PMS).

Premenstrual syndrome is a condition that occurs in some women about a week before menstruation. Symptoms include mood swings, tender breasts, bloating, lethargy, food cravings and lack of concentration. Giving in to cravings for carbohydrates and fats also can make blood sugar management more difficult.

High blood sugar can lead to other problems, such as:
- Vaginal yeast infections
- Irregular menstrual periods
- Loss of skin sensation around the vaginal area

What you can do

Keep a log. Record your blood sugar levels on a daily basis. Also jot down the day your period begins and the day that it ends.

Look for patterns in your blood sugar levels, especially the week before your anticipated period. Then talk with your diabetes care provider.

Your provider may recommend changes in your medication dose or schedule, or your eating or exercise regimens, to make up for hormone-related swings in your blood sugar.

DIABETES AND MENOPAUSE

Menopause — and the years leading up to it, called perimenopause — may present unique challenges if you have diabetes.

When 12 months have passed since your last period, you've reached menopause.

Menopause most often occurs between the ages of 45 and 55, but it can occur at younger or older ages. As women approach menopause, their ovaries gradually stop producing the hormones estrogen and progesterone.

How these hormonal changes affect blood sugar varies, depending on the individual. Many women notice that their blood sugar levels are more variable (increases and decreases) and less predictable than before. Hormonal changes as well as swings in blood sugar levels can contribute to menopausal symptoms such as mood changes, fatigue and hot flashes.

Similar symptoms

You may mistake menopausal symptoms such as hot flashes, moodiness and short-term memory loss for symptoms of low blood sugar. If you incorrectly assume these symptoms are due to low blood sugar, you may consume unnecessary calories to try to raise your blood sugar and cause it to go too high. The combination of menopause and diabetes can also cause other concerns, such as:
- *Vaginal dryness.* Decreased blood flow to the vagina causes its lining to become thin and dry.
- *Yeast infections.* Increased levels of glucose in vaginal mucus and vaginal secretions that are less acidic and protective increase susceptibility to such infections.
- *Urinary tract infections.* Thinning of the lining of the bladder increases susceptibility to infections.

Although it's easy to confuse the symptoms of menopause and diabetes and to treat your diabetes inappropriately as a result, you can take steps to reduce such problems.

What you can do

There are key steps you can take to manage your diabetes during menopause.

Measure your blood glucose frequently

You may have to check your blood sugar three or four times a day, and occasionally during the night. Consider keeping a log of your levels and symptoms. Sharing the log with your diabetes care team can help the team make necessary adjustments in your treatment.

Work with your diabetes care team to adjust diabetes medications

If your blood glucose levels increase, you may need to increase the dosages of your diabetes medications or take a new medication. This is especially likely if you gain weight or become less physically active. If your blood sugar decreases, you may need to reduce your dosages. Your need for insulin, for example, may significantly decline.

Ask if you need a cholesterol-lowering drug

If you have diabetes, you're at increased risk of heart and blood vessel (cardiovascular) disease. High levels of total and low-density lipoprotein (LDL) cholesterol add to this risk, as does menopause.

As a result, many people with diabetes need a cholesterol-lowering medication — usually a statin — to reduce their risk of heart attack, stroke and other cardiovascular diseases.

Get help for menopausal symptoms

You may want to see a gynecologist or women's health specialist for help with especially bothersome symptoms, such as intense hot flashes or painful vaginal dryness and thinning.

If you're having problems with vaginal symptoms, for example, your health care provider can prescribe treatments to help restore moisture. And antibiotics can help treat urinary tract infections. If weight gain is a problem — a concern for many women who reach menopause — consult with a registered dietitian nutritionist to help review your meal plans.

DIABETES AND ERECTILE DYSFUNCTION

It's estimated that more than half of men 50 and older living with diabetes experience some degree of erectile dysfunction, sometimes called impotence. But few of them talk about it with their doctors. This is too bad because if they did, chances are good that treatments — ranging from medications to surgery — could help restore sexual function for most.

Erectile dysfunction refers to the inability to achieve an erection of the penis or to maintain an erection long enough for sexual intercourse.

Causes of erectile dysfunction

Male sexual arousal is a process that involves many parts — the brain, hormones, emotions, nerves, muscles and blood vessels. If something affects any of these systems — or the balance among them — erectile dysfunction can result.

Erectile dysfunction can result from physical or psychological factors. The most common causes in men with diabetes are physical problems due to hard-to-manage blood sugar or long-term effects of the disease. Excess blood sugar can damage the nerves and blood vessels responsible for erections so that not enough blood reaches the penis to cause an erection.

Psychological factors that can produce erectile dysfunction include stress, anxiety, fatigue or depression. They can interfere with the body's typical production of hormones and how the brain responds to them, preventing erections from occurring. Certain medications also can cause erectile dysfunction, including some drugs used to treat high blood pressure, anxiety and depression.

When to seek help

It's not unusual to experience erectile dysfunction on occasion. But if this problem lasts longer than two months or is recurring, talk about it with your health care provider or your diabetes care team. They are professionals who are there to help you. Make sure your health care provider is aware of all of the medications that you take.

Several types of treatments are available. Which one's best for you depends on the cause and severity of your condition. Don't try to combine medications or treatments on your own, and don't take more than the prescribed doses. Find out if your insurance may help cover the cost of treatment.

Treatments include:
- *Oral medications.* Medications such as sildenafil (Viagra), tadalafil (Adcirca, Cialis), vardenafil (Levitra, Staxyn) and avanafil (Stendra) are successful erectile dysfunction treatments for many men. Talk to your health care provider to see if one of these might be right for you. Don't take these medications if you have heart disease, heart failure or low blood pressure or you take nitrate drugs (commonly prescribed for chest pain).
- *Other medications.* Synthetic prostaglandins can be placed into the penis, using a fine needle or a disposable applicator, to help relax smooth muscle tissue and enhance blood flow. Some people have erectile dysfunction that might be complicated by low levels of the hormone testosterone. In this case, testosterone replacement therapy might be recommended as the first step or given in combination with other therapies.

- *Pumps and implants.* If medications aren't effective or appropriate in your case, your health care provider might recommend a different treatment. A penis pump creates a vacuum that pulls blood into your penis, and a tension ring helps it stay firm during intercourse. Surgery to insert inflatable or bendable devices in the penis may help, too, when other methods aren't working.
- *Counseling.* Erectile dysfunction typically causes anxiety, stress, misunderstanding and frustration to both partners. Talk therapy with a psychiatrist, psychologist or other licensed therapist with experience in treating sexual problems can be a big help.

Pursuing both the psychological and physical factors of erectile dysfunction is very important to a successful treatment outcome.

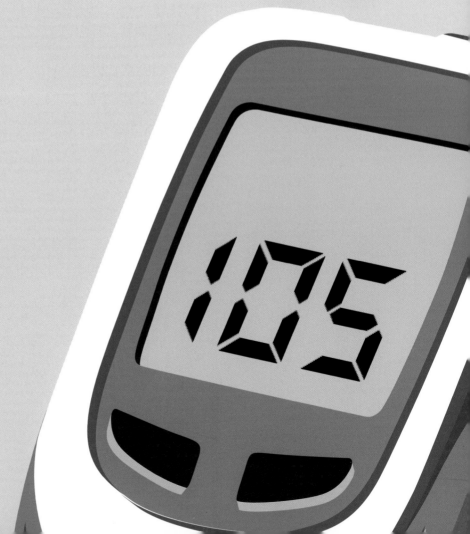

Traveling with diabetes

Many people who live with diabetes travel safely around the world and back. They enjoy everything from climbing the highest mountains to enjoying restful days on a beach. So can you!

Your experiences while traveling are valuable learning opportunities and contribute to your overall life experience. There's no reason your self-care routines, which keep you safe and healthy at home, can't do the same as you travel.

A rewarding successful trip can take a bit more preparation and care when living with diabetes. Remember that travel changes your location, routine, eating patterns, sleep schedules, physical activity and more. This doesn't need to stop you from travel, but rather it may encourage you to bring more mindfulness to your self-care needs.

The key to managing diabetes while traveling is to plan ahead and pack some mental flexibility along with your suitcases and camera. Work with your diabetes care team for support in making your travels safe and enjoyable.

PREPARATION

Location, location, location! When deciding your destination, be sure to consider elements such as climate, general security, food and water safety, and health care infrastructure. Knowing these things will allow you to plan and prepare for different scenarios and contingencies. The better prepared you are before you leave, the more you'll be able to relax and enjoy your destination.

Health care and vaccinations

Work with your health care provider or local travel clinic to make sure you have all the required vaccinations to enter as

---

TRAVEL TIP

Do your research before you go. Make note of local hospitals, clinics and pharmacies near your location that you can visit in case you need medical assistance while traveling. Also, check that your medication is available in that area, should you need an emergency supply.

Safety note: Concentrations of insulin and other medications may vary between countries. For your safety, be sure to confirm that any medication you purchase abroad is equivalent to what you use at home before use. Also inquire about previous storage of the medication to make sure that what you're receiving will be safe and effective.

well as safely travel within your destination. Make sure your vaccinations, your vaccination record and your written health record are all up to date, especially if you travel abroad. Bring copies with you on your trip, if needed.

It's a good idea to get a general physical exam and visit your dentist before you leave. This way you're minimizing health surprises away from home and you have a health baseline for when you return.

Travel insurance

When planning an international trip, travel health insurance is an important consideration for many travelers and especially for those living with diabetes or other chronic diseases. The Centers for Disease Control and Prevention (CDC) recommends considering three types of insurance:

- *Trip cancellation insurance.* This type of policy typically covers your flight,

---

PRE-DEPARTURE CHECKLIST

- Talk to your diabetes care team about your travel plans. Talk about whether you need to change your self-care plan while you travel.
- If you take insulin or glucose-lowering medications, ask about a glucagon emergency kit. Take one with you if recommended by your diabetes care team. If traveling with another person, your companion could carry a second kit for added safety, if desired.
- Bring a copy of your vaccination record and health record, if needed.
- Make sure that all medications you carry and all diabetes supplies have their prescription labels on them. If you use a daily or weekly medication-reminder pack, take the original prescription labels with you.
- Refill any prescriptions that may expire during your travel. *Outside of the United States, some medications are sold in different strengths.*
- Be sure you have your health insurance card with you at all times.
- Review your health insurance policy for travel information. Identify whether your travel destination is in your provider network. If it is not, learn what you need to do in order to have insurance coverage out of network. Also learn whether your policy gives you any special rights or opportunities if you get sick or injured far from home. Buying additional travel insurance also is an option to gain additional coverage. See top of this page for more on travel health insurance.
- If you use an insulin pump or a glucose sensor, check the manufacturer's website or call the customer service phone number for information about traveling. Some companies may loan products for use while traveling.

cruise or train tickets in the event you need to cancel your trip. Make sure it covers what you need, such as last-minute cancellations if you or a loved one gets sick or because of an international disease outbreak.

- *Travel health insurance.* If you have health insurance at home, ask whether it will cover health emergencies abroad.

If not, consider getting a short-term travel health insurance policy. If you need medical care abroad, you'll likely be asked to pay out of pocket. Even if your destination has universal health insurance, you probably won't be covered if you're not a citizen. The CDC recommends looking for a policy that will make payments directly to hospitals.

VISITING A TRAVEL CLINIC BEFORE GOING ABROAD

If you're planning a trip overseas, consider visiting a travel clinic before you leave. At a travel clinic, you meet with a health care provider who is knowledgeable about current health risks worldwide. The provider can help ensure that your trip is safe and you stay healthy. You may also be able to talk with a provider experienced in caring for travelers with conditions such as diabetes or who can coordinate recommendations with your own diabetes care provider.

Before your trip
Schedule a consultation well before you depart so that the travel clinic specialist can help you prepare. Your in-depth pre-travel consultation may include:
- Evaluation of your overall health in relation to travel.
- Identification of health risks in your destination, such as exotic infectious agents, altitude sickness or heat exhaustion.
- Administration of vaccines to prevent illnesses found around the world.
- Prescription of medications to prevent certain diseases such as malaria and to self-treat diarrhea if it occurs while traveling.
- Extensive education and counseling about the unique health and safety concerns for your travel itinerary. You will leave with a lot of helpful and up-to-date information.

After your trip
- Depending on where you're going and for how long, the travel clinic may recommend a routine follow-up evaluation after your return.
- The travel clinic can treat you if you acquire an infection on the trip.

- *Medical evacuation insurance.* If you're traveling to a remote area where medical care is not readily available, consider purchasing a policy that will pay for emergency transportation to a high-quality hospital.

You can find out more about the CDC's travel recommendations on its website at *www.cdc.gov/travel.*

Communication

Before you leave, make sure one or two of your family members or friends have a general idea of your plans, itinerary and possible needs in case of evacuation. You may also want to give them a copy of your driver's license, medical identification, passport, credit card contact numbers — anything you may need to replace or have quick access to if it's lost or stolen.

It might also be prudent to let your bank and credit card institutions know about your upcoming travel plans so that your transactions can proceed smoothly.

Be sure to always carry with you emergency contact numbers and your medical identification bracelet or tag.

To stay connected with people back home while overseas, consider getting a travel SIM card for your cellphone to save money

TIME ZONE CHANGES

When you travel across time zones, you'll need to adjust your medications and monitoring routines based on local time. Ask your diabetes care team if you need to create a medication regimen plan for when you return home or if you can simply go back to your typical diabetes management routine.

Medication regimen	Time zone adjustments
Oral and noninsulin injectable medications	Adjust next doses to local time.
Insulin therapies	Timing of injection(s) may need to shift progressively to local time. Work with your diabetes care team to create a safe plan.
Insulin pump therapy and smart insulin pen therapy	Adjust time on device to local time.

on cellular data rates. There are several options depending on how many countries you'll be visiting, including country-specific, regional and global SIM cards. Do a little research to find the best fit for your travel plans. Free Wi-Fi cafes are available around the globe for quick connections. Pay phones may also be available.

A GPS communicator doesn't require a cellular signal to communicate. And a personal locator beacon can send an SOS alert to local emergency services. Both are handy devices for backcountry or maritime travel.

Cultural perceptions and diabetes

Perceptions and the understanding of diabetes, whether type 1 or type 2, vary widely throughout the world and even throughout the United States. If you travel with an awareness of this and maintain a respect for local cultures, you're more likely to enjoy your trip.

Do continue to advocate for yourself, however, and take responsibility for your care. Most people around the world share a desire for good health and safety for themselves and those around them.

Ask questions and try to be open to others — as much as you feel is necessary — about living with diabetes and what your needs may or may not be.

TYPES OF TRAVEL AND ACTIVITIES

For some types of travel — such as traveling in a group or on your own, or going on an adventure trip — you may need slightly different strategies.

Group travel

Group travel is a great way to meet people or to create memories with friends and loved ones. Open communication with others about your diabetes is key for everyone to have an enjoyable experience.

Educate those around you regarding your needs and your usual routine. Let them know where your medications are as well

WORKING OVERSEAS

If you're working or volunteering in a different city or state or overseas, be sure to ask your employer about any resources your company may have for you as you begin your work in a new location. Resources might include, for example, coverage for moving costs or safe temporary housing, local language lessons, establishment with a local or virtual health care team, or discounts to a local fitness center.

as any emergency supplies you may have in case they need to locate these items. If you're at risk of low blood sugar (hypoglycemia), be sure your group or travel mates know the signs and symptoms as well as proper treatment (including how to use a glucagon emergency kit).

Solo travel

Solo travel can be a great way to meet people as well as venture out on your own. This type of travel can be incredibly rewarding and help you learn more about yourself and what you're capable of.

And solo travel can certainly be done safely. Again, open communication and self-advocacy are foundational to an enjoyable, safe experience. Help those you meet on your solo travels understand what it means for you to live with diabetes and how they can help if necessary.

Be sure your loved ones know your travel plans. Sharing an itinerary with them can be helpful in case they can't reach you.

Outdoor adventures

Living with diabetes doesn't mean you can't enjoy the great outdoors. With a few precautions, you can fully experience outdoor activities.

Canoeing or kayaking

When venturing out on the water, pack a waterproof flotation device for your

valuables such as your medications, cellphone, keys and other items. This way you'll be less likely to lose necessities that can interrupt your trip.

Also, consider what the temperatures will be like. This can help guide your packing. See temperature considerations under *What to Pack* on page 265.

Swimming

If you're on insulin pump therapy, you may need to disconnect from your pump while swimming. If you do, be sure to reconnect every hour and check your blood sugar (glucose) level to replace basal insulin losses, if needed.

Don't keep your medications, insulin pump or meter in the sun. Set up an umbrella or other shady spot to keep them in. Keep temperature-sensitive medications in a portable cooler or cooling bag (see page 266).

Hiking, cycling and more

Whenever you're increasing your physical activity, it's important to be prepared for changes in glucose levels. And if you're planning to be in higher altitudes, be sure to give your body time to adjust.

Follow these tips:
- Always keep pure glucose treatments and foods within reach in case your blood sugar level drops.
- Stay hydrated and avoid heat exhaustion.
- Protect yourself from sun or windburn.

- Monitor your feet for blisters, and know your physical limitations. Bring first-aid supplies with you.
- Plan to manage symptoms of altitude sickness, if necessary. These may include headache, nausea, dizziness or shortness of breath. If you begin to experience symptoms, descend to a lower altitude or wait until your body adjusts to the lower oxygen level before climbing higher.
- Know that some blood glucose meters and continuous glucose monitors (CGMs) are only tested for accuracy up to a certain altitude. Check with your device manufacturers prior to alpine travel.
- If needed, protect diabetes medications, testing supplies and technology devices from freezing by keeping them close to your body.
- See *Temperature-sensitive medications* on page 266 for tips on properly storing your medications while in hot or cold environments.

PLANES, TRAINS, CARS AND MORE

Whether you're traveling by plane, train, car or another method of transportation, it's important to be prepared for the time you'll be in transit.

Traveling by plane

Traveling by plane usually requires moving through airports and going through airport security checkpoints. Here's what you need to know for flying with diabetes.

Airport security

Give yourself extra time in airports. Some security screeners don't know about insulin-delivery devices and blood glucose monitoring. Delays can happen.

If you are wearing an insulin pump and you have diabetes supplies with you, tell the security staff that you have diabetes. If the screeners or other security staff question you, ask to speak with a supervisor if you feel it's necessary.

Ask your doctor to create a letter of medical need for your diabetes supplies and medications, in case you need proof of need. You may be able to have this printed in multiple languages, if needed.

Most diabetes technology systems (CGMs and insulin pumps) should not be exposed to airport X-ray machines. These include the luggage scanners and the body scanners at security checkpoints. Metal detectors, both the walk-through and wand styles, are safe, however.

You can request that your equipment be checked manually. You may need to undergo a pat-down check, according to airport security policies.

Check the website for the Transportation Security Administration (TSA). Learn about any rules for traveling with diabetes supplies and equipment. Look for information about using a blood glucose meter, insulin pump or CGM on a plane.

Also, check with your airport security's website prior to departure and arrival to make sure your experience is as smooth as possible.

Another tip: Check your technology manufacturers' recommendations for safe use while traveling and for assurance that no warranties will be voided due to exposure to different scanners or security equipment.

While in transit

Remain mindful of your blood sugar levels while in transit. Some people may experience higher or lower blood sugar levels depending on the size of the airport that they're navigating, the stress of making connecting flights, potential flight delays and other hiccups that may occur. Try to plan as best you can while keeping in mind that the unexpected may always occur.

While in the air

Be aware that air pressure changes may affect the pressure in your vials of insulin and other medications. Never place your diabetes medications or supplies in checked baggage. Always carry these in your carry-on luggage for safety and to avoid having your supplies and medications freeze or get lost. Be sure to check your medications prior to departure and upon landing.

Stay hydrated with plenty of water and get up and move every half-hour to an hour, if possible. Keep your medications, blood glucose meter and glucose treatments nearby if you're on medications that place you at risk of hypoglycemia.

Traveling by car, bus or train

When you're on the road, take special care to prevent hypoglycemia. If you're the one driving, take these precautions for your safety and the safety of others:

- Check your blood glucose before you go on a long drive. Check it regularly when you drive for more than one hour.
- In general, do not begin a long drive if your blood glucose is below 90. Treat it first and then recheck. Talk with your care team about what threshold is right for you.
- Bring with you testing supplies and snacks anytime you drive, travel in a car or operate any vehicle.
- Keep glucose treatments nearby if you are on medications that place you at risk of hypoglycemia.
- Stop driving right away if you or anyone with you notices signs and symptoms of hypoglycemia. Wait to resume until your blood glucose level is within your goal range and you no longer feel any symptoms.
- Take breaks to get out of the vehicle and move.

If you're a passenger in a car, a bus or a train, take every opportunity you can to get up and move about, whether getting out at a pit stop or getting up to stretch in the aisle. As with any travel, remember to stay hydrated and keep your medications and blood glucose meter handy, as well as any glucose treatments you might need if you're at risk of hypoglycemia.

Traveling by sea

When traveling by sea, check to see if your ship or boat will have an onboard medical staff. Complete any paperwork requested to ensure that the staff is informed of your needs.

Stay hydrated throughout your stay on the vessel. Use sunscreen regularly if you're spending a lot of time outside on the deck.

Follow the suggestions in *Temperature-sensitive medications* on page 266 to store your medical supplies safely.

Talk with your health care provider or local travel clinic about what to do in case you experience motion sickness. Your health care team can prescribe anti-motion sickness medications that you can take with you.

WHAT TO PACK

To have a safe and enjoyable trip, it's important to maintain your usual diabetes self-care routine as much as possible. Your health depends on having your diabetes medications and supplies with you at all times.

In your personal bag

Carry all of your medications and supplies with you to avoid loss or any delay in access. If you're flying, this also helps protect your medical supplies, such as insulin, from possible damage or freezing that might occur if you placed them in checked baggage.

Always keep some form of quick-absorbing glucose with you if you're on medications that place you at risk of hypoglycemia.

TRAVEL TIP

Be sure to talk to your diabetes care team about having a treatment plan in place for nausea, vomiting or diarrhea while traveling, regardless of mode of transportation. Vomiting and diarrhea increase your risk of dehydration, and having high blood sugar can increase it even more. This is why it's important to stay hydrated.

To minimize your risk of traveler's diarrhea, follow food and water safety precautions closely. Don't drink tap water if you're not sure it's safe to drink, and don't use ice cubes made from tap water. Stick to bottled water and be cautious with street food, raw or room temperature foods, and fruits and vegetables you haven't washed or peeled yourself. Visit the CDC's Travelers' Health site online for more information.

Choose nonliquid forms, such as glucose tabs, gels or candy.

In an airport, keep all medications and diabetes supplies in your carry-on bag until you get past security. If you're traveling with someone else, you can split your supplies between your bag and your companion's bag to minimize loss or theft. If you're traveling by yourself, be sure to never leave your luggage unattended. See the opposite page for a checklist of supplies for your personal bag.

Medications and administration supplies

Keep in mind that you are your own backup supplier for your medication needs. Bring enough diabetes supplies and medications to last longer than the length of your trip. In general, pack double of what you think you'll require. You'll need the extras if you have travel delays or lose some supplies. On some trips, you may want to take enough medication and supplies for an extra week or two.

If you monitor your blood glucose levels, be sure to pack additional testing supplies. You'll want to monitor your glucose more often while traveling than you usually do. If you're not sure how often to check, ask your diabetes care team before you travel.

If you use diabetes technology, bring additional supplies with you. Contact the manufacturer of the devices you use, as some companies provide loaner products to be used during travel.

Temperature-sensitive medications

If you're packing temperature-sensitive medications or supplies, pack them in a cooler or another temperature-regulating carrier. Cooler travel cases designed specifically for medicines — for example, Frio Insulin Cooling Cases — are available. They can keep your medication at the correct temperature for days at a time. These cooler packs are activated with water and can be regenerated every three days. Use them with caution in high-humidity environments, however, as they may not work properly in these conditions.

There are also smart thermometers (Med-Angel) that can monitor the temperature of your cooler case. These are remote temperature-monitoring devices that connect wirelessly to a smartphone application for real-time updates regarding the temperature of your medication, both during storage and carry modes.

You can keep some medications at room temperature when they are in use, such as insulin. Extra, unused supplies should be kept cool according to the temperature ratings on the product label.

Do be cautious when using hotel room refrigerators. These can experience high-temperature fluctuations and possibly damage your medications. Check with the staff at the place you're staying about possible solutions to maintaining key temperatures. When in doubt, pack your own temperature regulation tools and work with your diabetes care team to ensure you're protecting your medications.

Travel-sized sharps bin

If needed, plan to bring insulin needles, also known as sharps, in and out of your destination, unless you find a local pharmacy or clinic that can accept and dispose of them safely. Use a small, puncture-resistant plastic container that can be resealed. Needle safety is everyone's responsibility. Some regions in the world don't have the necessary infrastructure to safely remove these from public circulation; take safely stored used needles with you when you leave and

---

KEEP THESE SUPPLIES IN YOUR PERSONAL BAG

- Medical identification.
- Original prescription labels.
- A card or printout of your insulin pump settings. This can also be stored in your phone.
- Emergency phone numbers.
- Medical insurance card and travel health insurance documents, if purchased.
- Medications, insulin or both.
- Meter, strips, lancets and lancing device.
- Ketone testing strips, if directed by your diabetes care team.
- Syringes or pen needles. These are needed even if you're using an insulin pump (to have in case the pump fails).
- Sensor supplies, pump supplies or both.
- Backup pump, if feasible.
- Batteries for meter, pump and sensor.
- Food to help prevent low blood sugar (hypoglycemia) — in case you miss a meal. Examples include crackers, packaged cheese, peanut butter, fresh or dried fruit, nuts, or snack bars.
- Treatment for low blood sugar. Each example listed here has 15 grams of carbohydrate:
  - 4 glucose tablets
  - Tube of glucose gel
  - 4 ounces of fruit juice*
  - 4 ounces of sugar-sweetened soda* (not diet soda)
  - 15 small jelly beans (Jelly Belly size)
  - 15 Skittles
  - 8 SweeTARTS

* If you're flying, you can buy liquids after you pass through airport security.

dispose of them properly when you return home.

Other self-care products

Be sure to pack a first-aid kit with over-the-counter medications, bandages, sunscreen, personal hygiene products, earplugs, eyeglasses, charger cords for technologies, electrical outlet adapters or any other items you may need while traveling.

Clothing and footwear

Be sure to pack clothing that you know will keep you safe and comfortable in all expected local weather conditions. Take clothing you can wear in layers so that you can add or remove a layer as needed for your comfort.

Pack comfortable walking shoes that will prevent blistering. Consider taking an extra pair with you. Alternating footwear from one day to the next can also help prevent blisters from forming. Remain mindful of your overall foot safety and protect your feet from sunburn, puncture and other injuries.

When traveling abroad, security passport wallets and money belts can be used for money, credit cards, personal documents and medical records. They can also be used to store medications and diabetes technology.

Pack a hat or two to wear, to prevent unnecessary sun exposure. Some diabetes medications can place you at an increased risk of sunburn. Sunburn also can cause dehydration and high blood glucose levels. Talk with your diabetes care team about your medications and how to prevent potential weather hazards.

Be sure to wear some type of medical identification to alert those around you to your medical needs. Also, some health care institutions or online sites can help you create a medical card, written in the local language, that explains your diabetes and potential needs.

SAFE TRAVELS!

With some planning and preparation, you can enjoy many different travel experiences — from camping in your local state park to flying around the world. Be mindful of your needs and pack accordingly. And don't forget to lean on your diabetes care team for answers to your questions and support in finding the best resources for your trip. Enjoy!

ADVENTURES WITH DIABETES, *Anna L. Kasper, R.N., CDCES*

From a young age, I grew up traveling across the country each summer with my family. This exposed me to the excitement of learning about new environments and cultures other than my own home back in the Midwest. I was driven to see more. Travel is a powerful way to grow and learn. This is no less true while living with diabetes.

My type 1 diabetes diagnosis came in January 2007, two weeks before I was planning to travel to Spain on a class trip. That day, I was told — fortunately — that I would be able to travel but only if I started insulin therapy. They didn't have to tell me twice. Talk about motivation! I was determined that my diabetes wouldn't stop me from exploring and that has been the case ever since.

With a little extra flexibility and planning, there is no reason we can't care for ourselves away from home as safely as we do while in the comfort of our usual surroundings.

I don't want your diabetes to stop you from exploring. Start small, whatever that means to you, and build up to your travel goals.

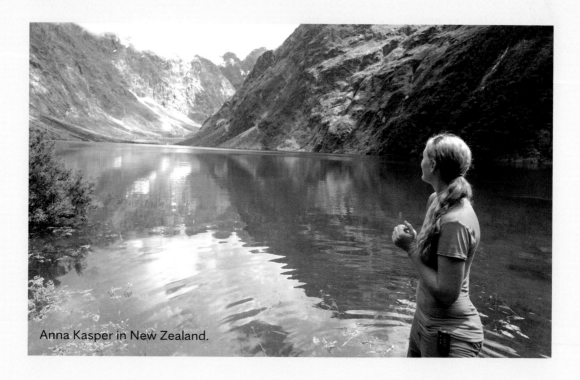

Anna Kasper in New Zealand.

Appendix

Mayo Clinic Healthy Weight Pyramid | 272

Mayo Clinic Healthy Dining Table | 273

Healthy recipes | 274

Sample glucose record | 296

Medical emergencies quick guide | 298

Noninsulin medications | 300

Insulin options | 302

How to inject insulin | 304

Using an insulin pen | 306

Additional resources | 308

MAYO CLINIC HEALTHY WEIGHT PYRAMID

The Mayo Clinic Healthy Weight Pyramid is designed to help you eat foods that provide a lot of weight and volume (bulk) but not many calories, so that you can feel full and still lose weight or maintain your weight. Vegetables and fruits are the foundation of the pyramid. You can eat virtually unlimited amounts of fresh or frozen veggies and fruits. Whole-grain carbohydrates, protein, dairy and unsaturated fats also are part of a healthy diet in limited amounts.

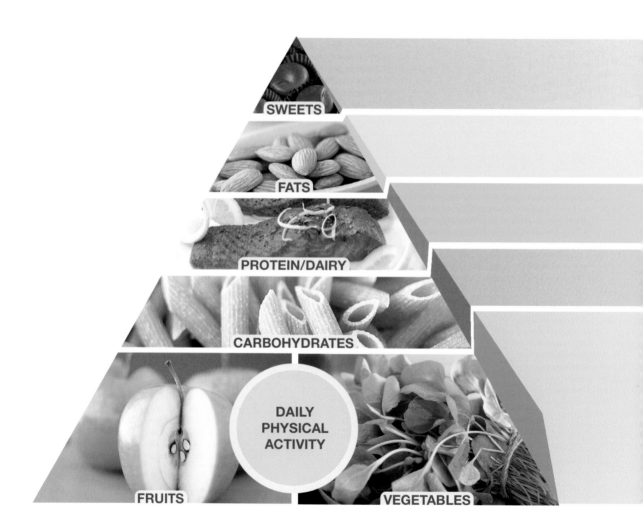

The graphic below helps you visualize what your meals should look like on your plate. It shows approximately how your servings should be divided at each meal. Keep in mind that your table setting will look different for other meals, such as breakfast and lunch, but use the graphic below to create a mental image of how much from each food group to eat.

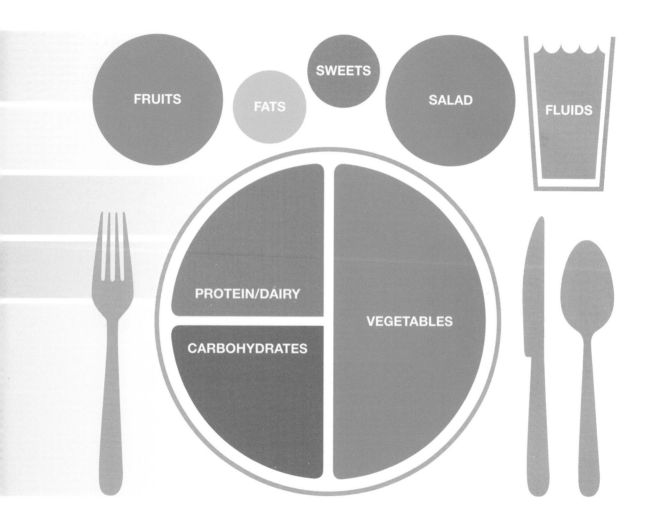

Healthy recipes

A diabetes diet simply means eating the healthiest foods, in moderate amounts, at regular mealtimes. This helps keep your blood sugar in your goal range and prevent damage to your nerves, kidneys and heart.

How do you eat well? It begins with enjoying a variety of foods, mostly plant-based but with room for meat, dairy and sweets, too. The recipes in this section give you a taste of how easy and enjoyable eating well can be.

DIABETES MEAL PLAN CHOICES

 = 1 serving nonstarchy vegetables

 = 1 serving fruits

 = 1 serving starches

 = 1 serving protein

 = 1 serving fats

Fresh fruit smoothie | 275

Cheesy poached egg sandwich | 277

Spinach frittata | 278

Quinoa cakes | 279

Tabbouleh salad | 280

Roasted squash soup | 281

Balsamic-glazed Brussels sprouts | 282

Butternut squash fries | 284

Parmesan crusted cauliflower | 285

Fish tacos with tomatillo sauce | 286

Baked salmon with soy marinade | 287

Tandoori chicken wrap | 288

Chicken & asparagus penne | 290

Baked chicken & wild rice | 291

Pork tenderloin with apples | 292

Beef & vegetable stew | 293

Apple-berry cobbler | 294

Strawberry shortcake | 295

Fresh fruit smoothie

SERVES 4 | DIABETES MEAL PLAN CHOICES:

1 cup fresh pineapple chunks
½ cup cantaloupe or other melon chunks
1 cup fresh strawberries
Juice of 2 oranges
1 cup cold water
1 tablespoon honey

Remove rind from pineapple and melon. Cut into chunks. Remove stems from strawberries. Place all ingredients in blender and puree until smooth. Serve cold.

NUTRITIONAL ANALYSIS PER SERVING (8 OUNCES): 72 calories, 0 g total fat, 0 mg cholesterol, 7 mg sodium, 17 g total carbohydrate, 1 g protein

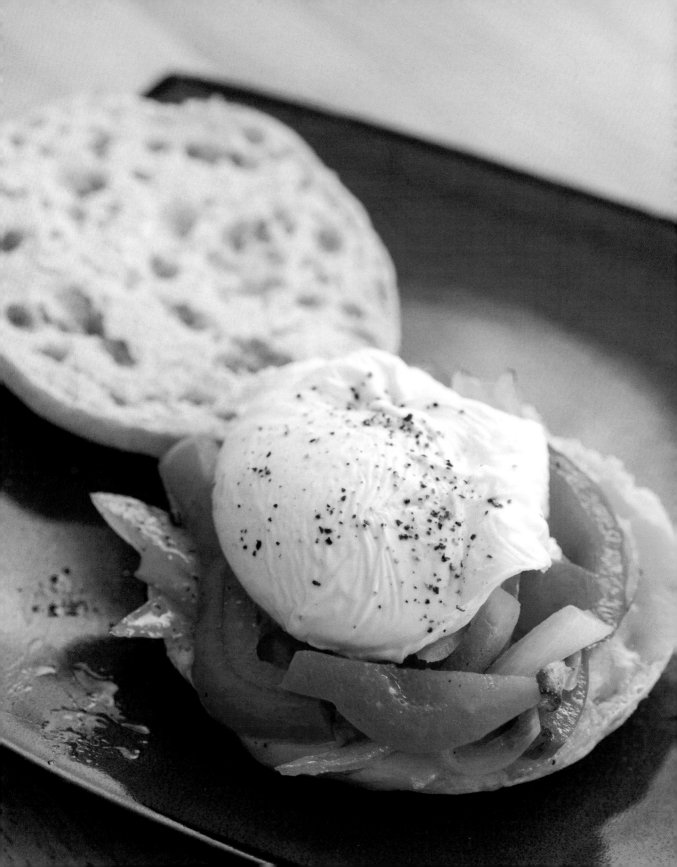

Cheesy poached egg sandwich

SERVES 6 | DIABETES MEAL PLAN CHOICES: **S** **P** ◣

1 cup chopped Roma tomatoes
¼ cup minced onion
1 tablespoon chopped fresh cilantro
1 jalapeno pepper, minced
1 lime, juiced
Pinch of salt
3 whole-wheat English muffins
3 ounces shredded sharp cheddar cheese
6 cups water
6 large eggs
1 tablespoon white vinegar
¼ teaspoon kosher salt

NUTRITIONAL ANALYSIS PER SERVING
(1 SANDWICH): 210 calories, 10 g total fat,
200 mg cholesterol, 360 mg sodium, 18 g
total carbohydrate, 13 g protein

Preheat oven to 425 F, or you can use a toaster oven. Prepare the tomatoes, onion, cilantro and pepper. In a medium bowl, combine tomatoes, onions, cilantro, pepper and lime juice. Add a pinch of salt to taste; set aside.

Cut the English muffins in half and top with cheese. Place on a baking sheet and bake in a toaster oven or in a regular oven for about 5 minutes.

To prepare the eggs, in a medium-shallow pan, bring water to a boil. Add the vinegar. Slowly crack the eggs and add to the pan one at a time; cook to desired doneness. Eggs that have runny yolks take about 3 to 4 minutes.

Using a slotted spoon, retrieve the eggs from the water. Place tomato mixture (pico de gallo) on each muffin half and top with egg. Sprinkle with salt.

Spinach frittata

SERVES 4 | DIABETES MEAL PLAN CHOICES:

1 teaspoon olive oil
1 garlic clove, minced
3 cups baby spinach leaves
3 whole eggs, plus 4 egg whites
¼ teaspoon freshly ground black pepper
½ yellow onion, chopped (about ½ cup)
¼ cup minced red bell pepper
2 waxy red or white potatoes, about ¾
    pound total weight, peeled and
    shredded
2 tablespoons chopped fresh basil
¼ cup shredded part-skim mozzarella or
    provolone cheese

NUTRITIONAL ANALYSIS PER SERVING
(1 WEDGE): 186 calories, 6 g total fat, 144
mg cholesterol, 176 mg sodium, 20 g total
carbohydrate, 13 g protein

Heat the broiler. Position the rack 4 inches from the heat source.

In a large, nonstick frying pan with a flameproof handle, heat ½ teaspoon of the olive oil over medium heat. Add the garlic and sauté until softened, about 1 minute. Stir in the spinach and cook until it wilts, 1 to 2 minutes. Transfer to a bowl. Set the frying pan aside.

In a bowl, whisk together the whole eggs, egg whites and pepper. Set aside.

Return the frying pan to medium heat and heat the remaining ½ teaspoon olive oil. Add the onion and sauté until soft and translucent, about 4 minutes. Stir in the bell pepper and the potatoes and cook until the potatoes begin to brown but are still tender-crisp, 4 to 5 minutes.

Spread the potatoes in an even layer in the pan. Spread the spinach evenly over the potatoes. Sprinkle with the basil. Pour in the beaten eggs and sprinkle evenly with the cheese. Cook over medium heat until slightly set, about 2 to 3 minutes.

Carefully place the pan under the broiler and broil until the frittata is brown and puffy and completely set, about 3 minutes. Gently slide onto a warmed serving platter and cut into 4 wedges. Serve immediately.

Quinoa cakes

3 sweet potatoes, peeled and cut into
  spears
1 cup uncooked quinoa
2 eggs
3 cloves garlic, minced
6 ounces Gruyere or Parmesan cheese,
  shredded
2 tablespoons finely chopped fresh
  parsley
1 teaspoon salt
¼ teaspoon ground black pepper
¼ teaspoon nutmeg
2 tablespoons olive oil

NUTRITIONAL ANALYSIS PER SERVING
(1 CAKE): 122 calories, 7 g total fat, 38 mg
cholesterol, 172 mg sodium, 10 g total
carbohydrate, 6 g protein

Heat oven to 375 F. Place the potatoes on a greased baking sheet. Bake for 45 minutes or until potatoes are completely soft. Meanwhile, cook quinoa according to package directions; set aside to cool.

In a large bowl, combine cooked potatoes, cooked quinoa, eggs, garlic, cheese, parsley, salt, pepper and nutmeg.

Heat 1 tablespoon of olive oil in a large saucepan. Form half of the quinoa mixture into ¼-cup patties and place in the pan; cook until cakes are golden brown. Place cooked patties on a baking sheet. Repeat process with remaining oil and quinoa mixture. Bake cakes in the oven for 5 minutes to ensure they are heated through.

Tabbouleh salad

1 ½ cups water
¾ cup bulgur (cracked wheat), rinsed and
    drained
1 cup diced, seeded tomatoes
1 cup chopped parsley
½ cup chopped scallions or green onions
1 teaspoon dill weed
4 black olives, sliced
¼ cup raisins
¼ cup lemon juice
2 tablespoons extra-virgin olive oil
Freshly ground black pepper, to taste

NUTRITIONAL ANALYSIS PER SERVING
(ABOUT ½ CUP): 108 calories, 4 g total fat,
0 mg cholesterol, 28 mg sodium, 16 g total
carbohydrate, 2 g protein

In a small saucepan, bring the water to a boil. Remove from heat and add the bulgur. Cover and let stand until the bulgur is tender and the liquid is completely absorbed, about 15 to 20 minutes.

In a large bowl, add the bulgur and the remaining ingredients. Toss gently just until the ingredients are evenly distributed. Cover and refrigerate for 2 hours to allow the flavors to blend. Serve chilled.

Roasted squash soup

1 small butternut squash, cut into half-
    inch pieces
2 teaspoons canola oil, divided
1 cup diced celery
1 ½ cups diced yellow onion
1 ½ cups spinach
2 cloves garlic, minced
1 cup diced carrot
4 cups unsalted vegetable stock
1 teaspoon sage
½ teaspoon nutmeg
1 teaspoon black pepper

NUTRITIONAL ANALYSIS PER SERVING
(ABOUT 2 CUPS): 213 calories, 5 g total fat,
0 mg cholesterol, 139 mg sodium, 37 g total
carbohydrate, 5 g protein

Heat the oven to 400 F. In a roasting pan, toss squash with 1 teaspoon of oil. Roast for 40 minutes or until brown. Set aside.

In a large pot, add the remaining oil, celery, onion, spinach, garlic and carrot. Saute over medium heat until vegetables are lightly browned. Add stock, sage, nutmeg, pepper and roasted squash to the pot, and simmer for a few minutes.

Carefully puree soup with a stick blender, or process soup in batches in a blender or food processor. Return pureed soup to pot and bring back to a simmer. Serve.

Balsamic-glazed Brussels sprouts

SERVES 6 | DIABETES MEAL PLAN CHOICES:

3 cups Brussels sprouts, cleaned and
  halved
1 cup coarsely chopped red onions
1 tablespoon olive oil
½ teaspoon kosher salt
½ teaspoon black pepper
2 tablespoons balsamic glaze

NUTRITIONAL ANALYSIS PER SERVING
(ABOUT ½ CUP): 60 calories, 2.5 g total fat,
0 mg cholesterol, 95 mg sodium, 8 g total
carbohydrate, 2 g protein

Preheat oven to 425 F. Lightly spray a
baking sheet with nonstick cooking spray.
Fill a medium pot with water and bring to
a boil.

Place a steamer basket over the boiling
water, add the Brussels sprouts and steam
approximately 3 to 5 minutes, depending
on size of sprouts. Remove the steamer
basket and drain off excess water from
Brussels sprouts.

In a large bowl, mix steamed Brussels
sprouts, red onions, olive oil, salt and
pepper. Toss well to evenly season the
Brussels sprouts and onions.

Roast 15 to 20 minutes, or until the
vegetables are golden brown in spots
(carmelized) and tender.

Drizzle the balsamic glaze over the
roasted Brussels sprouts and onions, and
serve.

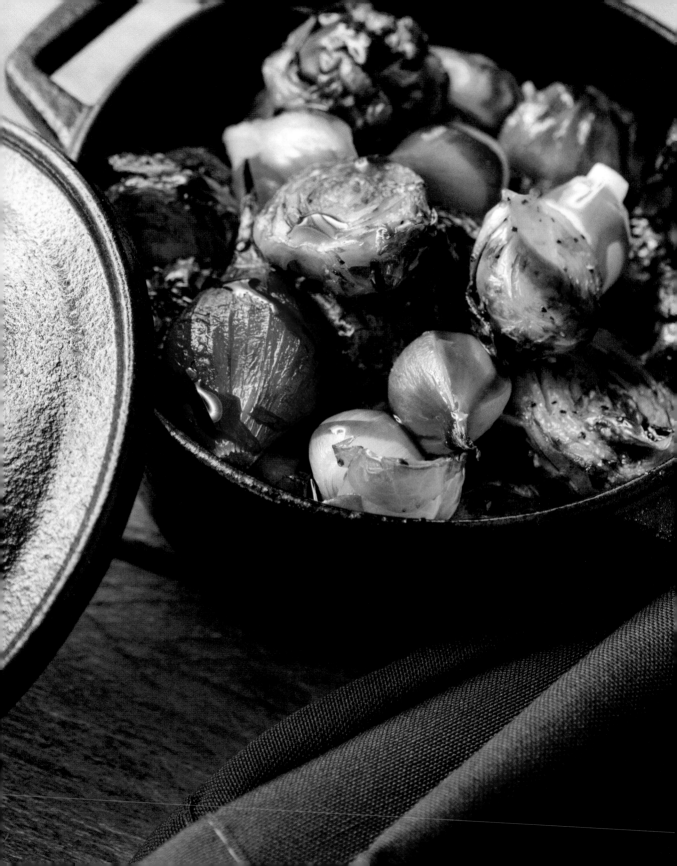

Butternut squash fries

SERVES 6 | DIABETES MEAL PLAN CHOICES:

1 medium butternut squash
1 tablespoon chopped fresh thyme
1 tablespoon chopped fresh rosemary
1 tablespoon olive oil
½ teaspoon salt

NUTRITIONAL ANALYSIS PER SERVING
(½ CUP): 50 calories, 2.5 g total fat, 0 mg
cholesterol, 160 mg sodium, 8 g total
carbohydrate, 1 g protein

Preheat oven to 425 F. Lightly coat a baking sheet with nonstick cooking spray. Peel the skin from butternut squash. Cut the squash into even sticks, about ½-inch wide and 3 inches long.

In a medium bowl, combine the squash, thyme, rosemary, olive oil and salt. Mix until the squash is evenly coated.

Spread the squash onto the baking sheet, place in the oven and roast 10 minutes. Remove baking sheet and shake to loosen the squash. Place the sheet back in the oven and continue to roast another 5 to 10 minutes until golden brown.

Parmesan crusted cauliflower

½ cup panko breadcrumbs
¼ cup fresh Parmesan cheese, finely
    grated (use fresh for the best flavor)
2 tablespoons olive or canola oil
1 teaspoon fresh lemon zest
1 teaspoon fresh basil, finely chopped or
    ½ teaspoon dried basil
¼ teaspoon paprika
3 cups cauliflower, chopped into 1 inch-
    wide florets

NUTRITIONAL ANALYSIS PER SERVING
(ABOUT ½ CUP): 100 calories, 6 g total fat,
0 mg cholesterol, 90 mg sodium, 10 g total
carbohydrate, 1 g fiber, 3 g protein

Preheat oven to 375 F. Lightly coat an 8x8-inch baking dish with nonstick cooking spray. Fill a medium pot with water and bring to a boil.

In a small bowl, add the panko, cheese, oil, lemon zest, basil and paprika. Use your hands to evenly combine the mixture.

Place the cauliflower in boiling water for 3 minutes; drain. Place the cauliflower in the baking dish, and sprinkle the bread-crumb mixture evenly over the top.

Bake approximately 15 minutes or until crust is lightly brown.

Fish tacos with tomatillo sauce

SERVES 4 | DIABETES MEAL PLAN CHOICES: **P** **P** **P** **V** **S**

12 ounces whitefish, such as cod or tilapia
Salt and pepper to taste (optional)
¼ head napa cabbage (1 ½ cups)
1 teaspoon cumin
2 teaspoons paprika
½ teaspoon chili powder
½ small yellow onion, diced (¼ cup)
2 tablespoons chopped cilantro
2 red Fresno peppers, diced
Zest and juice of 1 lime (½ teaspoon zest, 1 tablespoon juice)
4 tablespoons tomatillo salsa
4 wheat tortillas (6-inch diameter), lightly grilled or toasted

Season fish with salt and pepper if you like. Then bake fish at 375 F for about 20 minutes until internal temperature reaches 145 F. Or grill fish if you prefer.

Place remaining ingredients except tortillas in a mixing bowl and toss to combine. Flake fish and place on tortillas. Top with cabbage and salsa mixture. Serve immediately.

NUTRITIONAL ANALYSIS PER SERVING (1 FILLED TORTILLA): 187 calories, 3 g total fat, 39 mg cholesterol, 190 mg sodium, 21 g total carbohydrate, 19 g protein

Baked salmon with soy marinade

SERVES 2 | DIABETES MEAL PLAN CHOICES: Ⓟ Ⓟ Ⓟ Ⓟ Ⓕⓡ ◗

½ cup pineapple juice (no sugar added)
2 garlic cloves, minced
1 teaspoon low-sodium soy sauce
¼ teaspoon ground ginger
2 salmon fillets, each 4 ounces
¼ teaspoon sesame oil
Freshly ground black pepper, to taste
1 cup diced fresh fruit, such as pineapple,
    mango and papaya

NUTRITIONAL ANALYSIS PER SERVING
(1 FILLET): 247 calories, 7 g total fat, 157 mg
cholesterol, 192 mg sodium, 19 g total
carbohydrate, 27 g protein

In a small bowl, add the pineapple juice, garlic, soy sauce and ginger. Stir to mix evenly. Arrange the salmon fillets in a small baking dish. Pour the pineapple juice mixture over the top. Put in the refrigerator and marinate for 1 hour. Turn the salmon periodically as needed.

Heat the oven to 375 F. Lightly coat 2 squares of aluminum foil with cooking spray. Place the marinated salmon fillets on the aluminum foil. Drizzle each with ⅛ teaspoon sesame oil. Sprinkle with pepper and top each with ½ cup diced fruit. Wrap the foil around the salmon, folding the edges to seal. Bake until the fish is opaque throughout when tested with the tip of a knife, about 10 minutes on each side. Transfer the salmon to warmed individual plates and serve immediately.

Tandoori chicken wrap

SERVES 1 | DIABETES MEAL PLAN CHOICE: (P) (P) (P) (P) (V) (S) ◣

4 ounces boneless, skinless chicken breast
¼ teaspoon ground turmeric
¼ teaspoon ground cumin
¼ teaspoon minced garlic
¼ teaspoon ground white pepper
¼ teaspoon ground cayenne pepper
¼ teaspoon coriander seeds
¼ teaspoon ground nutmeg
2 ounces plain nonfat yogurt
1 piece flatbread (about 2 ounces)
1 cup chopped spinach (about 2 ounces)
¼ small cucumber, sliced (about 2 ounces)
Coarsely chopped basil, to taste

Season chicken with spices and let marinate in the refrigerator for 2 hours.

Heat gas or charcoal grill to medium high (or turn on broiler). Grill or broil chicken about 3 to 4 minutes per side or until the internal temperature is 165 F. Let cool.

Slice chicken and toss with yogurt. Build wrap with flatbread, sliced chicken and yogurt, spinach, cucumber and basil.

NUTRITIONAL ANALYSIS PER SERVING (1 WRAP): 343 calories, 6 g total fat, 85 mg cholesterol, 378 mg sodium, 29 g total carbohydrate, 41 g protein

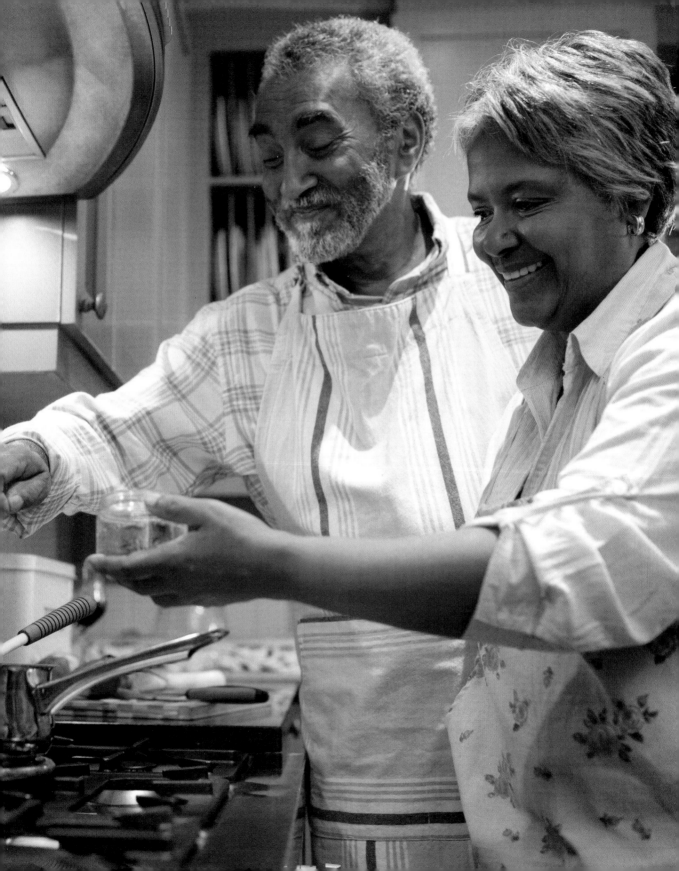

Chicken & asparagus penne

SERVES 2 | DIABETES MEAL PLAN CHOICES: **P P P V V V S S S**

1 ½ cups uncooked whole-grain penne pasta
1 cup asparagus, cut into 1-inch pieces
6 ounces boneless, skinless chicken breasts, cut into 1-inch cubes
2 cloves garlic, minced
1 can (14.5 ounces) diced tomatoes, no salt added, including juice
2 teaspoons dried basil or oregano
1 ounce soft goat cheese, crumbled (about 1 tablespoon)
1 tablespoon Parmesan cheese

NUTRITIONAL ANALYSIS PER SERVING (ABOUT 2 ½ CUPS): 433 calories, 9 g total fat, 75 mg cholesterol, 140 mg sodium, 54 g total carbohydrate, 34 g protein

Fill a large pot ¾ full with water and bring to a boil. Add the pasta and cook until al dente (tender), 10 to 12 minutes, or according to the package directions. Drain the pasta thoroughly. Set aside.

In a pot fitted with a steamer basket, bring 1 inch of water to a boil. Add the asparagus. Cover and steam until tender-crisp, about 2 to 3 minutes.

Spray a large nonstick frying pan with cooking spray. Add the chicken and garlic and sauté over medium-high heat. Cook until the chicken is golden brown, about 5 to 7 minutes. Add the tomatoes, including their juice, basil or oregano and simmer 1 minute more.

In a large bowl, add the cooked pasta, steamed asparagus, chicken mixture and goat cheese. Toss gently to mix evenly.

To serve, divide the pasta mixture between 2 plates. Sprinkle each serving with ½ tablespoon Parmesan cheese. Serve immediately.

Baked chicken & wild rice

SERVES 6 | DIABETES MEAL PLAN CHOICES: **P** **P** **P** **V** **S** **S**

1 pound boneless, skinless chicken breast halves
1 ½ cups chopped celery
1 ½ cups whole pearl onions
1 teaspoon fresh tarragon
2 cups unsalted chicken broth
¾ cup uncooked long-grain white rice
¾ cup uncooked wild rice
1 ½ cups dry white wine

NUTRITIONAL ANALYSIS PER SERVING (ABOUT 1 ½ CUPS): 313 calories, 3 g total fat, 55 mg cholesterol, 104 mg sodium, 38 g total carbohydrate, 23 g protein

Heat the oven to 300 F.

Cut chicken breasts into 1-inch pieces. In a nonstick frying pan, combine the chicken, celery, onions and tarragon with 1 cup of the unsalted chicken broth. Cook on medium heat until the chicken and vegetables are tender, about 10 minutes. Set aside to cool.

In a baking dish, stir together the rice, wine and remaining 1 cup chicken broth. Let soak for 30 minutes.

Add the chicken and vegetables to the baking dish. Cover and bake for 60 minutes. Check periodically and add more broth if the rice is too dry. Serve immediately.

Pork tenderloin with apples

SERVES 4 | DIABETES MEAL PLAN CHOICES: (P) (P) (P) (P) (Fr)

1 pound pork tenderloin
½ teaspoon white pepper
2 teaspoons black pepper
¼ teaspoon cayenne pepper
1 teaspoon paprika
2 teaspoons canola oil
2 apples, sliced
½ cup white wine or ½ cup unsweetened
    apple juice
¼ cup (about 1 ounce) crumbled blue
    cheese

NUTRITIONAL ANALYSIS PER SERVING
(ABOUT 4 OUNCES): 235 calories, 7 g total
fat, 79 mg cholesterol, 145 mg sodium, 17 g
total carbohydrate, 26 g protein

Heat oven to 350 F. Trim tenderloin of all fat and silvery membrane. Season with spices.

In a large skillet over medium-high heat, add oil and put tenderloin in the pan. Sear each side, using tongs to turn the meat. Transfer meat to a roasting pan and cook in oven for 15 to 20 minutes, until internal temperature reaches 155 F. Remove from oven and transfer tenderloin to a platter. Cover with foil and let rest.

Add apples to roasting pan and sauté on stovetop until dark brown. Add wine (or juice) and simmer until liquid is reduced by half.

Slice pork, spoon apples over top and sprinkle with blue cheese. Serve.

Beef & vegetable stew

1 pound beef round steak
2 teaspoons canola oil
2 cups diced yellow onions
1 cup diced celery
1 cup diced Roma tomatoes
½ cup diced sweet potato
½ cup diced white potato with skin
½ cup diced mushrooms
1 cup diced carrot
4 cloves of garlic, chopped
1 cup chopped kale
¼ cup uncooked barley
¼ cup red wine vinegar
1 teaspoon balsamic vinegar
3 cups low-sodium vegetable or beef stock
1 teaspoon dried sage
1 teaspoon minced fresh thyme
1 tablespoon minced fresh parsley
1 tablespoon dried oregano
1 teaspoon dried rosemary
Black pepper, to taste

Heat grill or broiler (medium heat). Trim fat and gristle from steak. Grill or broil steak 12 to 14 minutes, turning once. Don't overcook. Remove from heat and let rest while preparing vegetables.

In a large stock pot, saute vegetables in oil over medium-high heat until lightly brown, about 10 minutes. Add barley and cook an additional 5 minutes.

Pat steak dry with paper towels. Cut into half-inch pieces and add to pot. Then add vinegars, stock, herbs and spices.

Bring to a boil and simmer 1 hour, until barley is cooked and stew has thickened considerably.

NUTRITIONAL ANALYSIS PER SERVING (ABOUT 2 CUPS): 216 calories, 4 g total fat, 46 mg cholesterol, 138 mg sodium, 24 g total carbohydrate, 21 g protein

Apple-berry cobbler

SERVES 6 | DIABETES MEAL PLAN CHOICES:

For the filling:
1 cup fresh raspberries
1 cup fresh blueberries
2 cups chopped apples
2 tablespoons turbinado or brown sugar
½ teaspoon ground cinnamon
1 teaspoon lemon zest
2 teaspoons lemon juice
1 ½ tablespoons cornstarch

For the topping:
Egg white from 1 large egg
¼ cup soy milk
¼ teaspoon salt
½ teaspoon vanilla
1 ½ tablespoons turbinado or brown
    sugar
¾ cup whole-wheat pastry flour

NUTRITIONAL ANALYSIS PER SERVING
(ABOUT 2/3 CUP): 136 calories, trace total
fat, 0 mg cholesterol, 31 mg sodium, 31 g
total carbohydrate, 3 g protein

Preheat the oven to 350 F. Lightly coat 6 individual ovenproof ramekins with cooking spray.

In a medium bowl, add the raspberries, blueberries, apples, sugar, cinnamon, lemon zest and lemon juice. Stir to mix evenly. Add the cornstarch and stir until the cornstarch dissolves. Set aside.

In a separate bowl add the egg white and whisk until lightly beaten. Add the soy milk, salt, vanilla, sugar and pastry flour. Stir to mix well.

Divide the berry mixture evenly among the prepared dishes. Pour the topping over each. Arrange the ramekins on a large baking pan and place in oven.

Bake until the berries are tender and the topping is golden brown, about 30 minutes. Serve warm.

Strawberry shortcake

SERVES 8 | DIABETES MEAL PLAN CHOICES:

For the shortcake:
1 ¾ cups whole-wheat pastry flour, sifted
1/4 cup all-purpose (plain) flour, sifted
2 ½ teaspoons low-sodium baking powder
1 tablespoon sugar
¼ cup trans-free margarine (chilled)
¾ cup fat-free milk (chilled)

For the topping:
6 cups fresh strawberries, hulled and
    sliced
¾ cup (6 ounces) plain or vanilla fat-free
    yogurt

NUTRITIONAL ANALYSIS PER SERVING
(1 SHORTCAKE AND TOPPING): 218
calories, 6 g total fat, 1 mg cholesterol, 75
mg sodium, 36 g total carbohydrate, 5 g
protein

Heat the oven to 425 F. Spray baking sheet with cooking spray.

In a large mixing bowl, re-sift the flours, baking powder and sugar together. Using a fork, cut the chilled margarine into the dry ingredients until the mixture resembles coarse crumbs. Add the chilled milk and stir just until a moist dough forms.

Turn the dough onto a generously floured work surface and, with floured hands, knead gently 6 to 8 times until the dough is smooth and manageable. Using a rolling pin, roll the dough into a rectangle ¼-inch thick. Cut into 8 squares. Place the squares into the prepared baking sheet and bake until golden, 10 to 12 minutes.

Transfer the biscuits onto individual plates. Top each with ¾ cup strawberries and 1 ½ tablespoons yogurt. Serve immediately.

GLUCOSE RECORDS

Keeping track of your insulin doses and glucose values will help you see patterns and trends in your glucose levels. Here's a sample record form.

Day/date	Insulin type	Insulin Dosage				
		Breakfast	**Noon meal**	**Evening meal**	**Bedtime**	
Sunday						
	+/-					
Monday						
	+/-					
Tuesday						
	+/-					
Wednesday						
	+/-					
Thursday						
	+/-					
Friday						
	+/-					
Saturday						
	+/-					

Blood Glucose (BG) and Urine Ketone (UK) Test Results

		Breakfast		Noon meal		Evening meal		Bed-time	During night	Comments
		Before	After	Before	After	Before	After			
	Time									
	BG									
	UK									
	Time									
	BG									
	UK									
	Time									
	BG									
	UK									
	Time									
	BG									
	UK									
	Time									
	BG									
	UK									
	Time									
	BG									
	UK									
	Time									
	BG									
	UK									

HANDLING MEDICAL EMERGENCIES

If your blood sugar goes to extremes (too high or too low), you can have serious problems. Learn the signs below and what to do if they occur. If you have a medical emergency, take action immediately.

	Early signs and symptoms	Later signs and symptoms	
Low blood sugar (hypoglycemia)	• Sweating • Hunger • Shakiness • Dizziness • Blurry vision • Irritability • Nervousness • Nausea • Headache • Cold, clammy skin • Weakness	• Slurred speech • Drowsiness • Drunken-like behavior • Confusion	
Dangerously high blood sugar (hyperglycemic hyperosmolar state)	• Excessive thirst • Leg cramps • Dry mouth • Frequent urination • Dehydration	• Rapid pulse • Weakness • Confusion	
High ketones (diabetic ketoacidosis)	• High blood sugar • Dry mouth • Excessive thirst • Frequent urination	• Fatigue • Blurry vision • Nausea • Confusion • Vomiting • Loss of appetite • Abdominal pain • Weight loss • Shallow breathing • Weakness • Sweet, fruity odor on your breath • Drowsiness	

Emergency signs	What to do:
• Seizures • Coma, which can be fatal	If blood sugar is below 70 mg/dL, eat or drink something to raise your level quickly, such as hard candy (equal to 5 Life Savers), ½ cup regular (not diet) soft drink, ½ cup fruit juice, or 3 or 4 glucose tablets. If needed, repeat in 15 minutes. If there's no improvement, get medical help right away. If you use insulin, ask your diabetes care provider if you should have a glucagon emergency kit.
• Seizures • Coma, which can be fatal	If blood sugar is above 350 mg/dL and you feel ill or stressed, call your diabetes care team for advice. If it's 500 mg/dL or higher, see your diabetes care provider immediately. If your provider is unable to see you, go to the emergency department. Emergency treatment may correct the problem within hours. Without prompt treatment, the condition can be fatal. Older adults living with diabetes who don't get enough fluids are at particular risk.
• Seizures • Coma, which can be fatal	Check your ketone level, especially if blood sugar is persistently above 250 mg/dL. If the test strip color shows a moderate or high ketone level, call your diabetes care provider right away and ask how much insulin to take. Drink plenty of water to prevent dehydration. If your ketone level is high and you can't reach your diabetes care team, go to the emergency department.

NONINSULIN MEDICATIONS

Drug class – Drug name (brand name)	How they work	
Metformin (Fortamet, Glucophage, Glucophage XR, Riomet)	Reduce the amount of glucose your liver releases and the need for insulin; don't use if you have severe kidney failure or have had lactic acidosis	
SGLT-2 inhibitors empagliflozin (Jardiance), canagliflozin (Invokana), dapagliflozin (Farxiga), ertugliflozin (Steglatro)	Cause urinary loss of glucose and salt; not to be used if you've had ketoacidosis, have type 1 diabetes, or recurrent or severe urinary infections	
GLP-1 agonists injection: liraglutide (Victoza), lixisenatide (Adlyxin), semaglutide (Ozempic), dulaglutide (Trulicity), exenatide (Byetta, Bydureon); tablet: semaglutide (Rybelsus)	Increase insulin secretion when blood sugar levels rise; decrease appetite and increase satiety; not to be used if you've had pancreatitis, pancreatic cancer or medullary thyroid cancer	
DPP-4 inhibitors alogliptin (Nesina), linagliptin (Tradjenta), sitagliptin (Januvia), saxagliptin (Onglyza)	Increase insulin secretion when blood sugar levels rise; not to be used if you've had pancreatitis or pancreatic cancer	
Thiazolidinediones (TZDs) pioglitazone (Actos), rosiglitazone (Avandia)	Improve efficiency of insulin	
Sulfonylureas glimepiride (Amaryl), glipizide (Glucotrol, Glucotrol XL), glyburide (Diabeta, Micronase)	Release more insulin from pancreas	
Meglitinides nateglinide (Starlix), repaglinide (Prandin)	Release more insulin from pancreas	
Alpha-glucosidase inhibitors acarbose (Precose), miglitol (Glyset)	Slow down digestion and absorption of glucose from the intestine into your bloodstream after eating carbohydrates	
Pramlintide (Symlin)	Suppress glucagon (an anti-insulin hormone) and slow down emptying of stomach after eating	

	Main advantages	Main disadvantages/side effects
	Do not cause hypoglycemia; may promote weight loss; mostly inexpensive	Nausea, (typically resolves over time) and diarrhea; rarely vitamin B-12 deficiency
	At least some of these agents reduce the risks of heart attack, stroke, kidney failure, heart failure and death; possibly improve fatty liver	Increased frequency of urination, dehydration, urinary infection, genital yeast infection, diabetic ketoacidosis; can be expensive
	May reduce the risks of heart attack, stroke and death, and the progression of kidney disease; decrease hunger and snacking leading to 5-10 lb. weight loss; may improve fatty liver	Nausea, (typically resolves over time), vomiting and diarrhea; can be expensive
	Don't cause weight gain or hypoglycemia; tablets, once-daily dosing	May cause minor upper respiratory tract infection; caution using in people with autoimmune disease; can be expensive
	Convenient: tablet taken once a day; may reduce risks of heart attack and stroke; may improve fatty liver; mostly inexpensive	Weight gain; swelling (edema); heart failure; fractures; bladder cancer (pioglitazone)
	Convenient: tablet taken once or twice a day; inexpensive	Low blood glucose (hypoglycemia); weight gain (2-4 lb.); require home blood glucose monitoring
	Convenient: tablet taken with each meal; less likely than sulfonylureas to cause hypoglycemia	Rare low blood glucose (hypoglycemia)
	Convenient: tablet taken with each meal; blunt the rapid rise of blood glucose after meals; may promote weight loss	Abdominal bloating, gas and diarrhea
	Enhances the effects of short-acting insulin taken with the meals; can cause moderate weight loss	Injection taken along with a separate injection of meal insulin; nausea, vomiting, abdominal pain, headache, fatigue and dizziness; low glucose (hypoglycemia), especially in people with type 1 diabetes

INSULIN OPTIONS

Type of insulin	Insulin name (brand name)	Onset of action	Maximum effect	Duration	
Inhaled	insulin human (Afrezza)	Within 5 minutes	About 15 minutes	About 3 hours	
Very fast-acting	insulin aspart (Fiasp), insulin lispro-aabc (Lyumjev)	Within 5 minutes	About 1 hour	3-4 hours	
Rapid-acting	insulin aspart (NovoLog), insulin glulisine (Apidra), insulin lispro (Humalog, Admelog)	Within 15 minutes	1-2 hours	3-5 hours	
Short-acting	insulin regular (Humulin R, Novolin R)	30-60 minutes	2-4 hours	6-8 hours	
Intermediate-acting	NPH (Humulin N, Novolin N)	1-2 hours	4-12 hours	16-24 hours	
Long-acting	insulin detemir (Levemir)	2 hours	Up to 12 hours after injection	14-16 hours	
	insulin glargine (Lantus, Toujeo, Basaglar)	1-2 hours	Up to 18-24 hours after injection	24 hours	
Ultra-long-acting	insulin degludec (Tresiba)	4 hours	Spread over time	More than 48 hours	

*Follow the advice of your diabetes care provider. Onset, peak and duration times are estimates — times vary among individuals and are affected by the site of injection and other issues, such as when you last ate or exercised.

	How it's typically used*	Notes
	Inhale at the beginning of a meal	Not an injection, absorbed from the lungs; often used in addition to intermediate- or long-acting insulin
	Inject at the start of a meal or within 20 minutes after starting a meal	Absorbed promptly and very short-acting; often used in addition to intermediate- or long-acting insulin
	Inject 5-15 minutes before a meal	Absorbed quickly and effects wear off soon; often used in addition to intermediate- or long-acting insulin; commonly used in insulin pumps
	Inject 30 minutes before a meal	Works quickly, but effects don't last for long; usually used in addition to intermediate- or long-acting insulin
	Inject morning, evening (or bedtime), or both; does not have to be injected before a meal	Starts working slowly; effects last for about half a day; sometimes used in addition to shorter acting insulin
	Inject morning, evening (or bedtime) or both, about the same time every day; does not have to be injected before a meal	Takes several hours to start working; provides basal insulin needs for up to a day; sometimes used in addition to shorter acting insulin; may be used in addition to rapid- or short-acting insulin
	Inject once a day; does not have to be injected before a meal	Takes several hours to start working; provides basal insulin needs; often used in addition to shorter acting insulin

Getting ready

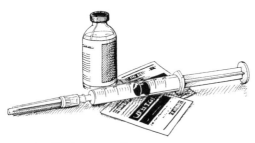

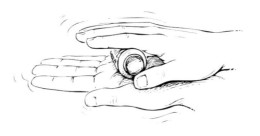

Step 1a. Gather supplies.
Step 1b. Wash hands.
Step 1c. Clean rubber membrane of vial
with an alcohol wipe.

Step 2. If using cloudy insulin, mix the
insulin: Gently roll bottle between palms 10
times, then tip bottle up & down 10 times.
All insulin should look cloudy.

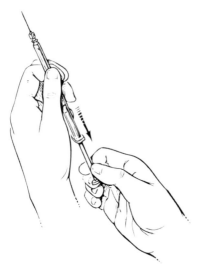

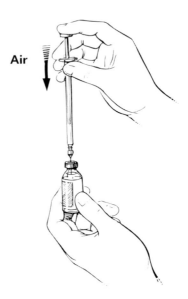

Air

Step 3. Draw air into syringe. The amount
of air you draw in should equal the amount
of insulin you will draw out in Step 5.

Step 4. Inject air into bottle.

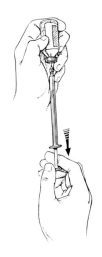

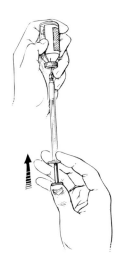

Step 5. Withdraw insulin.

Step 6. If there are air bubbles in the syringe, push all insulin back into bottle and repeat Step 5.

Injecting the insulin

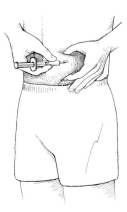

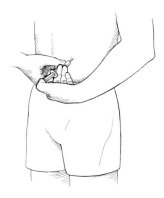

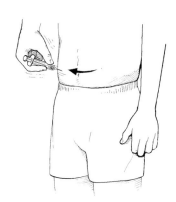

Step 1a. Pinch skin.
Step 1b. Insert needle.

Step 2. Push plunger in.

Step 3a. Remove needle.
Step 3b. Discard syringe properly.

1. Wash your hands with soap and water or put hand sanitizer on your hands.
2. Check the insulin pen label to make sure it is the correct type of insulin.
3. Take off pen cap.
4. Clean rubber membrane with an alcohol wipe.
5. Check the liquid in the pen. If the insulin is cloudy, gently role the pen between your hands 10 times. Then tip the pen up and down 10 times. The liquid should look consistently cloudy throughout.
6. Take protective tab off needle. With the outer needle cap on, screw the needle securely onto the insulin pen.
7. Pull off the outer needle cap. Save outer needle cap for later.
8. Carefully pull off the inner needle cap. Throw away this cap. *Do not let the needle touch anything.*
9. Do a safety test dose to remove any air. To do this, turn dose selector clockwise to dial 2 units. Hold pen with the needle pointing up as you push the injection button all the way in. A little insulin should come out of the needle. The dose indicator window should show "0." Remove your finger from the injection button.

   If insulin does not come out when you do the safety test dose, do the test again. If no insulin comes out after three tries, the pen has failed to prime and must not be used. Use a new needle.

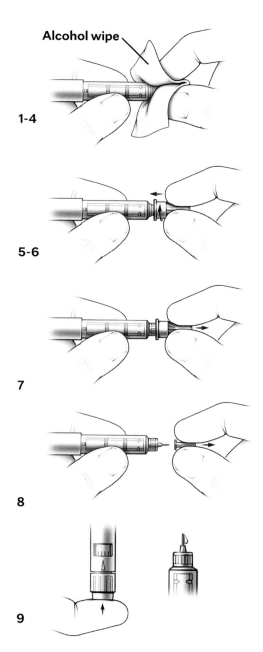

Alcohol wipe

1-4

5-6

7

8

9

10. Turn dose selector clockwise to dial the number of units you have been prescribed. If you set an incorrect dose, turn dose selector to the right or left until the arrow points to the correct number. You cannot set a dose larger than the number of units in the insulin reservoir.

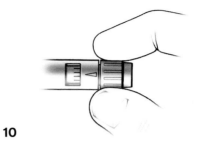

10

11. Select site for injection (back of arm, stomach, outer thighs). Remove clothing from the site.

12. Hold insulin pen in the palm of your hand. Keep the pen straight as you insert the needle straight into your skin. *Make sure the needle is inserted completely into your skin.*
Follow any directions from your health care team on whether to pinch your skin before you insert the needle into your skin.

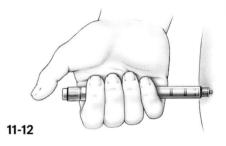

11-12

13. Use your thumb to push the injection button all the way in. For large doses, you may need to use the index finger of your other hand to push the injection button. *When the dose indicator window shows "0," slowly count to 10 as you keep the injection button pushed.*

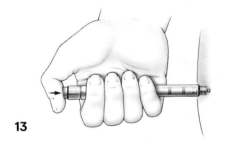

13

14. Remove the needle from your skin.

15. Carefully put the outer needle cap back on the needle.

16. Unscrew the needle from the pen. Throw away the covered needle in a puncture-resistant container.

17. Put the pen cap back on the insulin pen.

Additional resources

American Diabetes Association
800-342-2383
www.diabetes.org

American Heart Association
www.heart.org

Association of Diabetes Care & Education Specialists
800-338-3633
www.diabeteseducator.org

Centers for Disease Control and Prevention/ Diabetes
800-232-4636
www.cdc.gov/diabetes/index.html

International Diabetes Federation
www.idf.org

JDRF – Type 1 Diabetes Research Funding and Advocacy
www.jdrf.org

KnowDiabetesbyHeart
www.knowdiabetesbyheart.org
www.diabetesdecorazon.org (Spanish)

Mayo Clinic
www.mayoclinic.org

National Diabetes Prevention Program
www.cdc.gov/diabetes/prevention/index. html

National Institute of Diabetes and Digestive and Kidney Diseases
800-860-8747
www.niddk.gov

Index

A

acceptance, 243–245
activity trackers, 86
adapting to diagnosis, 198
adjusting insulin dosage. *See also* insulin
    (supplemental)
    about, 149
    correction dose, 155
    on I-C ratio, 154–155
    intermediate-acting insulin, 150–152
    long-acting insulin, 149–150
    safety considerations, 153
    short-/rapid-acting insulin, 152–154
advocacy groups, 219
aerobic activity, 81, 84–85. *See also*
    exercise
air travel, 263–264. *See also* traveling
    with diabetes
alcohol, 53
antibodies test, 177

anxiety, 207–208, 211
A1C test, 22–23, 177, 224–225
artificial sweeteners, 50–51
automated insulin delivery systems,
    171–173

B

balance, 96
balance exercises, 98–99
basal insulin, 167, 169
beverages, calories in, 79
blood and urine tests, 223
blood glucose monitors, 109, 112–113,
    118, 160
blood pressure check, 223, 229
blood pressure monitoring and goals,
    230–231
blood sugar (blood glucose)
    artificial sweeteners and, 50, 51
    exercise and, 103–105

blood sugar (blood glucose) continued
    insulin and, 57
    levels, stabilizing, 104
    raising quickly, 126
blood sugar management
    about, 108
    high blood sugar, 123–125
    low blood sugar, 125–128
    pregnancy and, 246–247
    staying within range and, 117–118
    steps in, 108
blood sugar monitoring
    about, 107, 108
    barriers, overcoming, 128–129
    children and, 182, 183–184
    information in, 116–117
    menopause and, 253
    negative response to, 107
    numbers game and, 116
    record-keeping, 114–117
    results, recording, 114–117
    test results signaling issues, 123
    testing frequency and, 108–111
    troubleshooting, 118–119
    type 1 diabetes in children, 178
blurred vision, 19–20
BMI (body mass index), 58–60
body scan meditation, 216
boluses, 167
breathing, relaxed, 240
burnout, diabetes, 205–206, 208

C

calf strengthening, 89
calf stretch, 95
calories, 46, 65, 67, 79
camps, diabetes, 194, 218–219
carbohydrates
    about, 38
    amount of, 38–39
    blood glucose and, 120

    counting, 47–49
    fast-acting, 104
    food labels and, 46
    healthy eating and, 38–39
    in Mayo Clinic Healthy Weight
        Pyramid, 66
    misconceptions, 38
    readily absorbable, 126
    serving size, 44
caregiver burnout, 206
care supplies, saving money on, 128
care team, diabetes
    about, 7, 217
    diabetes technology and, 161–162
    education and support, 159
    glucose goals and, 156
    importance of, 161–162
    in treatment selection, 132
celiac disease, 193
**certified diabetes care and education
    specialist,** 108, 111, 159, 212, 217
CGMs (continuous glucose monitors).
    See also technology, diabetes
    about, 25, 163
    accuracy and, 164, 165
    approaches of, 163–164
    children and, 178
    confirming levels and, 104, 164
    illustrated, 163
    looping systems and, 171
    noninvasive, 173
    skin sensitivity and, 165
    use decision, 164–165
change, expecting and accepting, 214
checkups, yearly, 222–223
chest stretch, 94
children with diabetes
    about, 175, 176
    achievement and, 190
    additional tests for, 192–193
    age groups, 184–185
    blood sugar monitoring, 192

camps and, 194, 218–219
child involvement and, 184–186
depression and, 187
dietary expectations and, 171
eating away from home, 189
emotional and social issues, 187
good habits for, 187–193
healthy eating and, 181–182, 188–189
insulin pumps for, 170–171
physical activity, 182, 190–192
puberty and, 180
smart choices and, 186
surviving sick days, 194–195
technology for, 162–163, 185
teenagers, eating disorders and, 188
type 1 diabetes, 175, 176–179
type 2 diabetes, 175, 179–186
cholesterol levels, 193, 225, 231
comatose condition, 25
combination pills, 138
combination therapy, 138
compassion, self, 204–205
coping skills, 213–215
coronary artery disease, 27–28
correction dose, insulin, 155
correction scale, 154, 155
counting carbs, 47–49
COVID-19 vaccine, 238

D

**DCCT (Diabetes Control and
 Complications Trial),** 151
depression, 187, 207–208, 211
diabetes. *See also specific types
 of diabetes*
 about, 12–14
 additional causes of, 18
 defined, 12–13
 LADA and MODY, 18
 long-term complications, 27–33

metabolic syndrome and, 21
 risk factors, 20–22
 signs and symptoms, 18–20
 statistics, 13
 tests to detect, 22–25
 types of, 15–18
 warning signs, 19
diabetes burnout, 205–206, 208
diabetes identification, 149
diabetes insipidus, 14
diabetes management
 blood sugar monitoring in, 114
 care team in, 161–162
 healthy-eating plan and, 34–55
 long-term benefits of, 157
 technology in, 158–173
 your role in, 162
diabetes mellitus, 14
diabetes self-management programs, 211
diabetic coma, 25
diabetic retinopathy (eye damage), 31–33
diagnosing diabetes, 12
diagnosis, adapting to, 198
dietitians, 42, 43
diets, fad, 72
distress, diabetes, 205
DKA (diabetic ketoacidosis), 26–27, 124
dosage, insulin
 adjusting, 149–155
 children and, 162
 correction, 155
 errors, 160
 higher vs. lower, 141
 on I-C ratio, 154–155
 for intermediate-acting insulin, 150–152
 for long-acting insulin, 149–150
 for meals, adjusting, 152–154
 options, 143–144
 right, finding, 149
DPP-4 inhibitors, 136–137

E

eating. *See* healthy eating; healthy-eating plan
eating triggers, 70–73
electric blankets, 235
emergency hypoglycemia treatment, 127
energy density, 68–69
energy drinks, 102
erectile dysfunction, diabetes and, 254–255
events, diabetes, 219
exams, tests, and quick checks, 229
exchange lists, 51–53
exercise
    aerobic, 81, 84–85
    after workout, 105
    benefits and risks of, 82
    best time for, 97
    blood glucose and, 121
    clothing and shoes for, 101
    complications from diabetes and, 91
    diabetes and, 82
    extreme temperatures and, 103
    gestational diabetes and, 90
    HIIT and, 92
    hydration and, 101–103
    injury avoidance and, 100–103
    insulin and, 97, 103
    intensity, gauging, 93
    ketones and, 104
    pregnancy and, 90
    rainy day workout, 100
    resistance training, 85–93
    safety, with diabetes, 103–105
    stretching/flexibility and, 93–96
    tai chi, 96–100
    walking, 83–84, 90, 191
    before workout and, 103–104
    yoga, 100
exercises
    balance, 98–99
    intervals, 92
    strengthening, 88–89
    stretching, 94–95
eye care, 228–233
eye damage (retinopathy), 31–33, 193
eye exams, 229, 232
eye photography, 233

F

family history, 14, 20
fasting blood glucose test, 24, 177
fats, 39, 40, 44, 72
fears, diabetes-related, 209
feet
    blood flow in, 234
    caring for, 233–236
    checking every day, 233
    diabetes and, 233
    keeping dry and clean, 233
    podiatrists and, 234
    protecting from injury, 235–236
    socks and, 235
    toenail trimming and, 235
fiber, 68
fitness, 83–84, 191–192
fitness water, 102
flu shot, 238
flu-like feeling, 18
food check, 223
food labels, reading, 46–47
food records, 70, 71
food(s)
    blood glucose and, 119–120
    children with diabetes and, 189
    as eating trigger, 70
    health relationship with, 211–213
    plant-based, choosing, 36
    power of, 71
    for sick days, children and, 195
fruits, 44, 66

G

gestational diabetes
    about, 17–18, 247, 248–249
    after delivery, 252
    exercise and, 90
    occurrence of, 249
    risk factors, 251
    screening and diagnosis, 18, 251
    signs and symptoms, 249
    treatment, 251
glaucoma test, 232
GLP-1 agonists, 135–136
glucagon emergency kit, 127
glucose sensors, 160–161
glycated hemoglobin test. *See* A1C test
glycemic index, 47
goals
    blood glucose, 117, 118
    daily calorie, 65, 67
    examples of, 64
    first steps toward, 65
    glucose, 156
    outcome, 62
    process, 62
    realistic, setting, 217–218
    reassessing and adjusting, 65
    reevaluating, 77–78
    SMART, 64, 217–218
    weight, setting, 62–65
    writing down, 65
group travel, 261
gums, red, swollen, tender, 20

H

HDL (high-density lipoprotein), 225, 231, 254
health education programs, 218
healthy eating
    about, 35, 36
    for all types of diabetes, 37
    carbohydrates and, 38–39
    children and, 181–182, 188–189
    concepts, 37
    consistency and, 42
    dietitians and, 42, 43
    family program for, 189
    fats and, 39, 40
    food labels and, 46–47
    meal plans and, 40–43
    plate method, 45
    protein and, 39
    rewards for, 55
    serving sizes and, 44–45
    setbacks, overcoming, 76–78
    snacks and, 52
    variety and, 43
healthy-eating plan
    cultural traditions and, 53–55
    exchange lists and, 51–53
    family/social life and, 54–55
    importance of, 35
    motivation for, 53–55
    for weight loss, 65–66
healthy weight. *See also* Mayo Clinic
    Healthy Weight Pyramid
    about, 57, 58
    determination of, 58–60
    eating triggers and, 70–73
    goals, 62–65
    habits for a lifetime, 78
    results, 60–62
    setbacks, overcoming, 76–78
    shopping and, 73–76
    willpower vs. self-control and, 77
heart attack, 28–29
herbal remedies, 136
HHS (hyperglycemic hyperosmolar state), 26,
    what to do, 298–299
high blood sugar. *See* **hyperglycemia**
HIIT (high-intensity interval training), 92
hiking and cycling, 262–263

hunger, shopping and, 73
hydration, exercise and, 101–103

hyperglycemia (high blood sugar)
    about, 25–26
    causes of, 123
    diabetic ketoacidosis (DKA) and, 124
    fear of, 209
    prevention steps, 125
    signs and symptoms, 123–124
    what to do, 124–125, 298–299
hypoglycemia (low blood sugar)
    about, 25, 125
    causes of, 125
    emergency treatment, 127
    fear of, 209
    glucagon injection and, 128
    missing early warning signs of, 24
    nighttime, 126
    prevention steps, 128
    signs and symptoms, 125–126
    what to do, 126–127, 298–299

I

I-C (insulin-to-carbohydrate) ratio,
    154–155
IDs, medical, 125
infection risk, 20, 33
inhaled insulin, 155
injections, insulin
    avoiding problems with, 147–149
    children and, 162
    insulin jet injector, 145
    methods of, 144–145
    process, 147, 304–305
    sites, selecting, 145, 146
    skin irritation and, 149
injury, avoiding, 100–103
insulin (hormone), 57, 131, 140, 141
insulin (supplemental). *See also* dosage,
    insulin

    adjusting to find right dose, 149–155
    appearance, changes in, 148
    children and, 179
    combination treatment, 156
    dosage options, 143–144
    exercise and, 97, 103
    frequency, 141–142
    inhaled, 155
    injecting, 145–149
    intensive therapy and, 156–157
    intermediate-acting, 150–152
    long-acting, 149–150
    pharmacy usage for, 148
    plan, 142–143
    premixed, 141
    rapid-acting, 152–155
    regimens, 142–143
    replacement plan, 143
    short-acting, 152–155
    storing, 148
    temperature and, 148, 266
    therapy, 140–157
    type 1 diabetes and, 179
    type 2 diabetes and, 142
    which is best for you, 142
insulin jet injector, 145
insulin pens, 144, 165–166
insulin pumps. *See also* technology,
    diabetes
    about, 166
    basal insulin and, 167, 169
    boluses and, 167
    for children, 170–171
    children and, 179
    considerations for use of, 169–170
    convertible, 173
    data, 168
    how it works, 167
    how to use, 168
    illustrated, 166, 167, 168
    as injection method, 144
    looping systems and, 171

sensor systems and, 161
tubeless-style, 168, 170
type 1 diabetes and, 131
use decision, 169–170
intensive therapy, 144, 156–157
intermediate-acting insulin, 150–152
intervals, exercise, 92

K

ketoacidosis, 26–27, 104
ketones test, 178
kidney disease (nephropathy), 30–31, 193
knee extension, 89
knee-to-chest stretch, 95

L

LADA (latent autoimmune diabetes of
    adults), 18
lancet and lancing device, 109
LDL (low-density lipoprotein), 225,
    231, 254
leisure activities, 245
lifestyle changes, 211
lipid panel, 225–226
liver, 13, 120–121
long-acting insulin, 149–150
long-term complications
    about, 27
    eye damage (retinopathy), 31–33
    heart/blood vessel disease, 27–29
    infection risk, 33
    kidney disease (nephropathy), 30–31
    nerve damage (neuropathy), 30
    stroke, 29–30
looping systems, 171
low blood sugar. *See* hypoglycemia

M

massage, 243
Mayo Clinic Healthy Weight Pyramid,
    66–70
meal plans, 40–43, 47
meal-replacement shakes/products, 78
meal routine, 74–75
medical emergencies, 25–27
medical evacuation insurance, 259–260
medical history, 60
medications. *See also* insulin
    (supplemental)
    about, 132–133
    children and diabetes, 182
    children sick days and, 194–195
    choice factors, 132–133
    combination pills, 138
    DPP-4 inhibitors, 136–137
    forgetting to take, 137
    GLP-1 agonists, 135–136
    metformin, 133–134
    SGLT-2 inhibitors, 134–135
    sulfonylureas, 139–140
    thiazolidinediones (TZDs), 138–139
    traveling with diabetes and, 266
meditation, 216, 242
menopause, diabetes and, 252–254
menstruation, diabetes and, 252
mental health
    anxiety and, 207–211
    burnout and, 205–206
    depression and, 207–211
    diabetes-related fears and, 209
    distress and, 205
    professionals, tips on finding, 210
    sharing the load and, 207
metabolic syndrome, 21
metaformin, 133–134
mindfulness practice, 215, 216
misconceptions, diabetes, 199–200

MODY (maturity-onset diabetes of youth), 18
monounsaturated fats, 39
mood disorders, 193
myths, diabetes, 199–200

N

needles, fear of, 209
nephropathy (kidney disease), 30–31, 193
nerve damage (neuropathy), 30
networks, diabetes, 218–219
neuropathy (nerve damage), 30
nonproliferative diabetic retinopathy, 32, 33
nutrition labels, reading, 73–76

O

omega-3 fatty acids, 41
optimism, nurturing, 213
oral glucose tolerance test, 24–25
outdoor adventures, 262–263

P

pancreas, 12–17, 18
personal bag, 265–266, 267
physical activity. *See also* exercise; exercises
    about, 81
    activity trackers and, 86
    balance and, 96
    benefits and risks of, 82
    blood glucose and, 121
    children and, 182, 190–192
    at home, 83
    importance of, 82
    Mayo Clinic Healthy Weight Pyramid and, 70
    at work, 83
plasma glucose levels, 114

plate method, 45
pneumonia vaccine, 238–239
podiatrists, 234
polyunsaturated fats, 39
prediabetes, 37, 181
pregnancy and diabetes. *See also* gestational diabetes
    about, 245
    after becoming pregnant and, 246–247
    expectations, 247–248
    first trimester, 247
    labor and delivery, 248
    planning and, 245–246
    second trimester, 247–248
    third trimester, 248
    unmanaged blood sugar complications, 250
premixed insulins, 141
process goals, 62
progressive muscle relaxation, 240–242
proliferative diabetic retinopathy, 32–33
protein and dairy, 39, 44, 66
psychotherapy, 211
pushups, wall or table, 88

R

rainy day workout, 100
random blood glucose test, 23, 176–177
rapid-acting insulin, 152–155
readiness, weight loss, 61, 62
recipes, adapting, 72–73
record-keeping, in blood sugar monitoring, 114–117
relationships
    misconceptions/myths and, 199–200
    navigating, 199–205
    positive support and, 200–203
    romantic, 203–204
    self-relationship and, 204–205
    words and, 201
relaxation, 240–241

replacement insulin plan, 143
resistance training. *See also* exercise
    about, 85–87
    benefits of, 85–87
    body as resistance and, 87–90
    exercises, 88–89
    guidelines for, 90–93
    muscle warmup/recovery and, 90
    process of, 87
    repetitions (reps) and, 90
    starting, 90
retinal exam, 232
retinopathy (eye damage), 193
risk factors, 17, 20–22, 251
romantic relationships, 203–204

S

saturated fats, 39, 40
seated hamstring stretch, 94
self-care inventory, 244
self-compassion, 204–205
serum creatinine test, 226–227
servings, determining number of, 70
serving sizes, 44–45, 70
SGLT-2 inhibitors, 134–135
sharps bin, travel-sized, 268
shifting weight side to side, 98
shoes. *See also* feet
    buying, 236
    exercise and, 85, 101
    foot care and, 235–236
    traveling and, 268
    walking, 85
shopping, 73–76
short-acting insulin, 152–155
sick days, children and, 194–195
signs and symptoms
    coronary artery disease, 28
    diabetes, 18–20, 24
    heart attack, 28–29

    hyperglycemia (high blood sugar), 123–124
    hypoglycemia (low blood sugar), 117–118, 125–126
    infections, 33
    nephropathy (kidney disease), 31
    neuropathy (nerve damage), 30
    proliferative diabetic retinopathy, 33
    stroke, 29–30
    type 1 diabetes in children, 176
    type 2 diabetes in children, 180–181
silent heart attacks, 28
sitting, reducing, 82–83
sitting meditation, 216
slit-lamp exam, 232
SMART goals, 64, 217–218
smart insulin pens, 165–166
smoking risks, 237
snacks, 52
sores, slow-healing, 20
sports drinks, 102
spot collection, 227
squats, 88
Steno-2 study, 151
strengthening exercises, 88–89
stress, 77, 121, 202, 239–240
stress management
    about, 239–240
    keeping your cool and, 243–245
    learning how to relax and, 240
    meditation and, 242
    progressive muscle relaxation and, 240–242
    relaxation techniques and, 242–243
stress response, 239
stretching, 93–96
stroke, 29–30
sugar alcohols, 50–51
sugar and sweets
    approach to, 49–50
    change in taste and, 51
    how to eat, 49

sugar and sweets *continued*
    in Mayo Clinic Healthy Weight
        Pyramid, 67
    reducing, in recipes, 72
    substitutes, 50–51
sugar-free products, 46
sulfonylureas, 139–140
supplemental insulin. *See* insulin (supple-
    mental)
supplies, care, 128
support
    asking for, 202–203
    care team, 159
    healthy eating, 212–213
    healthy weight, 76
    mental health, 206–207
    positive, family and friends and,
        200–203
support groups, 219
support system, 214
swimming, 262
syringes, 144, 145–147

T

tai chi, 96–100, 242
technology, diabetes
    about, 160
    alarm fatigue and, 215
    attachment considerations, 217
    automated insulin delivery systems,
        171–173
    benefits of, 159, 160
    continuous glucose monitors (CGMs),
        25, 104, 163–165
    decision on use of, 160–162
    diabetes care team and, 161–162
    future of, 173
    insulin pumps, 131, 144, 161, 166–171
    for kids, 162–163
    looping systems, 171
    thriving with, 215–217

    types of, 163–173
    using, 173
teeth, caring for, 236–237
test results, 114–117, 123
test strips, 109, 118
testing. *See also* blood sugar monitoring
    alternate site, 110
    basics, 111–112
    in dosage adjustments, 153
    expert tips, 113–114
    frequency, 108–111
    process, 111–114
    quality control test and, 118–119
    technique, checking, 119
    time of day for, 110
    tools needed for, 109
    troubleshooting, 118–119
    type 1 diabetes in children, 176–178
tests, living with diabetes
    A1C test, 224–225
    lipid panel, 225–226
    serum creatinine test, 226–227
    summary table, 229
    urine test for protein, 227
tests to detect diabetes
    about, 22
    A1C, 22–23, 224–225
    fasting blood glucose, 24
    oral glucose tolerance, 24–25
    random blood glucose, 23
    results, understanding, 23
thiazolidinediones (TZDs), 138–139
thirst, excessive, 18
thyroid hormone levels, 193
tingling feet and hands, 20
total cholesterol, 225
trans fats, 39
travel insurance, 258–260
travel medicine clinics, 259
traveling with diabetes
    about, 257
    by car or train, 264

care supplies and, 265–266
clothing and footwear and, 268
communication and, 260–261
cultural perceptions and, 261
group travel and, 261
immunizations and, 257–258
medications and, 265–266
movement and, 264
outdoor adventures and, 262–263
packing and, 265–268
personal bag and, 265–266, 267
by plane, 263–264
predeparture checklist, 258
preparation for, 257–261
research before, 257
by sea, 264–265
sharps bin and, 268
solo travel and, 262
story about, 269
time zone changes and, 260
treatment plan for, 265
working overseas and, 261
triglycerides, 225
trip cancellation insurance, 258–259
type 1 diabetes. *See also* diabetes
about, 15
as autoimmune disease, 15
exercise and, 82
family history and, 14
healthy eating for, 37
illustrated, 16
insulin (hormone) and, 141
pancreas and, 15, 16
pregnancy and, 247
resistance training and, 85–87
type 1 diabetes and children
about, 176
blood sugar monitoring, 178
insulin pump and, 179
insulin therapy, 179
multiple daily injections (MDIs), 179
signs and symptoms, 176

split-mixed program, 179
testing, 176–178
treatments, 178–179
type 2 diabetes. *See also* diabetes
about, 15–17
as epidemic, 11, 13
exercise and, 82
family history and, 14
healthy eating for, 37
herbal remedies and, 136
illustrated, 16
insulin (hormone) and, 141–142
insulin (supplemental) and, 142
pancreas and, 16, 17
pregnancy and, 247
risk factors, 17, 20–22
weight and, 58
type 2 diabetes and children
about, 179–180
blood sugar monitoring, 182, 183–184
care plan, creating, 182–186
child involvement and, 184–186
eating too much and, 120
exercise/physical activity and, 121
factors affecting, 119–123
food and, 119–120
four-hour fasting levels, 153
goals, 117, 118, 156
healthy eating and, 181–182
insulin and, 140
liver and, 120–121
medications and, 182
natural rise after eating, 117
pancreas and, 13
physical activity and, 182
plasma glucose levels and, 114
prediabetes and, 181
processing of, 13
screening, 181
signs and symptoms, 180–181
stress and, 121
treatment, 181–183

TZDs (thiazoldinediones), 138–139

U

UKPDS (United Kingdom Prospective Diabetes Study), 151
urination, increased, 18
urine test for protein, 227–228

V

vaccinations, 193, 237–239
vegetables, 44, 66
V-Go, 144
visual acuity test, 232

W

waist circumference, 60
walking, 84, 90, 191
walking in a line, heal to toe, 99
walking meditation, 216
walking shoes, 85
wall or table pushups, 88
water, 68, 102
weight, 19, 20–22. *See also* healthy weight
weight check, 223
weight loss. *See also* healthy weight
    amount for benefit, 58
    benefits of, 57
    energy density and, 68–69
    goals, 62–65
    healthy-eating plan for, 65–66
    readiness assessment, 61, 62
willpower vs. self-control, 77

Y

yoga, 100, 242–243

quarters the first time and this second time wasn't much better.

"I didn't know you cared. I hoped you did."

Winnie smiled. "Of course I care. You're like a puppy that needs lots of training."

"I was hoping for more than that."

"Oh yes, you stink. When was the last time you took a shower or did anything to clean yourself?"

"I believe it was the morning before I got my butt kicked by those two Nazis. Is it that bad?"

"Worse. I am now going to help you get out of bed and go down the hallway to the showers. You will clean up and you will put on fresh clothing. Then maybe we will go out in the sunshine."

"Will you shower with me?"

"Not in this lifetime," she said with a disarming smile that seemed to indicate that perhaps she didn't totally mean it. "I may pretend I'm a nurse and assist you but nothing more is going to happen. And I won't be shocked by what I see. I did have a brother. Actually, I'm afraid I might be disappointed."

"That hurts."

Winnie helped him to his feet. He was wearing GI boxer shorts and a T-shirt. She found clean clothing and helped him to the shower where he managed to undress himself. She did not leave as the hot water cascaded down his body. "You could change your mind and join me," he said.

"Not a chance. Sam might come in, and a couple of Dulles' guys are still staying here. Anybody could come in at any time. I like my privacy, thank you. Now, if you can manage to wash up without hurting yourself, I'll go and find you some clean sheets."

"Will you wash my back? I can't quite twist my arm around. It hurts too much."

She sighed. "That's the most original excuse I've ever heard." She took the washcloth and soap and leaned over far enough so she could do his back and the back of his legs without getting herself wet. He had a nice hard butt, which didn't surprise her. She realized that something else was getting hard.

"I see you're beginning to feel a whole lot better, so I'll leave you to your own devices."

"Wait just one minute," he said. He faced her and handed her the washcloth. "It won't take long."

She grinned wickedly and lathered the front of his body, taking special care to stroke his manhood. She hadn't played scrub-a-dub with a guy since her sophomore year in college with one of her brother's friends. Her brother had been really angry when he found out. The young man she'd cleansed had joined the Marines and gone on to fight on Guadalcanal. He'd come back with his body intact but his mind totally and horribly vacant. She'd gone to see him at the Bethesda Naval Hospital and been horrified. Her once vibrant friend who might have been a lover and even a serious suitor was nothing more than a vacant shell. His eyes were focused on something distant. Winnie had stayed for only a few minutes before leaving in tears. It was all the more reason to do what she could to end this damn war.

Ah well. It didn't take more than a minute or two before Ernie gasped and climaxed.

"I owe you," he said.

"And maybe someday I'll let you pay me back," she said. She was realizing that she was reconsidering Ernie and their relationship. So what if he was a puppy that needed a lot of training? She was a good trainer. She realized that she had compared Ernie to her brother and brought up his memory without feeling like crying. Maybe Ernie was good for her. "Now finish up and get out of there. You can buy me dinner."

Wally Oster had been as surprised as anyone when he'd been reclassified from 4-F to 1-A. His 4-F classification meant he had been rejected for military service because of his mental deficiencies. Even his grandfather said the boy was dumber than a stone. His family felt that his reclassification to 1-A, ready and eligible to be drafted, was due to several circumstances. First, the local draft board in their small west Texas town was under pressure to supply more warm bodies for the military. Thus, they had revisited a number of people whom they had deemed unqualified in the past. The second reason was that Wally had been caught vandalizing some of farms in the area that were owned by prominent citizens and even members of the board.

After being drafted, Wally had somehow muddled through basic training. The normally harsh and often brutal drill sergeants recognized that the lost and ignorant boy was a hopeless case, so they gave up trying and just passed him through. It was much like his teacher in the one-room schoolhouse out on the west Texas flatlands. She'd promoted him through to eighth grade and then he'd dropped out of school to work and earn pennies an hour as a laborer.

After basic, he'd been shipped directly to Europe where he'd wound up in the 105th Infantry Division.

He didn't realize it, but there were a number of former rejects like him in it and other divisions as the army began to scrape the bottom of the barrel and beneath.

Wally did like carrying a rifle. It made him feel powerful. So, when someone asked for a volunteer to take a German prisoner back to the stockade, he'd jumped at the chance. When he saw the scrawny young boy he was supposed to guard, he'd been disappointed. The boy was just a little smaller than he, scared, and not a threat and certainly not a superman. He'd giggled. The boy wasn't even Clark Kent. Wally liked the Superman stories. They were even better than Batman.

Someone had worked the kid over pretty thoroughly. His face was red and bruised, his eyes were swollen and his lower lip was split. Tough shit, thought Wally. He was a Nazi.

His orders were simple. Take him directly to the stockade and do not let him escape. Wally was given an M1 carbine and a fifteen round clip of ammunition. He loaded the carbine but was careful not to release the safety.

The prisoner was handcuffed with his hands to his front. He wondered why the people from Seventh Army who had come to interrogate him had waited until it was almost dark to send him back. Wally thought that they must know what they were doing since they were officers. His real concern was that he might miss dinner. He was one of a number who actually liked army food since it was so much better than what families back home had been able to afford. He'd gained weight on mess hall chow and even liked chipped beef on toast, which was always called shit on a shingle. Some of his friends laughed at him, but he didn't notice any of them skipping a meal. Since he spent much of his work day doing menial chores at the mess hall, he thought he could probably manage to scrounge up a meal.

They had gone about halfway when the boy announced that he had to pee. Wally had come from a German enclave in Texas and understood. "Why didn't you go before we started out?"

"I have to pee now," the boy announced and abruptly turned into an alleyway between several large tents.

Wally swore. He had no choice but to follow him. With astonishing quickness, the boy wheeled and yanked the carbine from Wally's grip and pointed it at him.

"Take off your uniform and boots."

Wally whimpered and complied. He had heard the slight click of the safety releasing. He was in grave danger. He also realized that the boy had somehow gotten out of his handcuffs. Damn. The boy had said they were too tight and one of the officers had loosened them. Damn.

"Lie down," Wally was ordered, and now crying openly, he obeyed.

"I don't want to die," he sobbed. "I want my mother."

"Coward," Hans Gruber said as he hit Wally in the head with the stock of his carbine. Wally tried to speak, but his world had become dark.

"Captain Tanner I presume."

Tanner laughed. They were outside a former school that had been designated as a hospital. "Doctor Hagerman, are you following me? Are you that concerned about my keeping my feet dry that you came all this way?"

The two men shook hands warmly. "No, I did not travel all the way from Belgium to see how your feet are doing. I got tired of treating GIs with penicillin for the clap and wanted to do some real doctoring."

Tanner pretended to be puzzled. "Clap? How on earth could our innocent soldiers get the clap since Ike has forbidden any contact between our horny GIs and equally horny German women?"

"Ike is doing as well with his nonfraternization rule as King Cnut did in trying to keep the tide from coming in. There are tens of thousands, maybe hundreds of thousands of German women who would like to make an arrangement with an American to provide them with food, shelter, and other basics. And so what if it means having sex with a stranger, or even several strangers? Does desperation make a woman a prostitute? I don't know. I'm not terribly religious, but I think I'll let God figure that out. Talk to a woman who would otherwise starve or her child would die if she didn't have sex with a GI, and then try to judge. I don't think anyone has a real idea how destitute the German people are, and many who do just don't give a damn."

"Obviously, you really feel strongly about this."

"Yes, and one last thing—When the savages from Russia rolled in, they gang-raped several million women. Most were German but the Reds really didn't care where they were from. Now, many of them are suffering from venereal diseases or unwanted pregnancies. I don't do abortions myself; they are illegal after all. But some of my associates do, and I'm not going to turn them in or criticize them."

Hagerman took a deep breath and smiled sheepishly.

"Sometimes I get worked up and I shouldn't. I understand that Ike is going to rescind that stupid and unenforceable nonfraternization policy. At any rate, you came here to see Private Oster, didn't you?"

The two men went down a hallway and into a ward where a curtain had been drawn around a bed. "Is he going to make it?" Tanner asked, suddenly worried. He'd been told that Oster had been wounded, but giving him such a degree of privacy was unusual if the wounds weren't grievous.

"He should recover nicely. His physical wounds aren't that serious. He's got a mildly fractured skull, if there is such a thing and, ah, one other problem."

Hagerman pulled the curtain and the two men stepped in. Oster was awake and looked at them in confusion. "Why are you here now? Did I do something else?"

There was a bandage wrapped around Oster's skull. "He doesn't need all this bandaging, but we're going to keep his head wrapped until we solve his problem. Private, I am now going to shift the bandage so Captain Tanner can see."

"No, I mean, no sir," Oster said.

"Yes you will," said Tanner, "but first tell me what happened."

Oster started to tear up. "I don't really know. One minute I'm walking with the prisoner and the next he's got my rifle and I'm on the ground. Then he hits me and then I wake up here and I've been cut."

Tanner thought he understood. The young Werewolf was still a Nazi fanatic. He either changed his mind, or something had changed it for him, or he'd been lying all along. Lena would not be happy at this turn of events. She had put so much emotion into changing the boy.

Of course, a big mistake had been made in giving this slow-witted American soldier any responsibility whatsoever. Now the Werewolves had an American uniform and an M1 Carbine along with at least one clip of ammunition.

Hagerman put his hand on Wally's shoulder. "Private Oster," he said firmly, "I am now going to pull off the bandage and show Captain Tanner what happened."

"Promise you won't tell anyone?"

They two men solemnly assured Wally that they wouldn't. Hagerman carefully pulled back the first bandage and exposed a second one covering a large patch of Oster's forehead. The young private was whimpering and not from pain. Tanner thought he knew what was coming next.

The second bandage was carefully pulled back, exposing a neatly gouged swastika in the middle of Wally Oster's forehead. Neither man said a thing. After a few seconds, Hagerman replaced the bandage. He thanked Wally, and the two men went outside where Hagerman lit a cigarette.

"Jesus, Doc, how are you going to get rid of that ugly thing? He can't go back with that obscene badge in the middle of his forehead."

"He won't have to. There's such a thing as plastic surgery. Good techniques were introduced in World War I, and there have been many improvements since then. He'll have a couple of minor operations to remove the swastika and then he'll have a small scar in the middle of his forehead that he can wear as a badge of honor showing that he'd been wounded in action. He's going to get a Purple Heart and maybe a trip home. I think I can convince some people that retarded boys who can barely read and write their own name should not be drafted and get him sent back home to West Crotch Rot, Texas. Who knows, maybe he'll thank me. What I would like to do is find out just who beat the crap out of the German."

"What?"

"Ah, something else you didn't know. Two guys came down from Seventh Army with permission from General Patch to question the prisoner after you were through with him. I understand that the questioning turned into interrogation and then torture to get him to give them information a fourteen-year-old kid probably didn't know in the first place. General Evans is absolutely livid and has complained upstream to Patch. It won't make a bit of difference since Patch is sick and going to be replaced. But at least we have some idea why our Werewolf recanted."

Staff Sergeant Billy Hill loved hunting. As a kid back home in Alabama, he'd take a rifle and hunt squirrels or rabbits. Back then he had a .22, and killing a squirrel was about all it would do. When he joined the army as a young adult he was already a highly skilled shooter with just about any kind of rifle or shotgun made.

Now what he really liked to do was hunt Germans. He had his own modified Garand M1 and it was fitted with a telescopic sight. He showed up at Sergeant Higgins' outpost unannounced but not unexpected. The two men had been friends for years and, since Hill's elevation to division staff, Higgins had extended an open invitation for Hill to go Nazi-hunting.

The crafty Higgins had his men build him a bunker that was well sited and camouflaged. "Do the Germans know about this place?" Hill asked.

"Not yet and I don't want them to. If you're gonna go hunting, don't draw attention to here."

"What are you worried about? One more attack on the German lines and they'll collapse like a house of cards."

Both men laughed harshly. "That's bullshit and you know it," said Higgins. "One more attack like the last one and this corps will be ruined and maybe the entire Seventh Army will cease to exist."

The 105th Infantry had recently been joined with the newly and partially arrived Tenth Mountain Division to form the Twenty-Fifth Corps. No commander had been designated so it had temporarily fallen on General Evans.

Hill grinned amiably at the handful of soldiers in the bunker. "Any of you brave men want to come with me?"

All but one looked away or lowered their heads. That one stared at him and shook his head. "What about you?" asked Hill, directing his question towards the man who was staring at him.

"No thank you, Sergeant. I'm not crazy."

Hill stiffened. "You implying that I am?"

The soldier, a PFC, wasn't intimidated. "Didn't mean that. I don't know what you're thinking and why you want to go out there and shoot people. I just don't. All I want to do is what's required of me and get home to my wife and kids."

Hill blinked. Kids? He'd known that fathers were being drafted, but this was the first time he'd run across one. No wonder the guy didn't want to volunteer. But that was just too bad. The guy was a soldier. "Are you saying you wouldn't obey a direct order to follow me out there into Nazi-land?"

"Of course I would. Just don't you go looking for any enthusiasm or any gung-ho and 'let's charge the machine gun' crap. First time somebody shoots at me, I go to ground and call for help."

"How old are you, Private?"

"Thirty-four and I want to reach thirty-five and be back home in Illinois when it happens."

"The Germans are our enemy, Private."

"With respect, Sergeant: says who? I'm part German and so is my wife. Some of the people you're going out to shoot could be my relatives. Fortunately, we don't have any Jap relations, so killing them's okay. My point is, Hitler's dead. Let's send in the diplomats and let them talk and end this thing."

"What about the Jews?"

"What about them? They're already dead and nothing can be done about it. Fact is, I don't totally believe all the bullshit they're feeding us about death camps and all that. I saw Dachau and it was a terrible place, but it still won't bring back anybody the Nazis killed. And if I get killed going out with you as some dumb volunteer, nobody's gonna bring me back either."

Angrily, Hill took his rifle and snuck out. He was perplexed by the man who didn't want to fight. Higgins had told him the password and countersign and pointed out the path through the barbed wire. Warnings about mines were also conveyed. The front had stabilized since the failed American attack.

It took hours of slow moving before Hill thought

he was in position to catch himself a German. He was covered with leaves and twigs and lay in a hollow part of ground. He would fire one round and then depart through a path he'd already figured out. In the meantime, he would simply be patient. He had no real choice. Haste didn't make waste. Haste could get a man killed.

He'd been waiting almost two hours and was beginning to think there would be no hunting today when, there it was. He saw a flicker of motion. A German soldier had stuck his head over his foxhole and was looking around. Hill thought that the poor boy's officer had probably told the soldier to see if any Americans were in sight. No, but they were within range.

Hill preferred killing officers, but none were around. He aimed at the soldier's exposed head and gently squeezed the trigger. The enemy soldier's head jerked back and disappeared. One more, thought Hill.

Seconds later, he was moving quickly through his escape route while machine guns and mortars fruitlessly sought him out. Another hour found him back in Higgins' bunker. That same older soldier looked at him. "Make a kill?" he asked.

"Damn right."

"Take his scalp, too?"

Hill turned red with anger. "Look, you little asshole, I'm out there fighting while you're in here hiding."

"Great, Sergeant, but tell me why we're fighting. We've got ninety percent of Germany, so who cares about this piddling little part called Germanica? The way I see it, the only real enemy we've got left is Japan. Germany didn't bomb Pearl Harbor, the Japs did. I say we pull out of here and let the few Nazis left do whatever they want while we get rid of the Japs."

"Private, are you saying you don't want to fight the Germans?"

"That's pretty much it, Sergeant. Are you gonna have me court-martialed? Maybe you'd like to see a picture of my kid. I want to be there when he grows up. I just don't want to die for something stupid and unnecessary."

Hill didn't answer. He took his rifle and headed back to the division's headquarters. He needed to talk to people about what he'd been told. Yeah, he had made a kill and he was proud of it. Or he thought he was. It was his fifteenth that he could confirm. It was a good kill. So why the hell did he feel so depressed?

CHAPTER 11

THE SIGHT OF GERMAN SOLDIERS MARCHING DOWN a street might not have shocked many people in Nazi-occupied Europe, but this was Arbon, Switzerland, not Poland or what had been Vichy France.

Ernie had been told to sit tight in Arbon, do nothing to aggravate anyone, especially the Nazis so close across the border, and observe. This morning he was sitting with Winnie and enjoying a coffee. She had just returned from another junket to Bern where she had met with Allen Dulles. He knew better than to ask why. Someday, he thought wryly, he'd have secrets to hold tightly as well.

She had also given up wearing her fat outfit, at least for this day, and was stylishly dressed in very modern slacks and a jacket, and Ernie greatly appreciated the fact. It was she who first saw the column of soldiers approaching.

"Ernie, look. Are they Swiss? They don't quite look Swiss."

Ernie turned and saw the coal-scuttle helmets. He

tried to remember if the Swiss wore them as well. After a moment, it didn't matter as the swastikas on the sides of their helmets became obvious. All he and Winnie could do was sit and stare in disbelief as the column marched by. The residents of Arbon were just as shocked. A few Germans tried to look stern but most of them were clearly enjoying themselves.

"Should we follow them?" Winnie asked. Ernie nodded and they let the column lead them to the very small train station that serviced Arbon. In recent weeks, a couple of spurs had been added and these led to fields just outside of town.

Along with a number of other people, they tried to get closer to where a locomotive pulling a number of freight cars had pulled up on one of the spur lines. Swiss police and German soldiers kept them at bay. Whoever or whatever was on the train was not for public view. The two of them pushed to the front of the crowd and presented their credentials proclaiming them as accredited diplomats. The Swiss police were adamant.

"Those documents will keep you from getting arrested, but not from being detained if I feel you are disobeying my lawful instructions," a police corporal said. When Winnie tried to say something, the policeman silenced her with a steely glance and a reminder that women in Switzerland were third-class citizens, and had not even risen to the level of second class. They could not vote and many jobs were closed to them.

"Will you stop me from taking pictures?" she asked.

"I wish you wouldn't," said the Swiss cop, "but I suppose I can't stop everyone." A number of Arbon's residents were taking their own photos of the incredible sight.

Ernie looked over the column of Germans and estimated their number at at least two hundred. "Is Switzerland being invaded?" he facetiously asked.

The policeman actually smiled. "I like to think it would take more than this to conquer my country."

A column of trucks was heard approaching. They arrived and pulled alongside the parked train. The doors on the freight cars were opened and the soldiers began unloading crates. Ernie always carried his binoculars and used them to see what was being moved. He also tried to see if any of the Krauts at the train were the ones who'd beaten him. He looked for any senior officers. When he thought he saw one, he pointed the person out to Winnie who snapped him with her telephoto lens.

The crates appeared to be carrying canned food and nothing more suspicious. Another freight car contained reasonably fresh produce and that was thrown into trucks.

"I have a question," Winnie asked. "Why did they make the soldiers walk here instead of letting them ride on the trucks?"

The police corporal paused for a moment and then laughed. "Because they're Germans, that's why. Germans always do things the difficult way."

The meeting between Allen Dulles and Alain Burkholter, the unofficial representative of the Swiss government, took place in a house in Arbon the next day. As usual, Burkholter was urbane and poised while Dulles was clearly agitated. They had before them a number of the photographs that Winnie had taken.

"We have nothing to hide," Burkholter said. "We said all along that we would support the Germanica government with those supplies needed to maintain their basic needs. We said that we would send them food and that is exactly what we are doing. Your photos show nothing in the way of military supplies. There were no rifles, no machine guns, no ammunition, and certainly no tanks. You would find, if we were to permit you to inspect these shipments, quantities of medical supplies as well."

Dulles smiled. "Are you saying that you would let us inspect the shipments?"

"Absolutely not. You read too much into my comment."

"But what if we were to somehow find that weapons and such were being shipped in? What would your government's stance be then, Mr. Burkholter?"

Burkholter simply shrugged. "I believe that I already stated the dilemma the Swiss government finds itself in. We dare not enrage the savage animal that is just outside our door. We have only a few planes and absolutely no tanks, so we cannot give the Germans any. But if they were to forcibly demand ammunition and small arms to include antitank and antiaircraft weapons, we would be hard-pressed to deny them."

"That and the fact that many citizens of Switzerland support the Nazis would also make it difficult to say no, wouldn't it?"

"I won't argue the point. By the way, if you are thinking of having your OSS people use their considerable skills at sabotage to stop or delay the shipments, please don't. We would be exceedingly angry, especially if Swiss citizens were either killed or injured. We would protest vigorously and consider taking very harsh action against the perpetrators."

With that and after traditional insincere pleasantries, the meeting ended. Burkholter departed by car and, after he was gone, Dulles signaled for Ernie and Winnie to join him.

Dulles lit up his pipe and puffed for a moment. It appeared to calm him. "I presume you heard everything."

"Clear as a bell," Ernie said. "The microphones were well placed."

"Good. We will make a copy here and send both separately to Washington. Now, I understand you heard what he said. But did you hear what he didn't say?"

"I don't understand," said a puzzled Winnie.

Dulles smiled tolerantly. He was very fond of Winnie. "Think. What are the rules of the game? What did he say about sabotage?"

Ernie understood first. "The rules are simple. Don't hurt anybody who's Swiss. Other than that, all options are open."

Tanner looked at the score or so of bedraggled and filthy men huddled in a classroom of what had been a school. They weren't particularly cold, but they were concerned about their immediate safety and their futures, which made some of them shiver. A couple of them tried to smile, signifying that they wanted to be friends despite the fact that they'd been shooting at Americans earlier this day.

"Are these today's trickles?" he asked Cullen, who nodded solemnly. The press had taken to saying that surrendering Germans were trickling in and the term had caught on.

Cullen was not happy. Responsibility for the loss of the young Werewolf and the wounding and mutilating of his guard had fallen on him. He had been the one to assign the job of guarding Gruber to the inept Oster and it had been he who had ordered the prisoner's handcuffs loosened. He'd actually believed Gruber's lament that they were so tight that they hurt. He'd had his tail reamed by General Evans along with having a formal reprimand in his file. If he'd been planning on making the army a career, those opportunities had gone. Fortunately, he too wanted nothing more than to go home.

Tanner counted heads. Twenty-three former enemy soldiers were looking at him. "Are they all Germans or are there any from elsewhere in the Reich?"

Cullen rolled his eyes. "Are you asking me if there are any Czechs in this small mob so you can bring Lena in here, the answer is yes, there is one and I've already sent for her."

Tanner felt himself flushing. "Am I that obvious?"

"Only when you speak. And, along with our one Czech, we have two Poles, a Frenchie and one lone Wop. God only knows how he wound up in Germanica, but we'll ask him and find out. A nickel says he got lost. And are you aware that several turncoat Russians have tried to surrender? We've gotten messages that, if we promise not to turn them over to the Reds, they will surrender. Otherwise, they will fight to the death and take as many of us as they can with them."

"How jolly," Tanner said. He understood the current policy was to turn over any captured Russians to the Reds. That they would execute them was not America's concern, he'd been told. He didn't agree. In fact, it sickened him, but he didn't have a voice in the matter.

The prisoners were all staring at him. They understood that their fate largely lay in his hands. They'd been told that the Americans usually respected the Geneva Convention regarding prisoners, but usually is not the same as always. There had been cases where Americans had considered prisoners a nuisance and had murdered them. This batch was terrified. The Americans could still kill them outright, or turn them back to the Nazis where they would be brutally executed, or worse, given to the Soviets even though they weren't turncoat Russians. Rumors of the horrors of Soviet captivity were beginning to circulate. It was highly unlikely that any German soldier taken by the Reds would ever see his home again. And even if he did, he would be old and crippled and mentally broken.

Lena arrived in her almost military outfit. She could have passed for someone from the Women's Army Corps. Tanner smiled and gestured to the man Cullen had identified as Czech. Lena took him by the arm and they walked away. Lucky Czech, thought Tanner. Lena had gained some much needed weight and it had affected her personality, which was now much more outgoing and even happy.

Tanner talked to the German POWs. They were all infantrymen and all enlisted. They looked gaunt. When asked how often they were getting fed, they'd laughed derisively. Not very often, was the response, and what food they did get was bad.

"We get to eat shit, while the fucking officers get the good stuff," said one German sergeant named Gunther. He stopped abruptly when he realized he was talking to one of the fucking officers he'd just disparaged. What Gunther had to say, however, was typical of the responses Tanner had been getting.

Tanner laughed and told him not to worry about rank and insulting German officers. This sergeant was particularly loquacious. He said that food deliveries were irregular and that they'd received no mail since arriving near the Alps. He said that many more would surrender if they had half the opportunity, but the diehards and SS fanatics were watching the men like hawks. A number of deserters had been hanged along with men who'd simply complained about their circumstances.

"The SS are fucking monsters. There might not be too many real Gestapo agents, but there are more than enough SS and that prick, Hahn, keeps them sniffing for the slightest hint of defeatism."

Another reference to Hahn, Tanner noted. He would really like to get his hands on that guy.

"You sound like you were a prisoner," Tanner said.

"Pretty much." Tanner had given the man an American cigarette and he was puffing on it with almost sexual pleasure. "But prisoners are not sent out with inadequate weapons and ammunition to get killed."

Tanner was intrigued. "You don't have enough ammo?"

"We were told not to waste it. Bullets don't grow on trees, you know. The same holds with rifles, machine guns, and anything else. We do have tanks. I've seen some of them dug in, but what we don't have is the fuel to run them. I could show you where a dozen Panzer IVs are dug in and immovable because their fuel tanks are practically dry. Petrol is almost non-existent. I talked to one crew leader and he said he could go about twenty miles on what his tank has. He was told not to expect any more. Not exactly the army that raced across France and Poland, is it?"

"Do you think those tanks are still there now?"

Gunther shrugged. "They were yesterday. And I've never seen any Panthers or Tigers, just Panzer IVs. I guess the good tanks are all shot up and gone. Is that worth another cigarette?"

It was, and Gunther took it eagerly. "Gunther, how about their trucks? How do they get the gasoline to get whatever supplies that do get to you?"

"In many cases, they don't use trucks. Human mules are used instead. But that won't last long, because the fools in the SS won't feed the slave laborers enough to keep them going. When all the slaves are either dead or too weak to work, I don't know how the front line soldiers will get anything. Of course, the bigwigs don't think of practical matters like that. I give it a couple of weeks before the slaves start dropping like flies."

"Gunther, did you always feel this way?"

Gunther was in his late thirties and looked wily. "Of course not, Captain. Your American phrase is 'bullshit,' so I will not bullshit you. When we were running all over Europe, we had anything we wanted. We had food, liquor, women, and warm beds, and most of the women were even willing. Life was good and Hitler was our God. Then we began fighting the Russians and then you people and it all went to hell. This war is over. Germany has lost and why can't idiots like Goebbels and Schoerner realize that? And oh yes, don't get me started on medical supplies. We may have invented aspirin but I haven't seen anything with the Bayer label on it in months."

Tanner smiled in a reassuring manner. "Gunther, I am now going to get you a map of the area and you are going to pinpoint the location of those tanks. Does it bother you that they are going to get bombed and that some of the men in those soon to be burning hulls were your friends?"

Gunther's expression was impassive. "A little, but this is war and I want to survive it. I think I deserve a bonus, don't you?"

Tanner handed him a full pack of Chesterfields, which Gunther grabbed and stuck into a pocket after making sure that none of his erstwhile comrades could see. Tanner walked away. There was nothing more to be gotten from the prisoners. Lena met him outside the interrogation center. "Did your Czech prisoner know anything?" he asked.

"About the German Army and its local dispositions, a little. About my father, nothing."

"I'm sorry."

"So am I, but I have no plans to stop looking. I will talk to every Czech I can find. I will either find that he is dead and at peace, or I will find him alive in some slave camp and get him out."

Her body shook and Tanner put his hands on her shoulders. She slipped against him and rested against his chest. "Sorry," she said softly after a few seconds. He slipped his arm around her and she did not resist.

"I'm not sorry at all. If you're hungry, we can get something to eat."

She looked at him in surprise and backed off.

"Did I say something wrong? If I did, I'm sorry."

She smiled at him. "There's nothing to be sorry about. I'm still not used to people being nice to me.

I think I'll get over it, and yes, you can find some place for us to eat even if it's just another mess hall. I've developed a taste for Spam or even that delicious dish called shit on a shingle."

Schafer and Sibre flew their heavily armed planes low down the valley that led to Innsbruck. Low and fast was one way to avoid the numerous antiaircraft guns that had been emplaced and were extremely well hidden. This morning, their target was a line of haystacks. Their orders were to kill those haystacks. Six other planes followed them and all were armed with semi-armor piercing rockets. To the best of their knowledge, theirs were the only P51s with rockets, although a number of P47s carried the weapons. They'd had a chance to practice with them and thought they were pretty damn good at hitting their targets.

"There," Schafer said. The line of haystacks was coming up quickly as was flak from antiaircraft guns. The various pilots peeled off and chose their targets. Sibre fired first and a pair of rockets streaked away. One missed by a few feet, but the second hit, sending hay and debris skyward. The explosion exposed a dug-in German tank and men were running away from it even though the tank didn't look badly damaged. A second pass and another hit. The tank blew up. Other tanks were dying as well. Napalm was dropped, turning wrecks into charnel houses. Both men later swore that they had flown so low that they could smell human flesh burning.

Their work done, they turned and headed for base. They counted noses. One P51 was smoking and the pilot would land first if he made it that far. Otherwise,